How the COVID-19 Pandemic Transformed the Mental Health Landscape

This book is a valuable historical record of how counselling psychologists responded to the COVID-19 pandemic around the globe. Volume I includes 14 chapters that address topics associated with transferring counselling practice online. Several chapters focus on transitioning to online therapy from face-to-face contact, including the effect of such a transition on the therapeutic relationship, and working with clients' emotional processes online.

Written by prominent researchers and clinicians in the field of counselling and psychotherapy, both the volumes together cover a wide range of perspectives and offer useful clinical recommendations related to effective telepsychotherapy practice. The chapters in these volumes were originally published as a special issue of *Counselling Psychology Quarterly*.

Shigeru Iwakabe is Professor of Clinical Psychology at Ritsumeikan University in Osaka, Japan. He conducts psychotherapy research on client emotional processes from an integrative perspective. His research interests include training and professional development in psychotherapy, case study research methods, psychotherapy integration, and cultural and social issues related to the practice of psychotherapy.

Sarah Knox is Professor in the Department of Counselor Education and Counseling Psychology at Marquette University, Milwaukee, WI, USA. The vast majority of her research is qualitative, and specifically uses consensual qualitative research (CQR). She focuses primarily on the psychotherapy relationship and process, training and supervision, and advising relationships and processes.

How the COVID-19 Pandemic Transformed the Mental Health Landscape

Transitioning to Telepsychotherapy Effectively, Volume I

Edited by

Shigeru Iwakabe and Sarah Knox

Routledge
Taylor & Francis Group
LONDON AND NEW YORK

First published 2023
by Routledge
4 Park Square, Milton Park, Abingdon, Oxon OX14 4RN

and by Routledge
605 Third Avenue, New York, NY 10158

Routledge is an imprint of the Taylor & Francis Group, an informa business

British Library Cataloguing in Publication Data
A catalogue record for this book is available from the British Library

ISBN13: 978-1-032-39963-8 (hbk)
ISBN13: 978-1-032-39968-3 (pbk)
ISBN13: 978-1-003-35221-1 (ebk)

DOI: 10.4324/9781003352211

Typeset in Myriad Pro
by Newgen Publishing UK

Publisher's Note
The publisher accepts responsibility for any inconsistencies that may have arisen during the conversion of this book from journal articles to book chapters, namely the inclusion of journal terminology.

Disclaimer
Every effort has been made to contact copyright holders for their permission to reprint material in this book. The publishers would be grateful to hear from any copyright holder who is not here acknowledged and will undertake to rectify any errors or omissions in future editions of this book.

Contents

Part II
Therapeutic Relationship

Part III
Working with Emotions

Citation Information

The chapters in this book were originally published in the journal *Counselling Psychology Quarterly*, volume 34, issue 3–4 (2021). When citing this material, please use the original page numbering for each article, as follows:

Foreword

Marshall McLuhan and the therapeutic importance of the telephone
Jesse D. Geller
Counselling Psychology Quarterly, volume 34, issue 3–4 (2021), pp. 319–320

Chapter 1

Telepsychotherapy: a leaflet for psychotherapists in the age of COVID-19. A review of the evidence
Barbara Poletti, Sofia Tagini, Agostino Brugnera, Laura Parolin, Luca Pievani, Roberta Ferrucci, Angelo Compare and Vincenzo Silani
Counselling Psychology Quarterly, volume 34, issue 3–4 (2021), pp. 352–367

Chapter 2

Transitioning to virtual programming amidst COVID-19 outbreak
Alejandra Sequeira, Adaeze Alozie, Melissa Fasteau, Alicia K. Lopez, Jennifer Sy, Karina A. Turner, Cali Werner, Elizabeth McIngvale and Thröstur Björgvinsson
Counselling Psychology Quarterly, volume 34, issue 3–4 (2021), pp. 538–553

Chapter 3

Mental-health care under threat: a pragmatic approach for ethical decision-making for practitioners in COVID-19
M. Bar, E. Fish and S. Mendlovic
Counselling Psychology Quarterly, volume 34, issue 3–4 (2021), pp. 525–537

Chapter 4

Psychotherapy at a public hospital in the time of COVID-19: telehealth and implications for practice
Zoe Silver, Mikaela Coger, Sebastian Barr and Rebecca Drill
Counselling Psychology Quarterly, volume 34, issue 3–4 (2021), pp. 499–507

Chapter 5

A brief transdiagnostic pandemic mental health maintenance intervention
Trisha Arnold, Brooke G. Rogers, Alyssa L. Norris, Anna Schierberl Scherr, Kayla Haubrick, Megan E. Renna, Shufang Sun, Margaret M. Danforth, Christina T. Chu, Elizabeth S. Silva, Laura B. Whiteley and Megan Pinkston
Counselling Psychology Quarterly, volume 34, issue 3–4 (2021), pp. 331–351

Chapter 6

Cultivating online therapeutic presence: strengthening therapeutic relationships in teletherapy sessions
Shari Geller
Counselling Psychology Quarterly, volume 34, issue 3–4 (2021), pp. 687–703

Chapter 7

Repairing alliance ruptures using supportive techniques in telepsychotherapy during the COVID-19 pandemic
Tohar Dolev-Amit, Liat Leibovich and Sigal Zilcha-Mano
Counselling Psychology Quarterly, volume 34, issue 3–4 (2021), pp. 485–498

Chapter 8

Grappling with our therapeutic relationship and professional self-doubt during COVID-19: will we use video therapy again?
Katie Aafjes-van Doorn, Vera Békés and Tracy A. Prout
Counselling Psychology Quarterly, volume 34, issue 3–4 (2021), pp. 473–484

Chapter 9

When distance brings us closer: leveraging tele-psychotherapy to build deeper connection
Cory K. Chen, Nicole Nehrig, Lauren Wash, Jennifer A. Schneider, Sagiv Ashkenazi, Elana Cairo, Angel F. Guyton and Amy Palfrey
Counselling Psychology Quarterly, volume 34, issue 3–4 (2021), pp. 554–567

Chapter 10

A methodology to improve eye contact in telepsychotherapy via videoconferencing with considerations for psychological distance
F. Grondin, A. M. Lomanowska, V. Békés and P. L. Jackson
Counselling Psychology Quarterly, volume 34, issue 3–4 (2021), pp. 586–599

Chapter 11

Let's face it: video conferencing psychotherapy requires the extensive use of ostensive cues
Shimrit Fisher, Timur Guralnik, Peter Fonagy and Sigal Zilcha-Mano
Counselling Psychology Quarterly, volume 34, issue 3–4 (2021), pp. 508–524

Chapter 12

Clinical recommendations for psychotherapists working during the coronavirus (COVID-19) pandemic through the lens of AEDP (Accelerated Experiential Dynamic Psychotherapy)
Hillary L. McBride, Andrew J. Joseph, Peter G. Schmitt and Brett M. Holtz
Counselling Psychology Quarterly, volume 34, issue 3–4 (2021), pp. 411–431

Chapter 13

Work with emotions in remote psychotherapy in the time of Covid-19: a clinical experience
Alexine Thompson-de Benoit and Ueli Kramer
Counselling Psychology Quarterly, volume 34, issue 3–4 (2021), pp. 368–376

Chapter 14

Emotion-focused and video-technology considerations in the COVID-19 crisis
Allan Abbass and Jasen Elliott
Counselling Psychology Quarterly, volume 34, issue 3–4 (2021), pp. 624–636

Notes on Contributors

Katie Aafjes-van Doorn, Clinical Psychology Doctoral Program, Ferkauf Graduate School of Psychology, Yeshiva University, New York, NY, USA.

Allan Abbass, Dalhousie University, Halifax, Nova Scotia, Canada; Private Practice, Calgary, Alberta, Canada.

Adaeze Alozie, McLean OCD Institute, Houston, TX, USA.

Trisha Arnold, Warren Alpert Medical School, Brown University, Providence, Rhode Island, USA; Department of Psychiatry, Rhode Island Hospital, Providence, Rhode Island, USA.

Sagiv Ashkenazi, Veterans Affairs New York Harbor Healthcare System, Manhattan Campus, Psychology Service, NY, USA.

M. Bar, Sackler School of Medicine, Tel Aviv University, Tel Aviv, Israel; Psychiatric Division, Sheba Medical Center, Ramat-Gan, Israel.

Sebastian Barr, Department of Psychiatry, Cambridge Health Alliance, Cambridge, MA, USA; Department of Psychiatry, Harvard Medical School, Boston, MA, USA.

V. Békés, Ferkauf Graduate School of Psychology, Yeshiva University, Bronx, NY, USA.

Thröstur Björgvinsson, McLean OCD Institute, Houston, TX, USA.

Agostino Brugnera, Department of Human and Social Sciences, University of Bergamo, Bergamo, Italy.

Elana Cairo, Veterans Affairs New York Harbor Healthcare System, Manhattan Campus, Psychology Service, NY, USA.

Cory K. Chen, Veterans Affairs New York Harbor Healthcare System, Manhattan Campus, Psychology Service, NY, USA; Department of Psychiatry, New York University School of Medicine, New York, NY, USA.

Christina T. Chu, Department of Medicine, Miriam Hospital, Providence, RI, USA.

Mikaela Coger, Department of Psychiatry, Cambridge Health Alliance, Cambridge, MA, USA.

Angelo Compare, Department of Human and Social Sciences, University of Bergamo, Bergamo, Italy.

Margaret M. Danforth, Department of Psychology, University of Massachusetts, Dartmouth, MA, USA.

Tohar Dolev-Amit, Department of Psychology, University of Haifa, Haifa, Israel.

Rebecca Drill, Department of Psychiatry, Cambridge Health Alliance, Cambridge, MA, USA; Department of Psychiatry, Harvard Medical School, Boston, MA, USA.

Jasen Elliott, Private Practice, Calgary, Alberta, Canada.

Melissa Fasteau, McLean OCD Institute, Houston, TX, USA.

Roberta Ferrucci, Department of Health Sciences, Università degli Studi di Milano, Milan, Italy.

E. Fish, Sackler School of Medicine, Tel Aviv University, Tel Aviv, Israel.

Shimrit Fisher, Department of Psychology, University of Haifa, Haifa, Israel.

Peter Fonagy, Research Department of Clinical, Educational and Health Psychology, University College London, London, UK.

Jesse D. Geller, Yale University Community Consultation Center, New Haven, CT, USA.

Shari Geller, Centre for MindBody Health, York University, Toronto, Canada.

F. Grondin, École de psychologie, Université Laval, Québec (QC), Canada; bCenter for Interdisciplinary Research in Rehabilitation and Social Integration (CIRRIS), Québec (QC), Canada; cCERVO Brain Research Center, Québec (QC), Canada.

Timur Guralnik, Department of Psychology, University of Haifa, Haifa, Israel.

Angel F. Guyton, Veterans Affairs New York Harbor Healthcare System, Manhattan Campus, Psychology Service, NY, USA.

Kayla Haubrick, Department of Psychiatry, Rhode Island Hospital, Providence, RI, USA.

Brett M. Holtz, Columbia University, New York, NY, USA.

Shigeru Iwakabe, Department of Psychology, Ritsumeikan University in Osaka, Japan.

P. L. Jackson, École de psychologie, Université Laval, Québec (QC), Canada; Center for Interdisciplinary Research in Rehabilitation and Social Integration (CIRRIS), Québec (QC), Canada; CERVO Brain Research Center, Québec (QC), Canada.

Andrew J. Joseph, AEDP Institute, New York, NY, USA.

Sarah Knox, Department of Counselor Education and Counseling Psychology, Marquette University, Milwaukee, WI, USA.

Ueli Kramer, Institute of Psychotherapy and General Psychiatry Service, Department of Psychiatry, University of Lausanne, Lausanne, Switzerland.

Liat Leibovich, Department of Psychology, University of Haifa, Haifa, Israel.

A. M. Lomanowska, École de psychologie, Université Laval, Québec (QC), Canada.

Alicia K. Lopez, McLean OCD Institute, Houston, TX, USA.

Hillary L. McBride, University of British Columbia, Vancouver, British Columbia, Canada.

Elizabeth McIngvale, McLean OCD Institute, Houston, TX, USA.

S. Mendlovic, Shalvata Mental Health Center, Hod Hasharon, Israel; Sackler School of Medicine, Tel Aviv University, Tel Aviv, Israel.

Nicole Nehrig, Veterans Affairs New York Harbor Healthcare System, Manhattan Campus, Psychology Service, NY, USA; Department of Psychiatry, New York University School of Medicine, New York, NY, USA.

Alyssa L. Norris, Warren Alpert Medical School, Brown University, Providence, Rhode Island, USA; Department of Psychiatry, Rhode Island Hospital, Providence, RI, USA.

Amy Palfrey, Veterans Affairs New York Harbor Healthcare System, Manhattan Campus, Psychology Service, NY, USA; Department of Psychiatry, New York University School of Medicine, New York, NY, USA.

Laura Parolin, Department of Psychology, University Milano Bicocca, Milan, Italy.

Luca Pievani, Department of Human and Social Sciences, University of Bergamo, Bergamo, Italy

Megan Pinkston, Warren Alpert Medical School, Brown University, Providence, RI, USA; Department of Medicine, Miriam Hospital, Providence, RI, USA; Department of Psychiatry, Duke University Medical Center, Durham, NC, USA.

Barbara Poletti, Istituto Auxologico Italiano, IRCCS, Department of Neurology and Laboratory of Neuroscience, Istituto Auxologico Italiano, IRCCS, Milan, Italy.

Tracy A. Prout, Clinical Psychology Doctoral Program, Ferkauf Graduate School of Psychology, Yeshiva University, New York, NY, USA.

Megan E. Renna, Ohio State University Wexner Medical Center, Institute for Behavioral Medicine Research & Comprehensive Cancer Center, Columbus, OH, USA.

Brooke G. Rogers, Warren Alpert Medical School, Brown University, Providence, RI, USA; Department of Medicine, Miriam Hospital, Providence, RI, USA.

Anna Schierberl Scherr, Warren Alpert Medical School, Brown University, Providence, RI, USA; Department of Psychology, Miriam Hospital, Providence, RI, USA; Department of Psychiatry, Duke University Medical Center, Durham, NC, USA.

Peter G. Schmitt, Karen Horney Clinic, New York, NY, USA; Kull Initiative for Psychotherapy, New York, NY, USA.

Jennifer A. Schneider, Veterans Affairs New York Harbor Healthcare System, Manhattan Campus, Psychology Service, NY, USA; Department of Psychiatry, New York University School of Medicine, New York, NY, USA.

Alejandra Sequeira, McLean OCD Institute, Houston, TX, USA.

Vincenzo Silani, Istituto Auxologico Italiano, IRCCS, Department of Neurology and Laboratory of Neuroscience, Istituto Auxologico Italiano, IRCCS, Milan, Italy.

Elizabeth S. Silva, Department of Medicine, Miriam Hospital, Providence, RI, USA.

Zoe Silver, Department of Psychiatry, Cambridge Health Alliance, Cambridge, MA, USA.

Shufang Sun, Warren Alpert Medical School, Brown University, Providence, Rhode Island, USA; Department of Psychiatry, Rhode Island Hospital, Providence, Rhode Island, USA.

Jennifer Sy, McLean OCD Institute, Houston, TX, USA.

Sofia Tagini, Istituto Auxologico Italiano, IRCCS, Department of Neurology and Laboratory of Neuroscience, Istituto Auxologico Italiano, IRCCS, Milan, Italy.

Alexine Thompson-de Benoit, Private Practice, Grandvaux, Switzerland.

Karina A. Turner, McLean OCD Institute, Houston, TX, USA.

Lauren Wash, Veterans Affairs New York Harbor Healthcare System, Manhattan Campus, Psychology Service, NY, USA.

Cali Werner, McLean OCD Institute, Houston, TX, USA.

Laura B. Whiteley, Warren Alpert Medical School, Brown University, Providence, RI, USA; Department of Psychiatry, Rhode Island Hospital, Providence, RI, USA.

Sigal Zilcha-Mano, Department of Psychology, University of Haifa, Haifa, Israel.

Foreword

Marshall McLuhan and the therapeutic importance of the telephone

Jesse D. Geller

ABSTRACT
A brief essay that discusses the significance of Marshall McLuhan's (1967) The Medium is the Massage in the context of online psychotherapy currently required in the pandemic of covid-19.

This week, all of my therapy sessions with my patients took place via an old-fashioned landline. Reflecting on how reliance on this medium restructured our conversations lead me to reread Marshall McLuhan's (1967) *The Medium is the Massage*. The central thesis of this pioneering text is that it is impossible to understand changes in social and cultural relationships without knowledge of the workings of electronic technology because, "Societies have always been shaped more by the nature of the media by which men communicate than by the content of the communication" (p.8).

In the psychotherapy seminar that I am now forced to conduct by Zoom, I asked my clinical psychology graduate students to think about whether and how the substance and style of their conversations with their patients have been altered by shifting from face-to-face dialogues to media mediated conversations. One recurrent theme has been the salience of conversations that revolve around the dynamic tension between intimacy and autonomy.

In my work with patients who are trying to reconcile the competing claims of pursuing creative and ambitious careers and being loving and attentive partners and parents, the Coronavirus has intensified their conflicts. When Patient R, an aspiring novelist, told me over the phone, "Trying to take good care of my bored son and being trapped in our apartment has destroyed my ability to work. I can't concentrate. I have the attention span of a gnat." Amongst other things, I normalized his experience by telling him that his favorite poet, Yeats, also experienced the conflict between work and love as an irreconcilable dilemma. The opening line of Yeats' poem "The Choice" is, "The intellect of man is forced to choose the perfection of the life or the work" (1968, p. 23).

By contrast, doing the work of therapy for me, in a world that reminds me of the therapeutic challenges that we faced during the early days of the AIDs crisis, is a sanctuary in which to distract myself from the engulfing presence of what one patient called "the plague." We therapists are fortunate that rather than being rendered obsolete by the digital revolution, our skills and services have become a crucial cultural resource.

Disclosure statement

No potential conflict of interest was reported by the author.

References

McLuhan, M. (1967). *The medium is the massage*. New York, New York: Bantam Books.
Yeats, W. B. (1968). *W. B. Yeats: Selected poetry*. London: Macmillan.

Preface

In response to the 2020 pandemic, the Co-Editors-in-Chief of *Counselling Psychology Quarterly* sought to contribute to the field of mental health at large by organizing two special issues of the journal that focused on *The practice of counselling and psychotherapy in the midst of pandemic: Surviving and thriving through the era of COVID-19*. *Counselling Psychology Quarterly (CPQ)* is an international and interdisciplinary peer-reviewed journal presenting papers that address theory, research, practice, and training related to the profession of counselling psychology. These special issues presented practice-oriented papers that supported the work of counsellors and counselling psychologists in a timely manner. This two-volume special issue series is now available as a two-volume book, *How the COVID-19 Pandemic Transformed the Mental Health Landscape*, that brings together 27 chapters documenting the profession's invaluable efforts and wisdom to cope and thrive through the early part of the pandemic.

The world was drastically transformed in 2020, as COVID-19 affected people across the globe. Those most vulnerable at the onset of this pandemic were the elderly and those with other health conditions and comorbidities. However, with the strategies to control the spread of the virus, everyone's daily activities were profoundly altered, including the closure of schools, businesses, and even hospitals to reduce the chance of infection. As a result, many people lost their jobs, leaving those from lower socioeconomic groups especially vulnerable. Whatever our individual circumstances, we likely all felt the effects of the pandemic, and thus the world was connected through our shared distress.

The fear of contagion, worsening medical and economic circumstances, extreme uncertainty, and changes to daily routines in all areas of life increased people's stress. The availability of the newest information on the Internet was a double-edged sword: We sought the most recent updates and reliable information to protect ourselves, but in doing so often also encountered misinformation, speculations, and catastrophic predictions. There was so much confusion and frustration: Our sense of security and safety was fundamentally altered.

During this unprecedented period, counselling psychologists and other mental health practitioners encountered many challenges to deliver services to their clients. Our work is based on human contact and an interpersonal relationship. Social distancing prevented us from meeting in person. The fear of contagion kept people away from one another, and mental health professionals were no exception. We were torn between our desire and natural inclination to approach and emphasize with our clients, and our instinctive need to withdraw and protect ourselves. Tele-psychology with recent web technology was available to move our services online. However, many of us still felt reservations, including how telemental health might alter the therapy relationship and boundary dynamics. We also knew that some clients did not have access to this technology to continue their treatment, and some therapists were not versed in these web technologies.

In seeking to speak to some of the challenges inherent in this unusual time, and as noted above, the special issues included a collection of chapters that addressed various practice-related concerns of delivering mental health services during the time of COVID-19. It was our hope that these issues would be a helpful resource to assist clinicians, and also that they would be historical documents of the work in which counselling psychologists and other mental health professionals engaged to continue to serve their clients.

In order to make these resources widely available, we increased the number of articles that could be accessed for free. We also used a more rapid review process to expedite the availability of the manuscripts to readers. The manuscripts may diverge from the format of more traditional papers, and may list useful practice tips in a more direct and simple form. The two-volume book, *How the COVID-19 Pandemic Transformed the Mental Health Landscape*, presents these efforts to address the challenges that counselling psychologists and counsellors encountered in an early period of the pandemic. The two-volume book includes all articles from the special issues of CPQ but organizes them thematically.

This volume (Part I) one includes 14 chapters that address topics associated with transferring counselling practice online. Several chapters focus on transitioning to online therapy from face-to-face contact, including the effect of such a transition on the therapeutic relationship, and working with clients' emotional processes online.

We would like to thank the authors who, in spite of the many stresses brought on by the pandemic, worked so hard to submit their work to *Counselling Psychology Quarterly* in a timely manner. We are also grateful that Editorial Board members accepted their fast-track review assignments to provide helpful comments. Finally, we would like to thank Alyse Taggart and the editorial team from Taylor and Francis, who made it possible for us to produce this special issue and make them available as a two-volume book.

August 2022
Co-Editors-in-Chief, *Counselling Psychology Quarterly*
Shigeru Iwakabe and Sarah Knox

Part I

Transitioning to Telepsychotherapy

Telepsychotherapy: a leaflet for psychotherapists in the age of COVID-19. A review of the evidence

Barbara Poletti, Sofia Tagini, Agostino Brugnera, Laura Parolin,
Luca Pievani, Roberta Ferrucci, Angelo Compare and Vincenzo Silani

ABSTRACT

COVID-19 outbreak imposes the adoption of extraordinary containment measures, including the strict necessity to limit interpersonal contact. Face-to-face psychotherapy collides with this requirement and, above all, it might endanger both therapists and patients' safety. Telepsychotherapy might come to the aid, ensuring therapeutic continuity and the possibility to reach people who might benefit of extra psychological support. Infectious outbreaks have been indeed associated with major psychopathological outcomes. The aim of the present work is to review the most recent experimental evidence about telepsychotherapy, focusing on its effectiveness, possible determinants of efficacy and therapists/patients' attitudes, to rapidly inform psychotherapists. Out of the 857 records found, 18 studies have been included in the review. Our results show that, despite therapists and public's skepticism, telepsychotherapy is a trustworthy alternative to be adopted, which can be used efficaciously to treat common mental-health disorders such as anxiety, depression and post-traumatic distress. As well as in the traditional setting, a higher number of sessions and the proper management of patients' expectations seem to be associated with better outcomes. On the contrary, low familiarity with web-based means of communication and technical issues might reduce specifically the effectiveness of telepsychotherapy.

Introduction

On December 2019, a pneumonia of unknown cause was first reported to the World Health Organization (WHO) in China. Lately, this disease was found to be caused by a new coronavirus (SARS-Cov-2) and was named COVID-19 (World Health Organization, 2020). Since then, the new coronavirus rapidly spread worldwide and on 11 March 2020 the WHO declared COVID-19 outbreak a pandemic. Accordingly, extraordinary containment measures have been adopted all over the World, including the obligation for any citizen to avoid unnecessary person-to-person interactions and social gatherings, as well as limiting movements only to mandatory necessities. Total isolation of individuals infected (or possibly infected) by SARS-Cov-2 was also imposed (e.g. Italian Ministerial Decree 8 March, 2020). The COVID-19 outbreak, thus, dramatically impacts on individuals' daily routine, including the possibility to carry out certain working-activities. When applicable, smart working from home was in fact encouraged.

Health-care professionals, including psychologists and psychotherapists, have been recognized to provide an essential service to the community, therefore allowed to continue their practice. However, in-person sessions endanger both therapists and patients' safety and collide with the requirement to minimize interpersonal contacts. On the other hand, the outbreak of an infectious disease has been associated with major psychological outcomes (Brooks et al., 2020; DiGiovanni, Conley, Chiu, & Zaborski, 2004; Hawryluck et al., 2004), not mentioning the need to support people in grieving. Ensuring therapeutic continuity and reaching vulnerable people who might benefit of extra psychological support seems, thus, mandatory in the present moment.

Telepsychotherapy might come to the aid (Van Daele, Karekla, Kassianos, Compare, & Haddouk, in press; Wind, Rijkeboer, Andersson, & Riper, 2020), especially given the unknown duration of the current containment measures. However, therapists might be unfamiliar or doubtful about the adoption of telepsychotherapy. Hence, the aim of the present work is to provide an updated review of the most recent experimental evidence about telepsychotherapy, to inform professionals in need to support people in this extra-ordinary moment of vulnerability. Specifically, we will focus on effectiveness, possible determinants of efficacy and therapists/patients' attitudes of any kind of individual or group psychotherapy delivered towards synchronous web technology (i.e. videoconference or chatrooms). We purposely focused *only* on telepsychotherapy, excluding non-psychotherapeutic on-line treatments (e.g. psychoeducational programs) and on-line self-help tools. These web-based interventions have been previously reported to be effective (Fiorini, De Giacomo, & L'Abate, 2015; Turvey & Roberts, 2015); nevertheless, their theoretical background, methodological approaches and depth of intervention are profoundly different than psychotherapy (e.g. concerning the amount of direct interaction and the relationship with the therapist). Thus, the inclusion of two different interventions might prevent from a clear understanding of treatment effectiveness and of its determinants. Furthermore, the mentioned on-line interventions are often delivered toward specific web-based platforms or complex interactive softwares, whereas telepsychotherapy requires only basic videoconferencing tools that can be accessed easily and quickly by the therapists.

Implications of the use of telepsychotherapy in the specific time of pandemic are discussed, as well as the possible psychological issues to deal with, according to the previously reported effects of infectious outbreaks on individuals' mental health (e.g. Brooks et al., 2020 for a review).

Methods

Research articles addressing the delivery of individual or group *psychotherapy* lead by a *licensed psychotherapist* towards *synchronous web technology* (i.e. videoconference or chatrooms) were considered eligible. Only studies involving adult participants (>18 years old) were included. Works concerning non-psychotherapeutic psychological treatments, as well as on-line self-help tools were excluded. Interventions in which the interaction between the psychotherapist and the patient was asynchronous (e.g. e-mails exchange) were also excluded since too different from the traditional psychotherapeutic setting.

Studies were identified by searching PubMed and Web of Science databases. We searched the terms "telepsychotherapy" and "psychotherapy" in combination with "distance" or "on-line"/"online" words, according to the most frequent definitions. The search was limited to studies written in English and published between 2015 and 2020. Time restrictions were imposed since both the efficiency of technological devices and people's familiarity towards web-based means of communication exponentially increase over time, possibly modifying individuals' attitudes towards telepsychotherapy and, eventually, its effectiveness (Etzelmueller, Radkovsky, Hannig, Berking, & Ebert, 2018). The last search was run on 30 March 2020.

The selection process is reported in detail in Figure 1. One reviewer performed the search and made a preliminary eligibility check based on titles and abstracts after removing duplicates. Then, the full text of the selected papers was analyzed, and eligibility discussed with a second reviewer. The reference lists of the selected papers were screened to identify additional pertinent articles.

Data were collected by one reviewer according to an extraction sheet previously developed. The following information was collected (when applicable): i) characteristics of the sample including diagnosis and sample size, ii) type of intervention, duration and number of sessions iii) the primary outcome considered, iv) main results. All data sought were found in the original articles, no additional research was needed.

Results

The search provided 857 (PubMed: 288, Web of Science: 569) citations. Two studies were detected by manually inspecting the reference lists of the full texts considered. One study, recently published, was found in a publicly available repository. After the removal of duplicates, 683 citations remained. All of them were screened for eligibility by title and abstract. A total of 576 records were excluded since they did not meet the eligibility criteria. The full text of the remaining 107 works was analyzed. Eighty-nine studies were excluded because they did not meet the inclusion criteria (see Figure 1 for further details on the exclusion reasons). A total of 18 studies were identified for inclusion in the review (see Table 1).

Ten studies investigated a variety of aspects related to the use of telepsychotherapy in depression (Catarino et al., 2018; Egede et al., 2015, 2016; Ekberg, Barnes, Kessler, Malpass, & Shaw, 2016; Ekberg et al., 2015; Etzelmueller et al., 2018), anxiety (Catarino et al., 2018; Théberge-Lapointe, Marchand, Langlois, Gosselin, & Watts, 2015), post-traumatic stress disorder – PTSD (Wierwille, Pukay-Martin, Chard, & Klump, 2016), panic attacks (Cipolletta, Frassoni, & Faccio, 2018) and bulimia nervosa (Zerwas et al., 2016). Eight works surveyed both the attitudes towards and the use of telepsychotherapy in the general public (Apolinário-Hagen, Vehreschild, & Alkoudmani, 2017; Hantsoo, Podcasy, Sammel, Epperson, & Kim, 2017), among psychotherapists (Gilmore & Ward-Ciesielski, 2019; Gordon, Tune, & Wang, 2016; Gordon, Wang, & Tune, 2015; Pierce, Perrin, & McDonald, 2019, 2020) and comparing health-care professionals and nonprofessionals (Schulze et al., 2019).

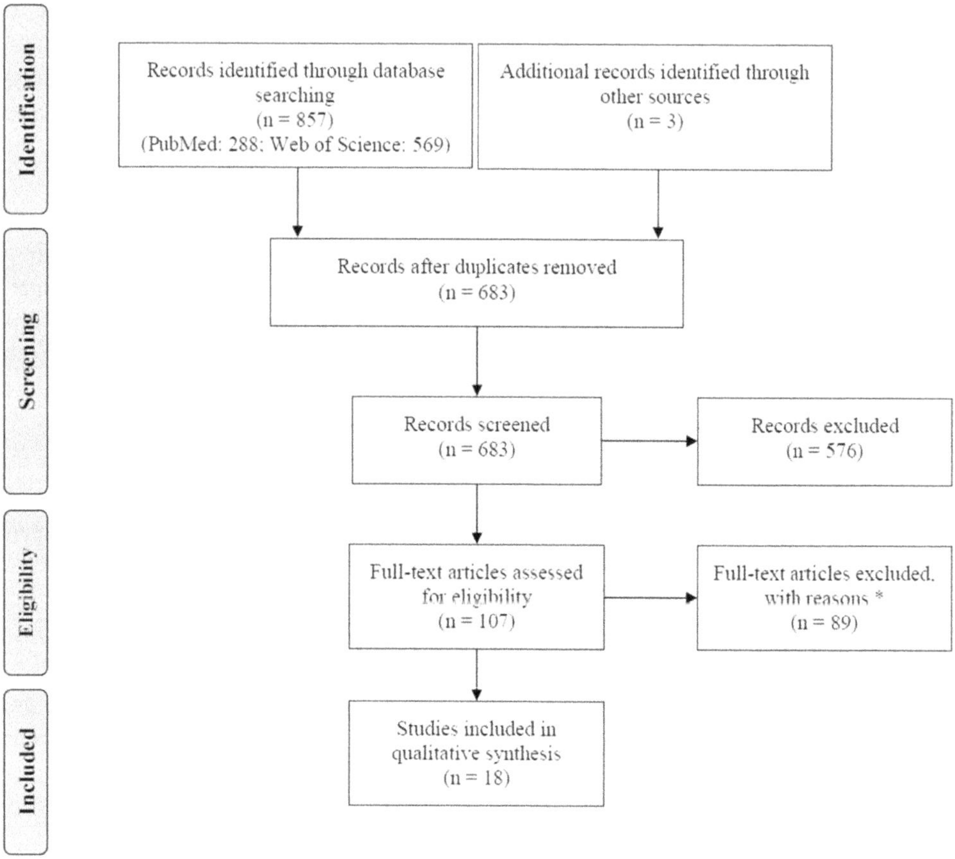

Figure 1. The flow diagram represents the studies selection process.

*main reasons of exclusion include treatments other than psychotherapy (e.g. self-help tools, psychological support or counseling, psychoeducational interventions); psychotherapy not lead by a licensed psychotherapist, questioning the reliability of the intervention; works other than original research articles (e.g, review, commentary or methodological papers); full text not available; studies focused on training or supervision of psychotherapists.

Cognitive/behavioral approaches were the most represented, including individual (Catarino et al., 2018; Egede et al., 2015, 2016; Etzelmueller et al., 2018; Théberge-Lapointe et al., 2015) and group (Zerwas et al., 2016) cognitive behavioral therapy – CBT, the behavioral activation therapy for depression (Ekberg et al., 2016), the brief strategic approach (Cipolletta et al., 2018) and the cognitive processing and prolonged exposure therapy (Wierwille et al., 2016). One of the survey-studies focused on the psychodynamic approach (Gordon et al., 2016, 2015); the others addressed attitudes towards telepsychotherapy in general (Apolinário-Hagen et al., 2017; Gilmore & Ward-Ciesielski, 2019; Hantsoo et al., 2017; Pierce et al., 2020; Schulze et al., 2019).

Effectiveness

A significant clinical improvement and symptom reduction were reported in patients affected by anxiety and depression following 6/8 weekly sessions of individual on-line CBT: a similar clinical improvement was observed in a severity-matched sample of

Table 1. The table illustrates the disorder treated, sample size, type of psychotherapy adopted, duration and frequency of sessions, and primary outcomes evaluated.

	Disorder Treated	Sample	Psychotherapeutic Approach	Duration	Primary Outcome Considered
Ekberg et al., 2015	Depression	TP: 183	CBT	55 min, up to 10 sessions	Management of patients' expectations during the first and second sessions
Egede et al., 2015	Depression	TP: 120 FFP: 121	Behavioral activation psychotherapy	8 x 60 min weekly sessions	Depressive symptoms (GDS; BDI; SCID)
Théberge-Lapointe et al., 2015	Anxiety	TP: 5	CBT	14 x 60 min weekly sessions	Anxiety (SIAD-IV) Worries (PSWQ, WW-II) Intolerance of uncertainty (IUS) Negative attitudes to problem (NPOQ) Cognitive Avoidance Strategies (CAQ)
Ekberg et al., 2016	Depression	TP: 183	CBT	55 min, up to 10 sessions	Management of patients' expectations during the first and second sessions in relationship to retention
Egede et al., 2016	Depression	TP: 120 FFP: 121	Behavioral activation psychotherapy	8 x 60 min weekly sessions	Quality of life (SF-36) Satisfaction (CPOSS) Treatment credibility Service delivery perceptions
Wierwille et al., 2016	PTSD	TP: 85 FFT: 136	Cognitive processing and prolonged exposure therapy	Not specified	PTSD (PCL-S) Depressive symptoms (BDI-II)
Cipolletta et al., 2018	Panic attacks	TP: 5	Brief strategic approach	3 x 50 min sessions	Relational dominance (conversation analysis)
Zerwas et al., 2016	Bulimia nervosa	TP: 16 FFP: 16	Group CBT	16 x 90 min weekly sessions	Abstinence from binge eating and purging
Catarino et al., 2018	Anxiety Depression	TP: 2211	CBT	6/8 weekly sessions	Anxiety and depressive symptoms (PHQ-9, GAD-7)
Etzelmueller et al., 2018	Depression	TP: 15	CBT	50 min, up to 25 sessions	Perceived patients' experience
Gordon et al., 2015	-	176 therapists	Survey on TP	-	-
Gordon et al., 2016	-	94 therapists	Survey on TP	-	-
Apolinário-Hagen et al., 2017	-	1558 general public	Survey on TP	-	-

(*Continued*)

Table 1. (Continued).

	Disorder Treated	Sample	Psychotherapeutic Approach	Duration	Primary Outcome Considered
Hantsoo et al., 2017	-	111 pregnant women 147 non-pregnant women 54 men	Survey on TP and FFT	-	-
Schulze et al., 2019	-	1000 non-professionals 96 physicians 36 therapists	Survey on TP	-	-
Pierce et al., 2019	-	1799 Psychotherapists	Survey on TP	-	-
Gilmore & Ward-Ciesielski, 2019	-	52 Psychotherapists	Survey on TP	-	-
Pierce et al., 2020	-	1791 Psychotherapists	Survey on TP	-	Demographic, organizational and clinical predictors of telepsychotherapy use

TP = telepsychotherapy; FFT = face-to-face therapy; CBT = Cognitive Behavioral Therapy; GDS = Geriatric Depression Scale; BDI = Beck Depression Inventory, SCID = Structured Clinical Interview for DSM-IV; SIAD-IV = Structured Diagnostic Interview for Anxiety Disorder; PSWQ = Penn State Worry Questionnaire; Why Worry II; IUS = Intolerance of Uncertainty Scale; NPOQ = Negative Problem Orientation Questionnaire; CAQ = Cognitive Avoidance Questionnaire; SF-36 = Short-Form Health Survey; CFOSS = Cognitive Avoidance Questionnaire; PCL-S = Post-Traumatic Stress Disorder Checklist – Specific; PHQ-9 = Patient Health Questionnaire; GAD-7 = General Anxiety Disorder Scale.

individuals attending the same mental-health promoting program but not involved in the study (between groups difference: *depression symptoms, d = 0.02; anxiety symptoms, d = 0.04)* (Catarino et al., 2018). Similarly, Théberge-Lapointe et al. (2015) reported that individual sessions of videoconferencing CBT (60-minutes weekly sessions for 14 weeks) determined a significant clinical improvement in patients with generalized anxiety disorder both at the end of the treatment and at 3-months follow-up (effect sizes for the factor *time* in a repeated measures ANOVA (η^2) range from 0.56 to 0.78 for the outcomes considered). Qualitatively, the effectiveness of telepsychotherapy was reported to be comparable to the overall efficacy of an in-person version of the same treatment, administered in a previous study (Dugas & Robichaud, 2007).

A significant clinical improvement in depressive symptomatology was reported during and after 8 weeks of individuals videoconferencing behavioral activation psychotherapy (60-minutes weekly sessions) (Egede et al., 2015). Notably, in this case, the effectiveness of telepsychotherapy was directly compared to a traditional in-person therapy, reporting that the two treatment modalities determined comparable clinical outcomes (between-groups differences in the percentage of patients who effectively responded to the treatment for the depressive symptomatology at 12-months follow-up were non-significant, ranging from − 5.09% [90% CI − 17.13 to 6.95] to 2.06% [90% CI − 7.46 to 11.58]), despite a slightly slower rate of improvement in the web-based delivery (Egede et al., 2015).

A significant, clinically relevant, reduction in PTSD and depressive symptoms was also reported in U.S. veterans after individuals videoconferencing cognitive processing and prolonged exposure therapy (Wierwille et al., 2016). The effectiveness of telepsychotherapy in this study was reported to be slightly lower than in-person treatment (73.2% of patients receiving telepsychotherapy achieved clinically significant improvement of post-traumatic distress at post-treatment versus the 82.9% of patients receiving a traditional therapy, x^2 (1) = 0.99, $p = 0.319$); however, the severity of PTSD at baseline was higher in the telepsychotherapy group, possibly explaining between-group differences at post-treatment (Wierwille et al., 2016).

Only one study (Zerwas et al., 2016) compared group psychotherapy in-person and *via* chatroom in a sample of individuals affected by bulimia nervosa. Both modalities were reported to be effective in terms of improved abstinence from binge eating and purging (i.e. the primary outcome); however, the improving rate was slower in the chatroom-based psychotherapy. Differences between groups in terms of abstinence from binge eating and purging were indeed reported at the end of the treatment, even though the size of the effect ($d = -0.18$) can be considered trivial (Cohen, 1988), but not at 12-months follow-up ($d = 0.07$). Furthermore, the two treatment modalities were reported to be similarly effective at both the post-treatment evaluation and follow-up also for overall symptom severity (post-treatment $d = 0.04$; follow-up $d = -0.12$), psychopathological comorbidity (*depressive disorder*: post-treatment $d = -0.11$, follow-up $d = -0.10$; *anxiety disorder*: post-treatment $d = 0.14$, follow-up $d = -0.04$), and overall quality of life (*Eating Disorders Quality of Life Questionnaire*: post-treatment $d = 0.01$, follow-up $d = -0.08$; *Short-Form Health State Classification*: post-treatment $d = 0.04$, follow-up $d = 0.14$) (Zerwas et al., 2016).

No differences in the perceived quality of life, satisfaction, credibility of the treatment and service delivery were observed between patients attending individual videoconferencing or in-person CBT (60-minutes weekly sessions for 8 weeks) at several timepoints from the beginning of the treatment (4 weeks, 8 weeks, 3 months and 12 months) (Egede et al., 2016). In line with these results, a qualitatively study evaluating the experience of 15 patients with depression attending individual videoconferencing CBT (50-minutes weekly sessions, up to 25 times) reported that a majority of them (80%) positively rated the intervention, expressing the possibility to establish a good working alliance (67%) and a close contact with the therapist (40%) (Etzelmueller et al., 2018). Many patients also emphasized the benefit of an individualized and flexible intervention (47% and 37%, respectively) reporting an improved understanding of their condition (60%) (Etzelmueller et al., 2018). Furthermore, on-line therapy was not perceived as less effective than a traditional face-to-face treatment (53%) (Etzelmueller et al., 2018). Finally, Cipolletta and colleagues (2018) qualitatively evaluated the dynamics of the therapeutic relationship during the first three sessions of a videoconferencing brief strategic therapy in 5 patients with panic attacks, reporting that they were similar to those observed in face-to-face interventions (i.e. asymmetric semantic and strategic dominance) (Lenzi & Bercelli, 2010).

Factors related to effectiveness

The post-treatment outcome among patients with anxiety and depressive symptoms was reported to be clinically relevant after at least five sessions of individual on-line CBT (Catarino et al., 2018). However, a higher severity of symptoms at baseline and comorbidity with long-term physical conditions were associated with lower clinical improvement (Catarino et al., 2018). Nevertheless, the effect of previous physical conditions might be an artifact since the psychopathological scales used for the assessment might have been too sensitive to the somatic symptoms related to anxiety and depression (Catarino et al., 2018).

Technical difficulties such as brief interruptions or complete breakdown have been claimed to be the most prominent drawback of videoconferencing psychotherapy (Cipolletta et al., 2018; Etzelmueller et al., 2018) since they favor misunderstandings that might compromise the therapeutic interaction (Cipolletta et al., 2018). Familiarity with web-technology, on the contrary, was perceived as promoting patients' compliance (67%) (Etzelmueller et al., 2018), while older age (average sample age: 36 years) was associated to a lower drop-outs rate and better clinical outcomes (Catarino et al., 2018).

Finally, an early and comprehensive management of patients' expectations about the structure of the whole therapy (i.e., on-line CBT) and the expected benefits were reported to be crucial to increment therapy retention (Ekberg et al., 2016), and eventually treatment effectiveness. Nevertheless, few therapists were reported to adopt this approach (20.5%), whereas most of them managed patients' expectations only concerning the first session of assessment (61.4%) or did not address patients' expectations at all (15.3%) (Ekberg et al., 2015).

Therapists and patients' attitudes

Survey-studies investigating attitudes towards telepsychotherapy reported that psychotherapists generally perceived videoconferencing treatments as possibly less effective than face-to-face therapies (Gordon et al., 2016, 2015; Schulze et al., 2019). Psychotherapists dealing with suicidal patients expressed specific worries about the impossibility of taking advantage of nonverbal and emotional cues during the patient's assessment and to exert a direct control over the patient if hospitalization is needed (Gilmore & Ward-Ciesielski, 2019). Similarly, psychotherapists treating conditions possibly related to acute patients' crises (e.g. grief [Odds Ratio – OR: 0.67], bipolar disorder [OR: 0.64], antisocial personality [OR: 0.50] and addiction [OR: 1.60]) were reported to adopt telepsychotherapy to a lesser extent (Pierce et al., 2020). Possible difficulties in dealing remotely with patients' crises were also pointed out by the psychodynamic therapists interviewed by Gordon et al. (2015). Psychodynamic therapists worried the most about the possibility of an efficacious exploration of patients' mental life and psychodynamic constructions (Gordon et al., 2016). On the contrary, they were less concerned about the prospect of working on transference towards the web (Gordon et al., 2016).

In line with these results, most of the therapists (80%) interviewed by Pierce et al. (2019) do not usually use telepsychotherapy. Furthermore, the authors reported that *other people*'s attitudes and expectations about telepsychotherapy were largely associated with therapists' own perception of usefulness and ease of use that, in turn, was associated with the actual use of telepsychotherapy.

Nevertheless, therapists recognized the possibility to reach remote patients as the main advantage of telepsychotherapy (Gordon et al., 2016, 2015). Additionally, both younger age and more years of working experience were reported to be positively associated with a higher use of telepsychotherapy (Gilmore & Ward-Ciesielski, 2019). Finally, the availability of clear institutional telepsychotherapy-supportive policies (OR: 2.25) and being specifically trained to use this treatment modality (OR: 8.74) were both predictors of a higher adoption of telepsychotherapy (Pierce et al., 2020).

The general public also seems doubtful about telepsychotherapy effectiveness (Apolinário-Hagen et al., 2017; Schulze et al., 2019), the quality of the therapeutic support delivered and the compatibility with every-day life conditions (Apolinário-Hagen et al., 2017). As a result, common people expressed a low willingness to use telepsychotherapy (Apolinário-Hagen et al., 2017; Hantsoo et al., 2017), though, people with no previous history of psychotherapy were generally more opened towards the use of telepsychotherapy (Hantsoo et al., 2017). On the contrary, accessibility and the possibility to reduce waiting-lists were recognized as main advantages, especially among those individuals who reported a higher perceived stress (Apolinário-Hagen et al., 2017). Similarly, pregnant women showed a high acceptability of internet-based psychotherapy (77.5% of the sample), and 30.6% of the sample also reported that they would prefer this type of therapy instead of in-person treatments (Hantsoo et al., 2017).

Discussion

The present work aims to summarize the most recent experimental evidence about telepsychotherapy to provide useful guidance for psychotherapists facing the challenge of COVID-19 outbreak. Overall, our results show that telepsychotherapy can be used to treat successfully common mental-health disorders. Telepsychotherapy effectiveness was indeed reported to be *comparable* to in-person treatment (Catarino et al., 2018; Egede et al., 2015; Zerwas et al., 2016) despite the rate of improvement might be slightly slower (Egede et al., 2015; Zerwas et al., 2016). Importantly, the experimental evidence specifically points to the possibility to treat efficaciously anxiety (Catarino et al., 2018), depressive (Catarino et al., 2018; Egede et al., 2015), and post-traumatic symptoms (Wierwille et al., 2016), which are the most frequent psychopathological outcomes associated to an infectious outbreak (Brooks et al., 2020).

Additionally, patients who were enrolled in telepsychotherapy treatments reported similar perceived quality of life, satisfaction, credibility of the treatment and service delivery opinions than patients attending in-person psychotherapy (Egede et al., 2016). In line with these results, patients receiving telepsychotherapy did not perceive the treatment as less effective than a traditional one (Etzelmueller et al., 2018). On the contrary, they reported good working alliance and close contact with the therapist, emphasizing the benefits of an individualized and flexible intervention in improving the understanding of their condition (Etzelmueller et al., 2018).

Different factors have been associated with telepsychotherapy effectiveness. Specifically, the length of the treatment was reported to be a crucial issue: more positive outcomes were indeed observed as the number of sessions increased (Catarino et al., 2018). This result might not be surprising and it mirrors the overall evidence of a positive relationship between the length of face-to-face interventions and the treatment effectiveness (Howard, Kopta, Krause, & Orlinsky, 1986; Knekt et al., 2008; Knekt, Lindfors, Sares-Jäske, Virtala, & Härkänen, 2013; Knekt et al., 2016; Lindfors, Knekt, Heinonen, Härkänen, & Virtala, 2015).

In this regard, a proper and comprehensive management of patients' expectations about the structure of the therapy and the benefits expected might encourage treatment retention (Ekberg et al., 2016). Additionally, in one study (Catarino et al., 2018) older age was associated with lower drop-outs rate, though the participants in that study were indeed quite young on average (i.e. 36 years old). Conversely, comorbidity with long-term physical conditions and higher severity of symptoms at baseline were reported to be related to lower clinical outcomes (Catarino et al., 2018). Notably, all these factors might conceivably affect also in-person psychotherapy. On the contrary, the experience of technical difficulties and low familiarity with the use of information technologies seem to affect specifically telepsychotherapy efficacy (Cipolletta et al., 2018; Etzelmueller et al., 2018).

Thus, the experimental evidence points to a reasonable telepsychotherapy effectiveness. In sharp contrast, both the general public and psychotherapists were reported to be doubtful about telepsychotherapy use and effectiveness (Apolinário-Hagen et al., 2017; Gordon et al., 2015; Schulze et al., 2019). In turn, they declared they would hardly choose it (Apolinário-Hagen et al., 2017; Hantsoo et al., 2017; Pierce et al., 2019). Nevertheless, this scenario was depicted when telepsychotherapy was an *option*. Now, it might be the only alternative. Attitudes and willingness to use telepsychotherapy seem indeed to be influenced by incidental needs. For instance, pregnant women who encountered mobility issues reported higher acceptability of telepsychotherapy than their non-pregnant counterparts (Hantsoo et al., 2017). Similarly, individuals with a higher level of perceived stress and, thus, possibly seeking treatments were more likely to adopt telepsychotherapy (Apolinário-Hagen et al., 2017). Accordingly, telepsychotherapy acceptability might be significantly shaped, and conceivably favored, by the ongoing COVID-19 outbreak. After all, the higher accessibility and the possibility to reach remote patients have been considered the main advantages of telepsychotherapy, even back when no one would have imagined a similar scenario (Apolinário-Hagen et al., 2017; Gordon et al., 2015).

However, the adoption of telepsychotherapy *during* a pandemic might also have some drawbacks, which need to be discussed. First, in the studies reviewed telepsychotherapy was adopted since the beginning of the therapeutic process. Conversely, the upsurge of an emergency forces the transition from face-to-face therapy to telepsychotherapy. An optimal use of telepsychotherapy implies the availability of appropriate equipment (including an efficient internet connection, suitable technological devices and videoconferencing tools) and of proper location where to conduct the therapy (Van Daele et al., in press). Because of the sudden shift to telepsychotherapy, both patients and therapists might not have immediate availability of the equipment needed; more importantly, if they have no access to dedicated and private space at home, it might be challenging to recreate that intimate, reassuring and safeguarded setting experienced in face-to-face sessions.

To the best of our knowledge, no previous study investigated the effect of this setting transition; however, both patients and therapists might experience it as destabilizing. Consequently, patients' adherence to the treatment and the therapeutic alliance might be endangered, as well as the therapy efficacy might be compromised. However, a solid pre-existing therapeutic alliance might work as protective factor, favoring a smooth transition.

Furthermore, therapists might not be specifically trained to deliver telepsychotherapy: this might threaten their perceived professional self-efficacy and self-confidence. Therapists who received a specific training on how to deliver telepsychotherapy are indeed more likely to adopt this treatment modality (Pierce et al., 2020). Therefore, training programs should take into high consideration the possibility of addressing these skills, at least briefly. Not surprisingly, younger and more expert therapists were reported to be more motivated to adopt telepsychotherapy (Gilmore & Ward-Ciesielski, 2019), possibly because they felt more confident in dealing with videoconferencing and about their professional capabilities, respectively.

Moreover, lack of clear policies and regulations about the delivery of telepsychotherapy (e.g. about how to protect the patients' privacy over the internet) has been reported to be a deterrent that may further discourage psychotherapists (Pierce et al., 2020). In this regard, therapists may refer to the guidelines provided by the European Federation of Psychologists'Associations (2001) and by the American Psychological Association (2013), as well as by the International Society for Mental Health Online (2000).

Last, but not least, also therapists must face the challenge of a pandemic, meaning that they might experience a significant level of distress too. As a result, therapists might struggle to accomplish adequately their professional duties towards telepsychotherapy. Thus, supervision might be even more crucial than usual. Interestingly, *telesupervision* was reported to be as much effective as in-person (Inman, Soheilian, & Luu, 2019; Jordan & Shearer, 2019; Martin, Lizarondo, & Kumar, 2018), even when switching the supervision modality in course (Tarlow, McCord, Nelon, & Bernhard, in press).

According to the previous considerations, we suggest that the effectiveness of telepsychotherapy *during* a pandemic should be further explored: the present moment represents indeed a unique opportunity of investigation. Specifically, the implications of the setting transition, of the possible difficulties to interact over the internet and of the therapists' professional preparedness should be addressed.

Finally, although most of studies focused on cognitive-behavioral approaches, many other kinds of therapy might be successfully implemented towards videoconferencing. Furthermore, many studies in literature reported successful on-line interventions other than psychotherapy, such as self-help tools or psychoeducational interventions (Manfrida, Albertini, & Eisenberg, 2017). These techniques might indeed be helpful to face the psychological consequences of COVID-19 outbreak; however, we decided to focus on psychotherapy as a more powerful form of psychological support, which can be easily and rapidly implemented by the therapists.

To conclude, telepsychotherapy represents a *trustworthy alternative* to be adopted, especially given the current necessity to limit face-to-face contact and, at the same time, the urgent need to provide effective support. As mentioned, infective outbreak might have a significant and specific impact on people's well being and mental health, including increased emotional difficulties, depressive symptoms, anxiety, irritability, insomnia, post-traumatic stress symptoms, fear and anger (e.g. Brooks et al., 2020; DiGiovanni et al., 2004), as well as sense of isolation (e.g. Hawryluck et al., 2004) and possibly grieving. Thus, all these issues should be specifically considered by (tele)psychotherapists currently delivering treatments. Additionally, certain individuals might be at higher risks than others to develop mental-health disorders, requiring extra care (Jiang et al., 2020). Above all, health-care professionals have been reported to be more affected by infectious outbreaks since their greater exposure to the disease and the higher risk of being infected (Reynolds et al., 2008). Furthermore, people who survived the infection or who experienced a bereavement conceivably represent higher-risk individuals.

Future studies should further address the investigation of telepsychotherapy effectiveness: the possibility to implement efficacious on-line treatments represents indeed an extraordinary opportunity to support most vulnerable individuals even in emergency circumstances, when face-to-face contact might be prevented.

Disclosure statement

No potential conflict of interest was reported by the authors.

ORCID

Barbara Poletti http://orcid.org/0000-0003-4398-2051
Sofia Tagini http://orcid.org/0000-0001-9888-7911
Agostino Brugnera http://orcid.org/0000-0002-4066-4552
Roberta Ferrucci http://orcid.org/0000-0001-5109-9483
Angelo Compare http://orcid.org/0000-0002-3336-7920
Vincenzo Silani http://orcid.org/0000-0002-7698-3854

References

American Psychological Association. (2013). Guidelines for the practice of telepsychology. *American Psychologist 68*(9), 791–800.

Apolinário-Hagen, J., Vehreschild, V., & Alkoudmani, R. M. (2017). Current views and perspectives on E-mental health: An exploratory survey study for understanding public attitudes toward internet-based psychotherapy in Germany. *JMIR Mental Health*, *4*(1), e8.

Brooks, S. K., Webster, R. K., Smith, L. E., Woodland, L., Wessely, S., Greenberg, N., & Rubin, G. J. (2020). The psychological impact of quarantine and how to reduce it: Rapid review of the evidence. *The Lancet*, *395*(10227), 912–920.

Catarino, A., Bateup, S., Tablan, V., Innes, K., Freer, S., Richards, A., ... Blackwell, A. D. (2018). Demographic and clinical predictors of response to internet-enabled cognitive–behavioural therapy for depression and anxiety. *BJPsych Open*, *4*(5), 411–418.

Cipolletta, S., Frassoni, E., & Faccio, E. (2018). Construing a therapeutic relationship online: An analysis of videoconference sessions. *Clinical Psychologist*, *22*(2), 220–229.

Cohen, J. (1988). *Statistical power analysis for the behavioral sciences*. (N. L. E. A. Hillsdale, ed.). (2nd ed.). Hillsdale. NJ: Erihaum.

DiGiovanni, C., Conley, J., Chiu, D., & Zaborski, J. (2004). Factors influencing compliance with quarantine in Toronto during the 2003 SARS outbreak. *Biosecurity and Bioterrorism: Biodefense Strategy, Practice, and Science*, *2*(4), 265–272.

Dugas, M. J., & Robichaud, M. (2007). *Cognitive-behavioral treatment for generalized anxiety disorder: From science to practice*. New York: Taylor & Francis Group.

Egede, L. E., Acierno, R., Knapp, R. G., Lejuez, C., Hernandez-Tejada, M., Payne, E. H., & Frueh, B. C. (2015). Psychotherapy for depression in older veterans via telemedicine: A randomised, open-label, non-inferiority trial. *The Lancet Psychiatry*, *2*(8), 693–701.

Egede, L. E., Acierno, R., Knapp, R. G., Walker, R. J., Payne, E. H., & Frueh, B. C. (2016). Psychotherapy for depression in older veterans via telemedicine: Effect on quality of life, satisfaction, treatment credibility, and service delivery perception. *The Journal of Clinical Psychiatry*, *77*(12), 1704–1711.

Ekberg, S., Barnes, R. K., Kessler, D. S., Malpass, A., & Shaw, A. R. G. (2016). Managing clients' expectations at the outset of online Cognitive Behavioural Therapy (CBT) for depression. *Health Expectations*, *19*(3), 557–569.

Ekberg, S., Barnes, R. K., Kessler, D. S., Mirza, S., Montgomery, A. A., Malpass, A., & Shaw, A. R. G. (2015). Relationship between expectation management and client retention in online cognitive behavioural therapy. *Behavioural and Cognitive Psychotherapy*, *43*(6), 732–743.

Etzelmueller, A., Radkovsky, A., Hannig, W., Berking, M., & Ebert, D. D. (2018). Patient's experience with blended video- and internet based cognitive behavioural therapy service in routine care. *Internet Interventions*, *12*(December2017), 165–175.

European Federation of Psychologists'Associations. (2001). *The provision of psychological services via the internet and other non-direct means*. Retrieved from http://ethics.efpa.eu/guidelines/

Fiorini, R. A., De Giacomo, P., & L'Abate, L. (2015). Towards resilient telehealth support for clinical psychiatry and psychology: A strategic review. In *Enabling Health Informatics Applications* J. Mantas et al., (Eds.), IOS Press (pp. 275–278).

Gilmore, A. K., & Ward-Ciesielski, E. F. (2019). Perceived risks and use of psychotherapy via telemedicine for patients at risk for suicide. *Journal of Telemedicine and Telecare*, *25*(1), 59–63.

Gordon, R. M., Tune, J., & Wang, X. (2016). What are the characteristics and concerns of high and low raters of psychodynamic treatment to Chinese students over VCON? What are the characteristics and concerns of high and low raters of psychodynamic treatment to chinese students over VCON? In *Psychoanalysis and Psychotherapy in China*, Routledge, *1*(November) (pp. 96-106).

Gordon, R. M., Wang, X., & Tune, J. (2015). Comparing psychodynamic teaching, supervision, and psychotherapy over videoconferencing technology with Chinese students. *Psychodynamic Psychiatry*, *43*(4), 585–599.

Hantsoo, L., Podcasy, J., Sammel, M., Epperson, C. N., & Kim, D. R. (2017). Pregnancy and the acceptability of computer-based versus traditional mental health treatments. *Journal of Women's Health*, *26*(10), 1106–1113.

Hawryluck, L., Gold, W. L., Robinson, S., Pogorski, S., Galea, S., & Styra, R. (2004). SARS control and psychological effects of quarantine, Toronto, Canada. *Emerging Infectious Diseases*, *10*(7), 1206–1212.

Howard, K. I., Kopta, S. M., Krause, M. S., & Orlinsky, D. E. (1986). The dose–effect relationship in psychotherapy. *American Psychologist*, *41*(2), 159.

Inman, A. G., Soheilian, S. S., & Luu, L. P. (2019). Telesupervision: Building bridges in a digital era. *Journal of Clinical Psychology*, *75*(2), 292–301.

International Society for Mental Health Online. (2000). ISMHO/PSI suggested principles for the online provision of mental health services. https://ismho.org/resources/archive/%0Asuggested-principles-for-the-online-provision-ofmental-%0Ahealth-services/

Italian Ministerial Decree 8 March. (2020). Ministerial Decree 8 March. Retrieved from https://www.gazzettaufficiale.it/eli/id/2020/03/08/20A01522/sg

Jiang, X., Deng, L., Zhu, Y., Ji, H., Tao, L., Liu, L., … Ji, W. (2020). Psychological crisis intervention during the outbreak period of new coronavirus pneumonia from experience in Shanghai. *Psychiatry Research*, *286*(February), 112903.

Jordan, S. E., & Shearer, E. M. (2019). An exploration of supervision delivered via clinical video telehealth (CVT). *Training and Education in Professional Psychology*, *13*(4), 323–330.

Knekt, P., Virtala, E., Härkänen, T., Vaarama, M., Lehtonen, J., & Lindfors, O. (2016). The outcome of short- and long term psychotherapy 10 years after start of treatment. *Psychological Medicine*, *46*(6), 1175–1188.

Knekt, P., Lindfors, O., Laaksonen, M. A., Raitasalo, R., Haaramo, P., & Järvikoski, A. (2008). Effectiveness of short-term and long-term psychotherapy on work ability and functional capacity — A randomized clinical trial on depressive and anxiety disorders. *Journal of Affective Disorders*, *107*(1–3), 95–106.

Knekt, P., Lindfors, O., Sares-Jäske, L., Virtala, E., & Härkänen, T. (2013). Randomized trial on the effectiveness of long- and short-term psychotherapy on psychiatric symptoms and working ability during a 5-year follow-up. *Nordic Journal of Psychiatry*, *67*(1), 59–68.

Lenzi, S., & Bercelli, F. (2010). *Parlar di sé con un esperto del sé. L'elaborazione delle narrative personali: Strategie avanzate di terapia cognitiva*. Eclipsi di IPSICO, Firenze.

Lindfors, O., Knekt, P., Heinonen, E., Härkänen, T., & Virtala, E. (2015). The effectiveness of short- and long-term psychotherapy on personality functioning during a 5-year follow-up. *Journal of Affective Disorders*, *173*, 31–38.

Manfrida, G., Albertini, V., & Eisenberg, E. (2017). Connected: recommendations and techniques in order to employ internet tools for the enhancement of online therapeutic relationships. Experiences from Italy. *Contemporary Family Therapy*, *39*(4), 314–328.

Martin, P., Lizarondo, L., & Kumar, S. (2018). A systematic review of the factors that influence the quality and effectiveness of telesupervision for health professionals. *Journal of Telemedicine and Telecare*, *24*(4), 271–281.

Pierce, B. S., Perrin, P. B., & McDonald, S. D. (2019). Path analytic modeling of psychologists' openness to performing clinical work with telepsychology: A national study. *Journal of Clinical Psychology*, 1–16. doi:10.1002/jclp.22851

Pierce, B. S., Perrin, P. B., & McDonald, S. D. (2020). Demographic, organizational, and clinical practice predictors of U.S. psychologists' use of telepsychology. *Professional Psychology: Research and Practice*, *51*(2), 184–193.

Reynolds, D. L., Garay, J. R., Deamond, S. L., Moran, M. K., Gold, W., & Styra, R. (2008). Understanding, compliance and psychological impact of the SARS quarantine experience. *Epidemiology and Infection*, *136*(7), 997–1007.

Schulze, N., Reuter, S. C., Kuchler, I., Reinke, B., Hinkelmann, L., Stöckigt, S., … Tonn, P. (2019). Differences in attitudes toward online interventions in psychiatry and psychotherapy between health care professionals and nonprofessionals: A survey. *Telemedicine and E-Health*, *25*(10), 926–932.

Tarlow, K. R., McCord, C. E., Nelon, J. L., & Bernhard, P. A. (in press). Comparing in-person supervision and telesupervision: A multiple baseline single-case study. *Journal of Psychotherapy Integration*.
Théberge-Lapointe, N., Marchand, A., Langlois, F., Gosselin, P., & Watts, S. (2015). Efficacy of a cognitive-behavioural therapy administered by videoconference for generalized anxiety disorder. *Revue Europeenne de Psychologie Appliquee*, *65*(1), 9–17.
Turvey, C. L., & Roberts, L. J. (2015). Recent developments in the use of online resources and mobile technologies to support mental health care. *International Review of Psychiatry*, *27*(6), 547–557.
Van Daele, T., Karekla, M., Kassianos, A. P., Compare, A., & Haddouk, L. (in press). Recommendations for policy and practice of telepsychotherapy and e-mental health in Europe and beyond. *Journal of Psychotherapy Integration*. doi:10.1037/int0000218
Wierwille, J. L., Pukay-Martin, N. D., Chard, K. M., & Klump, M. C. (2016). Effectiveness of PTSD telehealth treatment in a VA clinical sample. *Psychological Services*, *13*(4), 373–379.
Wind, T. R., Rijkeboer, M., Andersson, G., & Riper, H. (2020). The COVID-19 pandemic: The 'black swan' for mental health care and a turning point for e-health. *Internet Interventions*, *20*, 100317.
World Health Organization. (2020). Rolling updates on coronavirus disease. Retrieved from https://www.who.int/emergencies/diseases/novel-coronavirus-2019/events-as-they-happen
Zerwas, S. C., Watson, H. J., Hofmeier, S. M., Levine, M. D., Hamer, R. M., Crosby, R. D., … Bulik, C. M. (2016). CBT4BN: A randomized controlled trial of online chat and face-to-face group therapy for Bulimia Nervosa. *Psychotherapy and Psychosomatics*, *86*(1), 47–53.

Transitioning to virtual programming amidst COVID-19 outbreak

Alejandra Sequeira, Adaeze Alozie, Melissa Fasteau, Alicia K. Lopez, Jennifer Sy, Karina A. Turner, Cali Werner, Elizabeth McIngvale and Thröstur Björgvinsson

ABSTRACT

The COVID-19 pandemic prompted many mental health care providers to quickly reorganize their operations and services in an effort to continue serving their clientele while also ensuring the health and safety of their patients and staff. Over the course of five days (beginning 15 March 2020), the McLean OCD Institute at Houston (MOCDI-H) transitioned from providing three levels of care in-person to conducting intensive outpatient and traditional outpatient programming completely online. Through the teamwork of all members of the MOCDI-H staff and in collaboration with our patients and their families, we were able to develop virtual programming and make a smooth transition with minimal disruption to patient care. This article aims to describe how we facilitated our clinical transition in a quick and effective manner and became the first program within the OCD community to transition to teletherapy. An anecdotal exploration of the benefits and challenges experienced for patient care and providers is offered. Future directions and implications associated with the change from in-person sessions to teletherapy are discussed.

Obsessive-compulsive disorder and its treatment

Obsessive-Compulsive Disorder (OCD) is a chronic and debilitating disorder characterized by recurrent and unwanted thoughts, urges, or images that evoke anxiety and are experienced with or without compulsions, or repetitive behaviors or mental acts performed in an attempt to promptly relieve anxiety (American Psychiatric Association [APA], 2013). Untreated OCD is associated with poor quality of life and functional impairment in emotional, social, and occupational functioning (Swain & Behura, 2016); however, with appropriate evidence-based treatment, individuals with OCD often live with significant decreases in functional impairment (Burchi, Hollander, & Pallanti, 2018). Evidence-based treatment for OCD includes a form of Cognitive-Behavioral Therapy known as Exposure and Response Prevention (ERP) and medication management using Selective Serotonin Reuptake Inhibitors (APA, 2007). Research suggests that ERP attributes to a 61% reduction rate of symptoms (Collins & Coles, 2017). Despite the efficacy of these treatments for OCD, research suggests that stigma, cost of treatment, and limited adequately trained providers often prevents sufferers from obtaining treatment for OCD (Szymanski, 2012).

Our standard programming

At the McLean OCD Institute of Houston (MOCDI-H), previously known as the Houston OCD Program, our multidisciplinary team offers treatment across a continuum of care for patients with anxiety, OCD, and related disorders. We are a specialty clinic focused on providing evidence-based treatment to individuals who seek residential support, intensive outpatient, and outpatient programs. Our clinic typically operates with majority in-person services, though teletherapy is provided on occasion for those who need it, often as a means to help patients in their transition from our treatment program. Through our residential support and Intensive Outpatient Program (IOP), we can serve up to 15 adult patients per day, and our outpatient program can accommodate over 40 child, adolescent, and adult patients per day.

Our IOP includes patients participating in our traditional IOP day programming along with those who also receive residential support in addition to IOP services. All new patients undergo a required phone assessment with our Admissions Director (LPC) to screen for exclusion criteria and obtain appropriate releases of information to confirm with their recent outpatient providers their need for intensive treatment and fit for our programming. Once this process is completed, patients are admitted into our IOP program and assigned to a doctoral-level Behavioral Therapist (BT) who will provide their individual behavioral therapy throughout the course of their admission in our IOP.

Our day programming runs from 8:45 AM to 4:00 PM and is a combination of group therapy, staff supported exposure blocks, and individual sessions. Daily psycho-education groups are led by our BTs. Residential Counselors (RCs) are available throughout the day and evening to support patients' treatment. All patients receive three 45 to 50-minute individual sessions per week with their BT, one family therapy session a week with our Family Therapist (LMSW), and the option to receive psychiatric services from our Director of Psychiatric Services (D.O.).

Mental health during disasters

In March 2020, major disaster declarations occurred across the United States due to COVID-19 and its dangers to public health (Federal Emergency Management Agency, 2020). Previous literature exploring the influence of crises on psychological well-being found that during a crisis or disaster, individuals with preexisting mental health conditions may experience symptom exacerbation (Storch et al., 2019), are at a greater risk for suffering from decline in their mental health, and may also be at an increased risk for adverse physical health consequences (Clay, Goetschius, Papas, & Kendra, 2014; Grant, 2018; Witthauer, Gloster, Meyer, & Lieb, 2014). Specifically, a study found that with the Severe Acute Respiratory Syndrome (SARS) outbreak, individuals that were required to quarantine for nine days experienced anxiety, acute stress, sleep disturbance, and difficulty with making decisions as well as further isolated themselves from others immediately after their quarantine ended (Bai et al., 2004). An additional study examined the impact that a two week quarantine for exposure to the Middle East Respiratory Syndrome had for its 1,692 participants and found that during their period of isolation, 7.6% ($n = 176$) of individuals experienced symptoms of anxiety while 16.6% ($n = 275$) expressed anger (Jeong et al., 2016).

Despite the great need for mental health treatment both during and after a disaster, many individuals may be unable to get the care they need because of various barriers to care. For instance, a previous study found that individuals with preexisting mental health conditions may discontinue treatment post-disaster due to lack of access to and cost of care (Wang et al., 2008). Given the potential psychological impact associated with the current recommended COVID-19 precautions (i.e. quarantine, social distancing, working from home, etc.), it is critical for the mental health field to ensure quality, accessible, and cost-effective treatment for all.

Transitioning to teletherapy

Immediately upon the outbreak of the COVID-19 virus, our program recognized the importance of identifying ways to continue providing quality and evidence-based treatment to our patients. Initially, we implemented the Center for Disease Control's recommended cleaning, hygiene, and reduced contact protocols (Centers for Disease Control and Prevention, 2020). However, as the situation in America worsened, our treatment team determined that more action was needed in order to ensure the safety of our patients and staff. On Sunday, March15th, the program's leadership made the decision to close the residential support component of our programming. This decision was made because we do not have medical personnel on site that could handle a potential outbreak among our patients attending the residential support program or staff. Our team informed the patients on Monday, March 16th about the planned transition to telehealth so they could begin planning for their safe returns home no later than by the end of the day on Wednesday, March 18th.

A clinical staff meeting occurred the next day (Tuesday, March 17th) to discuss next steps for our on-site clinical work. As a review of the current literature revealed that internet-based treatment has been an effective method for providing evidence-based treatment to individuals with OCD (Andersson et al., 2012; Brand & McKay, 2012; Lenhard et al., 2017), the clinical staff determined that we would move to providing our outpatient and intensive outpatient services in a completely virtual format. Virtual outpatient sessions were encouraged to begin immediately (Tuesday, March 17th) and the Virtual IOP day programming, which the clinical staff developed in this meeting, was set to begin on Thursday, March 19th. With full participation from all members of our team, our clinic was able to successfully make this move to teletherapy as planned.

Our ability to act quickly yet collectively contributed to MOCDI-H becoming the first (or among the first) programs specializing in OCD to transition intensive specialty care to a fully virtual format. Other specialty OCD intensive programs made the switch to the virtual format at later dates. For instance, the McLean OCD Institute in Boston opened their virtual Partial Hospitalization Program on April 28th, 2020, Rogers Memorial Hospital began offering their intensive outpatient options in a virtual format during the week of March 30th, and the Neuro Behavioral Institute moved to virtual programming on March 23rd.

Description of our virtual intensive programming

Our Virtual IOP began at 8:45 AM on Thursday, March 19th and was provided primarily over the Zoom platform, with individual sessions offered through our electronic record system's

(Theranest) teletherapy services. Due to licensing requirements, we initially limited participation to current IOP patients who resided or were located in the state of Texas. Our Virtual IOP mirrored our standard IOP as closely as possible, with only minor adjustments or changes due to the new delivery format. With regards to the schedule, the clinical staff elected to remove one afternoon psycho-educational group, which reduced our scheduled programming by an hour (8:45am to 3pm versus 4pm). This decision was made after consultation with the patients and clinical team to support group logistics. Please refer to Table 1 for a full description of our standard and Virtual IOP schedules.

Additionally, the Virtual IOP offers an increase in the number of sessions with BTs for the same price as our standard IOP. Further, we built additional flexibility into the care delivery model by providing the opportunity for patients to participate in our virtual IOP group only, for a reduced rate, with the option to meet with their BT and Family Therapist as needed through our standard outpatient fee for service model. Table 2 provides more information about the cost of and services provided with each program.

Our BTs were able to successfully transfer the content of their psycho-educational groups to a virtual format. Zoom's screen-sharing ability allows BTs to continue using the visual aids (i.e. videos, photos, websites, worksheets) they use when leading in-person groups as well as the ability to write out or draw the key points, graphs, and models they would typically illustrate on our Smart Board. BTs can also use the group chat to send patients direct links to online resources. Peer interactions and group discussions remained an integral part of our groups as Zoom allows each participant to see and speak with other members of the group throughout the session.

Considerations for the development of our virtual IOP

Financial considerations

Although we are a private pay mental health clinic, we support our patients' efforts to file for reimbursement from their insurance companies. Patients who wish to file for

Table 1. Comparison between our standard and virtual IOP treatment day schedules.

	Pre-Virtual		Post-Virtual
Time	Activity	Time	Activity
8:45–9:00	Goals Group	8:45–9:00	Goals Group
9:00–9:45	Psychoeducational Group	9:00–9:45	Psychoeducational Group
9:45–10:00	ERP Check-In	9:45–10:00	ERP Check-In
10:00–11:45	ERP	10:00–11:45	ERP
12:00–1:00	Lunch	12:00–1:00	Lunch
1:00–2:00	Psychoeducational Group	1:00–2:45	ERP
2:00–3:45	ERP		

Table 2. Comparison of standard and virtual IOP fees and services.

	Standard IOP	Full Virtual IOP	Virtual IOP-Group Only
Cost Per Day	$675	$675	$300
Sessions with BT	3 Hours/Week	1.5 Hours/Day	Not Included
Sessions with Family Therapist	1 Session/Week	1 Session/Week	Not Included
Support from RCs	Provide Support Throughout Treatment Day	Provide Support Throughout Treatment Day	Provide Support Throughout Treatment Day

reimbursement independently receive a superbill after the service is rendered. For patients who would like additional support with this endeavor, we connect them with SJ Health Insurance Advocates (SJHA), a firm with whom we partner to help our patients navigate the insurance process, obtain reimbursement, and negotiate single case agreements as needed and when possible. A single case agreement is a contract between a health insurance company and an out-of-network provider, such as our clinic, that allows a specific patient to utilize their in-network benefits while receiving treatment from MOCDI-H.

When we moved to teletherapy, we collaborated with SJHA to verify the move to our Virtual IOP would not interrupt our patients' ability to receive reimbursement. Fortunately, due to the circumstances surrounding COVID-19, most insurance companies relaxed their regulations around telemedicine coverage. This helped prevent some of our patients from having to terminate or postpone treatment due to financial restrictions.

Admission requirements

Admission to our Virtual IOP continues to be limited to only those individuals living in Texas, with some exceptions for patients who have a pre-existing therapeutic relationship with our team and live in a state whose laws allow our BTs to provide temporary treatment during this pandemic (Association of State and Provincial Psychology Boards, 2020). Although we continue to follow our program's standard screening process, our patient admission into the program has changed slightly. Instead of patients starting all services on the day of admission, as is the typical protocol for our standard IOP, we are now requiring patients to engage in outpatient sessions with their assigned BT prior to beginning the Virtual IOP.

We made this decision for a couple of reasons. First, we wanted our BTs to complete an intake evaluation to further assess a patient's fit for our virtual intensive programming. We also wanted to ensure the BTs had adequate time to introduce the patient to our program, develop a behavioral plan the patient can use to guide their two daily exposure blocks, and provide appropriate psycho-education, which has been found to enhance treatment adherence (APA, 2007). Further, this change allows BTs to obtain a sufficient understanding of the patient to help inform the RCs of the best ways to support the patient throughout the virtual treatment day. This additional process in admissions is not necessary in our standard IOP because our staff is generally able to interact with the patient in-person throughout the day, which allows us to get to know the patient in a more accelerated way that is not feasible through teletherapy. To date, both RCs and patient experiences have been positive. While patients indicate their desire to return for in-person services, benefits such as support with OCD exposures in their home environments have been noted by several of our patients.

Data from the first month of virtual programming

Table 3 provides a summary of the pre-and post-virtual programming. Data are displayed by service types offered at our clinic. The no service type listed in the table indicates non-billable services. These service types are often registered for patients in our intensive programming where services are bundled. Our program's cancellations policy indicates a cancellation occurring at least 24 hours in advance of the scheduled appointment will not be charged for the session. Late cancellations indicate cancellations that took place within 24 hours of the scheduled appointment time, which are subject to billing per our program's policy. No shows indicate the patient neither attended the session, nor cancelled/rescheduled it. These no shows are also subject to billing.

Prior to our transition to teletherapy, our average daily program census from 17 February 2020 through 17 March 2020 (excluding weekends for a total of 22 weekdays) was 5.3 residential support patients, 3.6 IOP patients, and 19.7 outpatients. Post-transition, our average daily virtual program census from 19 March 2020 through 18 April 2020 (excluding weekends for a total of 22 weekdays) was 3.3 IOP patients and 22.4

Table 3. Comparison between pre-virtual (02.18.2020–03.15.2020) and post-virtual appointments (03.18.2020–04.15.2020).

Service Type	Service Type (n)		Appointments Retained (n)		Cancellations (n)		Late Cancellations (n)		No Shows (n)	
Outpatient	Pre	Post	Pre	Post	Pre	Post	Pre	Post	Pre	Post
Doctoral	384	478	330	421	40	31	10	11	4	15
Masters	17	10	14	9	2	1	1	0	0	0
LMSW	4	2	4	2	0	0	0	0	0	0
LPC	6	10	6	9	0	1	0	0	0	0
LPC-I	3	8	3	4	0	4	0	1	0	0
Total	414	508	357	445	42	36	11	12	4	15
IOP										
Doctoral	19	11	18	10	0	0	1	0	0	1
Masters	0	0	0	0	0	0	0	0	0	0
LMSW	0	0	0	0	0	0	0	0	0	0
LPC	8	5	2	0	0	1	0	0	1	1
LPC-I	2	1	1	0	0	0	0	0	0	0
Total	29	17	21	10	0	1	1	0	1	1
Family Therapy										
LMSW	8	6	7	5	0	0	0	0	0	0
Total	8	6	7	5	0	0	0	0	0	0
Phone Assessment										
Doctoral	2	0	1	0	1	0	0	0	0	0
Masters	0	0	0	0	0	0	0	0	0	0
LMSW	0	0	0	0	0	0	0	0	0	0
LPC	20	11	19	9	0	1	0	0	1	1
LPC-I	0	0	0	0	0	0	0	0	0	0
Total	22	11	20	9	1	1	0	0	1	1
Diagnostic Evaluation										
Doctoral	20	7	18	4	2	2	0	0	0	1
D.O	3	2	3	1	0	1	0	0	0	0
Masters	0	0	0	0	0	0	0	0	0	0
LMSW	2	0	2	0	0	0	0	0	0	0
LPC	2	0	1	0	1	0	0	0	0	0
LPC-I	0	0	0	1	0	0	0	0	0	1
Total	27	9	24	6	3	3	0	0	0	2
Psychiatry Appointments										
Intake	3	2	3	1	0	1	0	0	0	0
Follow-Up	16	13	16	9	0	4	0	0	0	0
Total	19	15	19	10	0	5	0	0	0	0
No Service Type										
Doctoral	114	106	114	106	0	0	0	0	0	0
D.O	18	15	17	10	1	5	0	0	0	0
Masters	0	0	0	0	0	0	0	0	0	0

(Continued)

Table 3. (Continued).

Service Type	Service Type (n)		Appointments Retained (n)		Cancellations (n)		Late Cancellations (n)		No Shows (n)	
Outpatient	Pre	Post	Pre	Post	Pre	Post	Pre	Post	Pre	Post
LMSW	39	16	39	16	0	0	0	0	0	0
LPC	0	0	0	0	0	0	0	0	0	0
LPC-I	0	0	0	0	0	0	0	0	0	0
Total	171	137	170	132	1	5	0	0	0	0
Sliding Scale										
LMSW	18	10	18	9	0	0	0	0	0	1
LPC	0	0	0	0	0	0	0	0	0	0
LPC-I	5	0	5	0	0	0	0	0	0	0
Total	23	10	23	9	0	0	0	0	0	1

Pre = Pre-Virtual; Post = Post-Virtual; Doctoral providers include 6 PhD/PsyD, a PhD licensed as LMSW, and a doctoral candidate.

outpatients. These numbers indicate a slight decrease in IOP patients (−0.3/per day) and an increase in outpatients seen per day (+2.7/per day).

It is important to note that some of our IOPs were unable to participate in our Virtual IOP due to its limitation of availability to those living in Texas. Similarly, many of our IOPs, particularly those in our residential support program, elected to step down to our outpatient program until we are able to return to in-person treatment. As our patient census to date continues to rise for our IOP and outpatient programs, we are projecting that our transition to teletherapy will facilitate a growth in our clientele. We base this projection on the growth in our outpatient tele-sessions, which is surpassing our average in-person outpatient sessions per day. This growth seems to indicate that there is an increasing need for virtual mental health services, particularly for those struggling with OCD and anxiety disorders, during this time.

It is also important to note that amid the COVID-19 pandemic, many families are now faced with a burden of extra responsibilities, such as balancing working from home, increasingly more active participation in their children's education, as well as trying to keep up with their family's various commitments. This increased workload can overwhelm a family and may be translating to an increase in missed appointments and late cancellations. However, we are confident that this will become less of an issue moving forward as families are starting to establish a new routine in the light of this crisis and have more ability to adjust to the demands of the virtual program.

Anecdotally, issues with technology have led to delayed starts to sessions, thus causing an increase in extended sessions or reschedules. Consistent changes in patients' schedules have presented a challenge for setting regular standing appointments times, which we have found to be helpful in enhancing appointment adherence. However, this problem was solved through the flexible nature of working from home as BTs are able to provide additional options for scheduling appointments within their standard clinical day. We find that these real-life challenges are providing a valuable opportunity to discuss time management, work/life balance, and self-care with patients as well to demonstrate flexibility and effective problem-solving skills.

During our normal programming, individuals in our residential support and intensive outpatient programs are asked to complete a variety of self-report measures upon admission and discharge, with a shortened version of these assessments administered on a weekly basis. This protocol remains the same during virtual programming. The following measures were used for this paper. Of note, for all measures, higher scores represent greater symptom severity.

Yale-Brown Obsessive-Compulsive Scale (Y-BOCS; Goodman et al., 1989), a ten-item measure designed to assess the severity of an individual's OCD-related obsessions and compulsions. The Y-BOCS is scored on a five-point scale ranging from 0 (no symptoms) to 4 (extreme symptoms) and overall severity is measured on a scale from 0–40. Due to its sound reliability and validity, the Y-BOCS is considered the gold standard assessment for measuring OCD-symptomology (Deacon & Abramowitz, 2005). Additionally, it has been found to be sensitive to medication-related changes, with score reductions specifically demonstrating improvements in OCD-symptoms (Goodman et al., 1989).

The Center for Epidemiologic Studies Depression Scale (CES-D; Radloff, 1977) is a twenty-item assessment designed to measure symptoms and severity of depression. The CES-D is scored on a four-point scale from 0 (rarely or none of the time) to 3 (most or all of the time) and overall severity is measured on a scale from 0–60. It has been found to have a high internal consistency, with Cronbach's alpha coefficients between.85 and .90, and to be a reliable assessment for measuring symptoms of depression across gender, age, and racial classifications (Radloff, 1977).

The General Anxiety Disorder-7 (GAD-7; Spitzer, Kroenke, Williams, & Lowe, 2006) is a seven-item measure used to identify and monitor anxiety symptoms throughout treatment. The GAD-7 is scored on a four-point scale from 0 (not at all) to 3 (nearly every day), with overall severity measured on a scale from 0–21. It was initially validated as a diagnostic assessment for Generalized Anxiety Disorder in a sample of 2,149 patients and found to have 89% sensitivity, 82% specificity, and a intraclass correlation coefficient of .83 (Spitzer et al., 2006).

The Distress Intolerance Index (DII; McHugh & Otto, 2012) is a ten-item designed to measure the inability to tolerate negative states. The DII is scored on a five-point scale from 0 (very little) to 4 (most or very much) and overall scores are based on a scale from 0–40. It has been found to have strong internal consistency, reliability, and validity (both convergent and discriminant), as well as to be correlated with other measures of distress intolerance (McHugh et al., 2014; McHugh & Otto, 2012).

For the purpose of this paper, data were analyzed from our Virtual IOP's first survey, which was taken the day they began our virtual programming and was compared to the most recent survey they had completed on May 11th. Table 4 provides a description of our patients' demographic characteristics and Table 5 provides a summary of their first and most recent assessments (May 11th).

Data suggest overall trends in reductions of scores of the Y-BOCS, CES-D, GAD-7, and DII across all patients. This finding seems to indicate that our virtual programming has been effective in reducing symptoms of OCD, anxiety, and depression. Although we recognize that more information, from a larger number of individuals and over a longer span of time is required to understand how effective our Virtual IOP truly is in treating individuals with OCD, anxiety, and depression, we believe this finding demonstrates that our current patients are benefitting from this Virtual IOP. We plan to continue gathering data to further determine the treatment effectiveness delivered through teletherapy.

Table 4. Demographic characteristics.

	N	%
Race/Ethnicity		
Caucasian (White, Not of Latino or Asian descent)	4	80.0
Biracial	1	20.0
Gender		
Female	2	40.0
Male	3	60.0
Parent Age		
17–24	3	60.0
25–34	2	40.0
Primary Diagnosis		
OCD	3	60.0
Other	2	40.0

N = 5.

Table 5. Treatment variables.

Treatment Variables	Mean	SD	N
Starting Y-BOCS	23.0	2.7	3
Current Y-BOCS	20.3	4.0	3
Starting CES-D	18.8	8.0	5
Current CES-D	15.2	8.9	5
Starting GAD-7	22.0	5.6	5
Current GAD-7	19.0	3.7	5
Starting DII	28.0	7.0	5
Current DII	26.0	7.2	5

Identified benefits of our virtual programming

Throughout the process of converting to teletherapy, our team witnessed the emergence of several changes we perceive as being beneficial to both the staff and patients. One key benefit was our quick and efficient transition to teletherapy, which was done while maintaining our standard quality of care and with minimal to no disruption of service to our patients. Another benefit we identified was the ability to expand our services to most of our currently established patients who live outside of Texas. The loosening of state licensing laws seen throughout the United States provided us this unique opportunity to offer continued evidence-based services to more patients. This ability has allowed us to overcome this geographic barrier, which is one of the most prevalent barriers to treatment for individuals with OCD. The Virtual IOP, particularly our Virtual IOP group only option, also provided a cost-effective, highly accessible treatment option for individuals who otherwise may not be able to afford treatment, spend several weeks away from work or school, or be away from their responsibilities at home.

Furthermore, through our virtual programming, BTs are now able to assist with in-home exposures without the patients having to pay the additional travel related costs associated with home visits. In-home support can be incredibly beneficial to patients because an individual's home is often the location in which their OCD is especially triggered (Baruah et al., 2018; Rosa-Alcázar et al., 2019; Selles et al., 2018); however, finances tend to inhibit many patients from being able to receive this support. Teletherapy offers a solution that reduces this expense.

Similarly, we have noticed an increase in the number of outpatient sessions retained and a decrease in the number of outpatient appointments cancelled with more than 24 hours' notice (the treatment program required time to cancel appointments). We attribute these changes to teletherapy's ability to enable patients who typically have difficulty leaving work or school as well as those with long travel times to the clinic to better access therapy sessions on a more consistent basis. Eliminating the travel and schedule related barriers to care may have helped many patients obtain the appropriate therapy dosage that was previously difficult to receive. This is a significant improvement since frequency of sessions is often predictive of treatment outcome for ERP (Abramowitz, 2006; Freedman, Hoffenberg, Vorus, & Frosch, 1999).

Additionally, given that most, if not all, members of our patients' family are at home during this COVID-19 quarantine, we are noticing that family members are more likely to be available to participate in treatment sessions when applicable. This allows for increased social support for the patient and the opportunity for families to learn more effective ways to respond when their loved one is struggling. Family education can be helpful when the patient transitions out of intensive treatment and steps down to outpatient therapy (Goetter, Herbert, Forman, Yuen, & Thomas, 2014; Netter et al., 2018). Additionally, family therapy with important members of the patients' support team can help reduce inter-family related stressors that may be impacting the patients' symptoms, as well as equip family members to eliminate their collusion with the patient's OCD symptoms (APA, 2007).

Providers are noting improvements to the psychological services they are able to provide. Teletherapy helps BTs gain a better understanding of their patients' home environment, which provides unique opportunities for exposures. For instance, understanding the layout and location of triggering areas in a patient's home allows the BT to generate more effective exposures for spaces protected by OCD (e.g. "clean" zones). We are finding that teletherapy allows patients to confront their OCD in the areas in which it is most triggered, rather than practicing the exposures in more neutral or "safe" areas, such as a BT's office. This practice has been found to be helpful to the treatment of OCD (Goetter et al., 2014).

Challenges associated with virtual programming

While there have been many benefits during the transition to teletherapy, it is not without its challenges. First, we found that some patients with low treatment motivation prior to the transition appeared to be less willing to attend sessions through teletherapy. Maintaining the structure and consistency of therapy sessions within a home setting has also been challenging for some patients. We are noticing that some patients have struggled to sustain their focus as their home has more sources of distraction than does the BT's office. For instance, participating in a teletherapy session has caused some patients to become distracted by emails, texts, or other notifications that pop-up on their screens. Additionally, background noise and interruptions from members of the patients' family have been a distraction for many individuals. Although we have recommended that patients ensure they are participating in sessions in a quiet, private space that is free from distractions, we cannot ensure distractions do not occur.

Ensuring confidentiality is of the utmost importance for providing effective and ethical standards of practice; however, teletherapy presents new challenges for managing confidentiality and patient privacy. For instance, while BTs have control over who enters and exits a therapy office, they are unable to do so through teletherapy. As BTs can only see what is in view of the camera, they are often unable to verify that others are not listening in on the patient's session. A breach in confidentiality may occur if, for example, a family member who does not have permission to participate in treatment is in the same room or nearby and overhears confidential information.

Measures have been taken to maintain confidentiality to the best of the clinician's ability. Specifically, in accordance with the American Psychological Associations' telepsychology guidelines (APA, 2013), our BTs discussed the limits of confidentiality that are unique to teletherapy at the outset of this transition and asked patients to review and sign our Informed Consent Checklist for Telepsychological Services (see in Appendix A) prior to their first teletherapy session. BTs ensure patient confidentiality on their end by working in a private and quiet location with a door that closes. Many BTs have also used sound machines to ensure members of their family cannot listen in on sessions. To help ensure confidentiality on the patients' end, BTs request patients attend therapy sessions in a closed room, free from noise and distraction. At the beginning of the first teletherapy session, patients are informed that unless otherwise instructed by the patient, the BT will stop talking if they notice another person or voice in the room. These measures have been taken to best address confidentiality concerns as well as to maintain a high-quality care.

Similarly, using technology to facilitate therapy sessions introduces new challenges for potential breaches in internet security. Using non-secure telecommunications platforms for sessions makes them vulnerable to internet hackers and issues with unreliable internet connections. To resolve this issue, BTs are instructed to use the Health Insurance Portability and Accountability Act- compliant video-conferencing software offered through our electronic health record system as a first choice for individual teletherapy. This offers the most security because access to the session is limited as the patient either has to obtain the unique URL for the session through their patient portal account or the BT has to send the URL to them directly. The session can only begin once the therapist starts the session on their end.

While this system has been successful overall, two key obstacles have been identified. First, the system does not allow for the group sessions we require in order to facilitate our Virtual IOP. Similarly, some patients have experienced difficulties with logging into the system and maintaining consistent visual and audio connection throughout the session. When difficulties occur, and in our Virtual IOP, the Zoom video-conference software is used. Unfortunately, the potential for Zoom-bombing threatens confidentiality. To address this problem, strict measures were implemented and include requirements such as sending patients a new Zoom code, with a unique password, for each individual session. Our Zoom meeting includes a waiting room feature that ensures no one is allowed into the session unless given permission by their BT. Once the session begins, the BT locks the Zoom session so no one else may enter the video conference.

Internet and technology can provide their own challenges to treatment, as the internet can unpredictably stop working, causing the session to unexpectedly end. This can cause disruption to treatment, as the patient and therapist may miss pieces of what was said or body language if the screen freezes or lags. Although this is an ongoing challenge, we found that it is often ameliorated with the BT calling the patient on their phone and continuing the session as best as possible. Those who are less technologically inclined have required extra help with beginning sessions on time. These patients have been reminded to log into their computer 10 minutes prior to their session to problem solve technological issues and obtain support from relatives to set up cameras and video sessions. However, over time, we have noticed that our patients have become accustomed to these technologies and are able to login with more ease.

Some patients who transitioned from our standard IOP to our Virtual IOP found that the virtual model does not allow for the same level of social interaction with peers and staff with which they are accustomed. That is, our IOP patients have grown accustomed to a cohort of others and miss the camaraderie and social support gained through the natural group process of our standard IOP. We have made several efforts to help overcome this difficulty by offering additional virtual support groups after the treatment day. Additionally, we are providing patients with a list of local and national support groups in which they can also participate.

Other ERP-specific challenges have been identified anecdotally through the transition to teletherapy. Patients with OCD benefit most from ERP, which involves confronting feared thoughts, images, and situations directly without engaging in any compulsions to reduce the anxiety and/or neutralize the threat. We have found that since our transition, some patients are delaying the practice of more difficult exposures. Most of these delays are not forms of avoidance; rather, they seem to be attributed to the increased distress the individual is experiencing as a result of this quarantine. For example, many patients are experiencing increases in their anxiety related to the various changes in their schedule, workload, and resources. Other patients are also noticing increases in their depressive symptoms, which is most often caused by lack of social interactions with others. ERP is therefore being interrupted to address these stressors.

During in-person sessions, BTs provide a supportive and structured role for assisting patients through their challenging exposures. Many patients benefit from a gradual approach to ERP in which they watch the BT model the exposure first and then engage in the exposure with the BT, prior to working on it independently. This approach, which is typically used with patients that are new to ERP, has been difficult to replicate via telehealth. The encouragement for individuals to stay in place is also presenting a challenge to creating and completing effective exposures, particularly for individuals with contamination fears, agoraphobia, and social anxiety. Fortunately, we are able to substitute in-vivo exposures with imaginal exposures and internet-based exposures such as looking at triggering pictures or watching triggering videos online. Research shows that these options are also effective for treating OCD and phobias (Foa, 2010). Patients with social anxiety have been able to continue their treatment by using virtual methods to meet and communicate with other people.

For providers and patients, boundaries offer a sense of structure and security. Typical boundaries that ensure professionalism are more challenging to implement as communicating online lends itself to less formal interactions. For example, patients can now see their BT's home, potentially observing family pictures, furniture, and religious paraphernalia that reveal information not otherwise shared with the patient. Due to this added level of intimacy, our BTs are taking purposeful steps towards maintaining professional boundaries with patients. One such step is that BTs are being selective of where and how they conduct teletherapy sessions. Specifically, our leadership has encouraged BTs to continue dressing in business-casual attire and to sit in front of a blank or non-distracting wall. For BTs who do not have access to an area that provides a professional background for sessions, they are encouraged to use the background feature of Zoom to help remove distractions and limit patients' exposure to personal items. Additionally, to combat boundary issues, BTs strive to maintain professional hours with patients so as to ensure a healthy work-life balance. Our team has ensured that our BTs continue to have their standard one-hour peer-supervision meeting each week in which they can discuss challenging cases and circumstances with their colleagues. This peer-supervision has become even more valuable as we navigate the various challenges of teletherapy.

Future directions

While the changes in our mental health system amidst this COVID 19 pandemic have created a considerable amount of challenges for providers and patients, it has also allowed us to explore a treatment modality with which many clinicians did not have previous experience. The unique challenges presented by the current global crises have compelled the mental health community to adapt to and overcome barriers (e.g. accessibility, confidentiality, treatment adaptations) for the dissemination and implementation of quality evidenced-based care offered in a virtual format. Our transition to teletherapy has taught us a number of lessons that we, as a mental health community, can use to enhance accessibility to effective and evidence-based care to individuals requiring traditional and intensive outpatient programming. Successful implementation of, satisfaction with, and demonstrated benefit from teletherapy may inspire a significant improvement in access to care throughout the country.

Teletherapy is not currently a standard of care in many mental health programs for a variety of reasons. One of these reasons is clinicians' beliefs about teletherapy. Current research notes clinicians' hesitations (e.g. reimbursement rates, resistance to change, and cultural concerns) towards the integration of teletherapy keeps them from introducing it into their practice (McClellan et al., 2020; Scott-Kruse et al., 2018). Licensing restrictions also greatly limit the use of teletherapy.

Anecdotal evidence appears to suggest that virtual intensive therapy may be a more feasible and cost-effective option for some individuals. However, solutions to the various challenges to teletherapy listed in previous sections are necessary in order to ensure we are able to provide the most effective care possible with the least amount of restrictions and disruptions. Future research is needed in order to further inform the screening and admission processes for virtual intensive programming. Moving forward, targeted screening protocols should be established to identify which individuals could benefit from participating in teletherapy. Additionally, future research should focus on exploring what factors can be used to determine if a patient is appropriate for or can benefit from intensive teletherapy.

Further exploration of other uses of telecommunication services to support patients' treatment is strongly recommended. Specifically, future studies should explore how virtual accountability check-ins, used as an adjunct to traditional in-person therapy, may provide continued intensive treatment for individuals with OCD in a more cost-effective and accessible manner. This information has the potential to significantly benefit individuals who are unable to participate in the full treatment day. Many patients exhibit improvements while in our standard IOP, but express anxiety about being able to apply the skills they learned in the program once they return to their work and home environment. It would be helpful for the field to conduct future studies on whether a virtual IOP can function as a step-down option from in-person residential or IOP programs for OCD and anxiety. The combination of virtual check-ins and exposure planning sessions could help these patients transition back to their responsibilities and practice independence while still having accountability and in-the-moment support as they navigate the transition.

Telehealth creates the ability to offer specialized, evidence-based treatment to a larger geographic area, thus increasing access to care. However, as it stands, most psychologists are required to obtain licenses in multiple states if they wish to provide services across state lines. The COVID-19 outbreak in the United States has temporarily given rise to an experiment in the flexibility of interjurisdictional practice and other existing statutes. In light of this global pandemic, it is prudent for mental health licensing boards to consider developing a national licensure as a means to facilitate the dissemination of evidenced-based treatment to individuals across the country. This is especially important for specialty mental health care which is limited geographically. Further research is needed to determine whether this increase in flexibility has resulted in improvements in access to care, treatment outcomes, and patient satisfaction. Such information can help advocates and legislatures understand the need for changes in our mental health system and take steps towards eliminating barriers to care.

Overall, while COVID-19 has certainly had its negative impacts on individuals with mental health symptoms, continuation of care has been possible for many. The use of teletherapy may have provided benefits to patients that are not otherwise accessible. While the transition to teletherapy for our programming was unexpected and expedited, our ability to transition quickly and efficiently has allowed our patients an opportunity to continue to maintain and improve their anxiety, OCD and related symptoms. The integration of teletherapy to our programming has reinforced the significant benefits this treatment modality offers to patients, especially in times of crisis when in-office visits are not possible or recommended. We plan to continue developing solutions to the challenges we face and look forward to expanding our knowledge of and comfort with teletherapy.

Disclosure statement

No potential conflict of interest was reported by the authors.

ORCID

Alejandra Sequeira http://orcid.org/0000-0001-9545-6235
Jennifer Sy http://orcid.org/0000-0002-9045-553X
Elizabeth McIngvale http://orcid.org/0000-0001-6063-0483

References

Abramowitz, J. (2006). The psychological treatment of obsessive—compulsive disorder. *The Canadian Journal of Psychiatry*, *51*(7), 407–416.

American Psychiatric Association (APA). (2007). *Practice guideline for the treatment of patients with obsessive-compulsive disorder*. Retrieved from http://www.psych.org/psych_pract/treatg/pg/prac_guide.cfm

American Psychiatric Association (APA). (2013). *Diagnostic and statistical manual of mental disorders* (5th ed.). Washington, DC: American Psychiatric Association.

American Psychological Association (APA). (2013). Guidelines for the practice of telepsychology. *American Psychologist*, *68*(9), 791–800.

Andersson, E., Enander, J., Andrén, P., Hedman, E., Ljótsson, B., Hursti, T., ... Rück, C. (2012). Internet-based cognitive behaviour therapy for obsessive–compulsive disorder: A randomized controlled trial. *Psychological Medicine*, *42*(10), 2193–2203.

Association of State and Provincial Psychology Boards. (2020). *Temporary/telepsychological practice and COVID-19*. Retrieved from https://cdn.ymaws.com/www.asppb.net/resource/resmgr/covid19/temporary_interjuisdictional.pdf

Bai, Y., Lin, C. C., Lin, C. Y., Chen, J. Y., Chue, C. M., & Chou, P. (2004). Survey of stress reactions among health care workers involved with the SARS outbreak. *Psychiatric Services*, *55*(9), 1055–1057.

Baruah, U., Pandian, R. D., Narayanaswamy, J. C., Math, S. B., Kandavel, T., & Reddy, Y. J. (2018). A randomized controlled study of brief family-based intervention in obsessive compulsive disorder. *Journal of Affective Disorders*, *225*, 137–146.

Brand, J., & McKay, D. (2012). Teletherapy approaches to obsessive-compulsive related disorders. *Psychotherapy Research*, *22*(3), 306–316.

Burchi, E., Hollander, E., & Pallanti, S. (2018). From treatment response to recovery: A realistic goal in OCD. *International Journal of Neuropsychopharmacology*, *21*(11), 1007–1013.

Centers for Disease Control and Prevention. (2020, March 20). *Steps healthcare facilities can take now to prepare for COVID-19*. Retrieved from https://www.cdc.gov/coronavirus/2019-ncov/hcp/steps-to-prepare.html

Clay, L. A., Goetschius, J. B., Papas, M. A., & Kendra, J. (2014). Influence of mental health on disaster preparedness: Findings from the behavioral risk factor surveillance system, 2007–2009. *Journal of Homeland Security and Emergency Management*, *11*(3), 375–392.

Collins, L. M., & Coles, M. E. (2017). Sudden gains in exposure therapy for obsessive-compulsive disorder. *Behaviour Research and Therapy*, *93*, 1–5.

Deacon, B. J., & Abramowitz, J. S. (2005). The yale-brown obsessive compulsive scale: Factor analysis, construct validity, and suggestions for refinement. *Journal of Anxiety Disorders*, *19*(5), 573–585.

Federal Emergency Management Agency. (2020). *COVID-19 disaster declarations*. Retrieved from https://www.fema.gov/coronavirus/disaster-declarations

Foa, E. B. (2010). Cognitive behavioral therapy of obsessive-compulsive disorder. *Dialogues in Clinical Neuroscience*, *12*(2), 199–207.

Freedman, N., Hoffenberg, J., Vorus, N., & Frosch, A. (1999). The effectiveness of psychoanalytic psychotherapy: The role of treatment duration, frequency of sessions, and the therapeutic relationship. *Journal of the American Psychoanalytic Association*, *47*(3), 741–772.

Goetter, E. M., Herbert, J. D., Forman, E. M., Yuen, E. K., & Thomas, J. G. (2014). An open trial of videoconference-mediated exposure and ritual prevention for obsessive-compulsive disorder. *Journal of Anxiety Disorders*, *28*(5), 460–462.
Goodman, W. K., Price, L. H., Rasmussen, S. A., Mazure, C., Fleischmann, R. L., Hill, C. L., ... Charney, D. S. (1989). The yale-brown obsessive compulsive scale: I. Development, use, and reliability. *Archives of General Psychiatry*, *46*(11), 1006–1011.
Grant, C. (2018). *Disaster preparedness to reduce anxiety and post-disaster stress* (K4D Helpdesk Report). Brighton, UK: Institute of Development Studies
Jeong, H., Yim, H. W., Song, Y. J., Ki, M., Min, J. A., Cho, J., & Chae, J. H. (2016). Mental health status of people isolated due to Middle East respiratory syndrome. *Epidemiology and Health*, *38*, e2016048.
Lenhard, F., Andersson, E., Mataix-Cols, D., Rück, C., Vigerland, S., Högström, J., ... Serlachius, E. (2017). Therapist-guided, internet-delivered cognitive-behavioral therapy for adolescents with obsessive-compulsive disorder: A randomized controlled trial. *Journal of the American Academy of Child and Adolescent Psychiatry*, *56*(1), 10–19.
McClellan, M. J., Florell, D., Palmer, J., & Kidder, C. (2020). Clinician telehealth attitudes in a rural community mental health center setting. *Journal of Rural Mental Health*, *44*(1), 62.
McHugh, R. K., Kertz, S. J., Weiss, R. B., Baskin-Sommers, A. R., Hearon, B. A., & Björgvinsson, T. (2014). Changes in distress intolerance and treatment outcome in a partial hospital setting. *Behavior Therapy*, *45*(2), 232–240.
McHugh, R. K., & Otto, M. W. (2012). Refining the measurement of distress intolerance. *Behavior Therapy*, *43*(3), 641–651.
Netter, A. L., Hessler, J. B., Diedrich, A., Lehr, D., Berking, M., Pfeuffer, S., & Voderholzer, U. (2018). Usability and naturalness of videoconference-based exposure and response prevention for obsessive–compulsive disorder at the patients' homes: A pilot study. *Journal of Cognitive Psychotherapy*, *32*(4), 303–314.
Radloff, L. S. (1977). The CES-D scale: A self-report depression scale for research in the general population. *Journal of Applied Psychological Measurement*, *1*(3), 385–401.
Rosa-Alcázar, Á., Rosa-Alcázar, A. I., Olivares-Olivares, P. J., Parada-Navas, J. L., Rosa-Alcázar, E., & Sánchez-xMeca, J. (2019). Family involvement and treatment for young children with obsessive-compulsive disorder: Randomized control study. *International Journal of Clinical and Health Psychology*, *19*(3), 218–227.
Scott-Kruse, C., Karem, P., Shifflett, K., Vegi, L., Ravi, K., & Brooks, M. (2018). Evaluating barriers to adopting telemedicine worldwide: A systematic review. *Journal of Telemedicine and Telecare*, *24*(1), 4–12.
Selles, R. R., Belschner, L., Negreiros, J., Lin, S., Schuberth, D., McKenney, K., ... Stewart, S. E. (2018). Group family-based cognitive behavioral therapy for pediatric obsessive compulsive disorder: Global outcomes and predictors of improvement. *Psychiatry Research*, *260*, 116–122.
Spitzer, R. L., Kroenke, K., Williams, J. B., & Lowe, B. (2006). A brief measure for assessing generalized anxiety disorder: The GAD-7. *Archives of Internal Medicine*, *166*(10), 1092–1097.
Storch, E. A., Shah, A., Salloum, A., Valles, N., Banu, S., Schneider, S. C., & Goodman, W. K. (2019). Psychiatric diagnoses and medications for hurricane Harvey sheltered evacuees. *Community Mental Health Journal*, *55*(7), 1099–1102.
Swain, S. P., & Behura, S. S. (2016). A comparative study of quality of life and disability among schizophrenia and obsessive-compulsive disorder patients in remission. *Industrial Psychiatry Journal*, *25*(2), 210.
Szymanski, J. (2012). Using direct-to-consumer marketing strategies with obsessive-compulsive disorder in the nonprofit sector. *Behavior Therapy*, *43*(2), 251–256.
Wang, P. S., Gruber, M. J., Powers, R. E., Schoenbaum, M., Speier, A. H., Wells, K. B., & Kessler, R. C. (2008). Disruption of existing mental health treatments and failure to initiate new treatment after hurricane Katrina. *The American Journal of Psychiatry*, *165*(1), 34–41.
Witthauer, C., Gloster, A. T., Meyer, A. H., & Lieb, R. (2014). Physical diseases among persons with obsessive compulsive symptoms and disorder: A general population study. *Social Psychiatry and Psychiatric Epidemiology*, *49*(12), 2013–2022.

Mental-health care under threat: a pragmatic approach for ethical decision-making for practitioners in COVID-19

M. Bar, E. Fish and S. Mendlovic

ABSTRACT

It is difficult to overstate the global impact of Coronavirus disease (COVID-19) outbreak. From lockdowns to resource scarcity, the effects of the virus have been widespread and felt by all. Less obvious, but equally severe, is the impact on the practice of psychology. In this time of crisis, complex ethical challenges arise daily in our practice, many of which likely to remain with us for years to come. Thus, there is a pressing need for a pragmatic ethical framework that psychologists can use to navigate the conflicting duties and rapidly changing demands during this time of crisis. To that end, we suggest utilizing the Georgetown principles, four pragmatic ideals developed by biomedical ethicists which can aid clinicians in framing and managing ethical dilemmas. In this work, we show how these principles can be applied to complex ethical conflicts typical of clinical practice in the era of COVID-19. We will discuss ways in which the Georgetown principles are echoed in the Psychologists Code of Conduct, emphasizing items in the Code that are directly relevant to the COVID-19 pandemic. Our goal is to leave the reader with a practical ethical methodology that can be used for quick, effective, and morally sound decision-making. The goal of this paper is not to tell clinicians what decisions they should make; rather, herein we will provide clinicians with tools that will enable them to make ethically-informed decisions on their own.

It is difficult to overstate the impact that Coronavirus has had, and will continue to have, on countries around the world. Coronavirus Disease 2019 (COVID-19) is a highly contagious infectious disease associated with high morbidity and mortality rates. The World Health Organization (WHO) has declared the outbreak to be a public health emergency of international concern (World Health Organization, 2020, January 20), and on 11 March 2020 recognized it as a global pandemic (World Health Organization, 2020, March 11). Efforts to prevent the virus from spreading have led many countries to adopt strong preventive measures, including national or regional lockdowns, self-quarantines, curfews, travel restrictions, and extensive facility closures (Chinazzi et al., 2020), causing severe socioeconomic disruption (Brooks et al., 2020). Public administrations worldwide have encouraged health care facilities, including institutions of mental health, to suspend or minimize any nonessential services, including the cancelation of elective procedures, transfer and discharge of existing clients, and replacement of in-person visits with telemedicine (e.g., Centers for Disease Control & Prevention, 2020, February 29; Centers for Medicare & Medicaid Services, 2020, March 30). During a crisis of this magnitude, the day to day functioning of all health care organizations is inevitably disrupted in ways that make fulfilling the traditional standard of care extremely challenging, if not impossible (Phillips, Knebel, & Johnson, 2009).

In the face of emergency ethical questions about allocation of scarce resources, ensuring equal treatment of those subject to discrimination, continuity of care, and a host of other issues arise daily (Calain, Fiore, Poncin, & Hurst, 2009). For psychologists, such dilemmas are particularly relevant, as they touch on some of the core ethical grounds of psychological practice (Hanson, Kerkhoff, & Bush, 2005). These include, among others, the obligation to provide care, the issue of dual agency prioritization of clients, boundaries of competence, and conflicts of interest. Moreover, the unprecedented conditions and restraints of the COVID-19 crisis have immediate and far-reaching consequences for day-to-day practice, including the necessity of changing the setting in which therapy is conducted as well as its duration and goals. In times of profound crisis, such issues are often overlooked (Van Heugten, 2014, p. 139). As such, there is an urgent need for a pragmatic framework that can assist practitioners in navigating ethical decision-making processes rapidly arising in the field. Thus, we hereby propose a simple approach to assist psychologists in facing complex ethical issues relevant to the clinical practice of COVID-19 era, while effectively balancing the conflicting demands of the client, the healthcare institution, and the law. To meet that end, we would suggest turning to the adjoining field of biomedical ethics.

Ethical considerations of psychological practice in times of crisis

The American Psychological Association (APA) defines five general principles that constitute the highest ideals of the profession: beneficence and nonmaleficence, fidelity and responsibility, integrity, justice, and respect for people's rights and dignity (American Psychological Association, 2017). As psychologists, we use these principles every day to guide our decisions and to help us do what is right for our clients, our profession, and society as a whole. However, the conditions of the current pandemic pose novel challenges for the implementation of these principles.

Ethical pitfalls may take different forms. While psychologists always seek to safeguard the welfare and rights of those with whom they work, in times of crisis, public policy and organizational demands may preclude or override the standard professional mandate. As a result of the need to reconcile different responsibilities and obligations, psychologists are at high risk of ethical missteps and even outright malpractice (Lowman, 2006). These might include, but are certainly not limited to, biased prioritizing of clients, unfair discrimination, and premature treatment termination due to reallocation of resources. At the same time, practitioners might not be able to obtain the training necessary to ensure the competence and integrity of their services (Hanson et al., 2005). Even experienced practitioners might be required to quickly acquaint themselves with new and unfamiliar techniques or populations, stretching their professional boundaries. In these conditions, professional and peer supervision are often limited or nonexistent, further impacting practitioners' clinical discretion and performance. Moreover, many authors also provide examples of therapeutic boundary crossing in mental health interventions at these times, including unavoidable breaches of the clinical setting, violations of confidentiality, and undue disclosures of the therapist's personal information (Loewenberg, Dolgoff, & Harrington, 2000). These are just a few examples of the myriad possible issues that arise during a global calamity of this scale. Countless other challenges will likely arise. Each of these novel situations will require careful attention, formulation, analysis, and solution as they arise.

Navigating the unique challenges of COVID-19 era

The ethical challenges psychologists currently face stem from the unique medical and socioeconomic conditions of the COVID-19 pandemic. These include: (1) global crisis on an unprecedented scale; (2) a continuous (versus circumscribed) event, with unknown duration; (3) real, life-threatening danger; (4) fear of contagion, which significantly limits human interaction; (5) a rapidly changing reality; (6) a state of extreme uncertainty in all life domains; (7) dramatic changes to the usual habits and routines of daily life; (8) social-distancing constraints and regulations; (9) decreased availability of social support systems; and (10) the spread of panic and misinformation by the media and authority figures (e.g., Karabag, 2020). Experts predict that the post-COVID-19 era will present its own challenges, including economic depression, overwhelmed healthcare systems, and worsening socioeconomic disparities (Platje, Harvey, & Rayman-Bacchus, 2020). Specifically, in the field of psychology, issues related to remote treatment delivery, identification of high-risk populations and prioritization of care, and the determination of diagnostic threshold for what constitutes a "normal" reaction to an abnormal situation, will require special attention (Ho, Chee, & Ho, 2020; Ransing et al., 2020; Wind, Rijkeboer, Andersson, & Riper, 2020). Thus, to make sustainable ethical decisions during and after the current pandemic, the likely repercussions of such unique circumstances should be considered.

As with clinical decisions, arriving at sound ethical decisions is often best accomplished through a systematic, logical process (Bush, 2019). However, such in-depth processes are usually more to the concern of public administrations, regulators, professional liability insurance carriers, and ethical committees. In the current work, we ask to focus on practicing psychologists, who are required to address concrete and immediate ethical dilemmas involving his or her clients. To obtain ethical guidance, practitioners often turn to professional codes. Most jurisdictions have ethical codes. In the field of psychology, the most commonly used ethical codes in English speaking countries are the APA's Ethical Principles of Psychologists and Code of Conduct (hereinafter referred to as the Ethics Code; American Psychological Association, 2017) and the British Psychological Society (BPS) Code of Ethics and Conduct (British Psychological Society, 2018). These are official and enforceable guidelines intended to provide a common set of principles and standards to cover situations frequently encountered by therapists. However, they are not exhaustive, and leave a great deal of room for practitioners' discretion. As stated by Bush (2019), "*Professional ethic codes* [. . .] *are intended to provide guidance across psychological activities, contexts and specialties. As such, they must, by necessity, be rather general in nature* [. . .]. *Despite the value of these principles and directives, psychologists commonly need more specific guidance for establishing and maintaining ethical practices in their specific professional contexts*". This is especially true in times of crisis, when conditions do not allow for thorough and careful discussion as commonly advised. Both Ethical Codes address the ethical complexity of practicing under unexpected conditions, but only to some extent, while encouraging therapists to exercise professional judgment in ethical decision-making and taking into account the unique circumstances in which that decision is being made (British Psychological Society, 2018, p. 2).

Although both organizations mentioned above have recently published short guides advising practitioners during the current crisis ("*COVID-19 and psychology services: How to protect your clients and your practice*"; American Psychological Association, 5 March 2020; "*Guidance for psychological professionals during the Covid-19 pandemic*"; British Psychological Society, 28 March 2020), they do not address in detail the complex ethical challenges that psychologists are likely to face in their everyday practice, nor the available tools that might help them navigate such difficult situations. Thus, the aim of the current paper is to provide psychologists with further practical guidance, allowing them to effectively manage ethically complex dilemmas while under substantial pressure. Importantly, our proposition to apply the Georgetown principles to common ethical dilemmas in psychology is not intended to replace the existing Ethical Codes. On the contrary, it is meant to assist therapists in behaving ethically and in accordance with accepted codes of conduct during these trying times.

The Georgetown principles of biomedical ethics

"The Georgetown principles" (also referred to as "The Georgetown Paradigm", "The Georgetown Mantra" and "The Four Principles") are known to be the most read bioethics textbook in the history of the United States (Holm, 1995), with nine revised editions addressing the developing nature of the field. It is largely regarded as the mainstay of applied ethics and moral reasoning in the healthcare setting (Gillon, 2003; Macklin, 2003). The principles combine the Kantian imperative to behave in accordance with the purest moral principles with Bentham and Mill's arguments in favor of the greatest good for the greatest number. They were originally developed by Beauchamp and Childress (Beauchamp & Childress, 1979/2001), who asserted that the following four principles lie at the core of moral reasoning in healthcare: respect for autonomy, beneficence, non-maleficence, and justice.

Respect for autonomy refers to one's capacity to be a "rational agent" in making decisions for oneself, without undue pressure, coercion, or other forms of persuasion exerted by the healthcare practitioner. This principle is the basis for the notion of "informed consent", which is the permission individuals give prior to taking part in a proposed medical or psychotherapeutic procedure. It is contrasted with paternalism, which characterizes a situation in which healthcare providers overrule the wishes of the client, believing that they know what is in the client's best interest better than the client does. Notably, respect for autonomy is sometimes limited in cases where clients are deemed legally incapable of making informed decisions regarding their treatment. However, the Georgetown perspective rightly reminds us that an individual cannot be deemed wholly competent or incompetent to make all possible decisions, and competence must be reassessed with regards to every choice involved in care (Beauchamp & Childress, 1979/2001).

Beneficence describes the obligation of healthcare providers to act in ways that are in the interest of an individual client or of society as a whole. A beneficent action is one that achieves the highest possible good out of a range of possibilities. The benefits of that action should outweigh the risks and costs.

Non-maleficence requires one to refrain from deliberate harm, either through acts of commission (i.e., imposing a careless or unreasonable risk) or omission (i.e., intentionally failing to perform actions that would be of known benefit to a client).

Lastly, ***justice*** describes the duty of healthcare providers to ensure equal treatment and fair distribution of goods. Central to the principle of justice is the issue of distributive justice, which is the question of how to best allocate goods and services when they are in limited supply.

Beauchamp and Childress strongly emphasize the fact that these four principles have no intrinsic hierarchy and should not necessarily be prioritized over other ethical considerations (Beauchamp & Childress, 1979/2001, p. 57). Instead, they form a pragmatic framework by which practitioners facing complicated ethical dilemmas can organize their thoughts and deliberations. Indeed, behind the four principles lies the authors' negation of ethical foundationalism (i.e., an approach that presume there is fundamental ground for moral judgement, for instance, in truths about human nature or human reason; Hutchings, 2010, p. 67), and of getting lost in abstract debate during medical decision-making processes. The four principles draw their power from their simple and pragmatic nature, which makes them applicable to real-world ethical dilemmas (Hain & Saad, 2016).

Ethical dilemmas in clinical practice in of COVID-19 era

The following section consists of four ethical dilemmas emerging from the unique conditions typical of clinical practice in the era of COVID-19. These were chosen out of many possible challenging situations, and serve to demonstrate how practitioners can use the four Georgetown principles to successfully navigate the conflicting duties and standards imposed on them at this time of crisis.

Dilemma #1

> *A 40-year-old nurse, who is exposed to corona clients daily, is in long-term and intensive (twice a week) therapy. His therapist is in his early seventies, and out of concern for his age, is taking precautions to avoid COVID-19 exposure. The therapist is afraid to continue therapy. Given that this is an ongoing situation and that he is unfamiliar with teletherapy, he cannot consider conducting therapy through this medium. Is the therapist allowed to deny care?*

This dilemma directly concerns the issue of Unfair Discrimination (Standard 3.01; APA, 2017). In their work-related activities, practitioners are not to refrain from treating clients based on age, gender identity, race, ethnicity, culture, national origin, religion, sexual orientation, disability, or socioeconomic status. Denying client care because of the client's profession, especially while the therapeutic process is ongoing, is expected to cause deliberate harm and would, therefore, violate the *nonmaleficence* principle. The issue of

Personal Problems and Conflicts is also relevant to this case (Standard 2.06; American Psychological Association, 2017). This standard requires psychologists to refrain from initiating an activity when they know (or should know) that there is a substantial likelihood that their personal problems will prevent them from performing their work-related activities in a competent manner. When they become aware of such a conflict, they must either limit, suspend, or terminate these duties; which of these three options they choose is up to their discretion. Indeed, therapists who are dealing with overwhelming personal issues may have a difficult time being available to their clients (Sussman, 1995). In the aforementioned dilemma, the psychologist might feel unsafe, might worry about his health, and might feel resentment towards the client who has become a live threat. These feelings may limit his ability to effectively conduct therapy.

When the *beneficence* principle is considered, it is very likely that the costs of continuing this treatment would outweigh the benefits. The potential damage of intense negative countertransference could be, for some clients, irreparable, and might prevent them from seeking treatment in the future (Kächele & Schachter, 2014). Thus, one ethically informed choice would be to immediately suspend treatment, while openly and honestly communicating the reasons for this decision to the client. Although psychologists are often warned about the proper extent of self-disclosures given in therapy, in this case the therapist would be encouraged to disclose his feelings and doubts insofar as they relate to the current situation. Moreover, according to the *autonomy* principle, the client is also to be offered a choice to wait until the outbreak subsides, in order to resume treatment, or alternatively, start a new treatment with another therapist. However, for him to be able to make a decision for himself, he should be given information regarding possible consequences of his choice, such as the possibility that he will be put back on the clinic waiting list if he is unable to find a new therapist on his own.

Dilemma #2

> *A client who works in a nursing home calls his therapist to cancel tomorrow's session. During the call, he discloses the fact that his wife has tested positive for COVID-19, and because he is a close personal contact he too should be self-quarantining; however, he has decided to ignore this requirement and continue working. Although he is fully aware of the risks he presents to elders living in the home, he fears that he cannot afford the financial costs of unpaid sick leave from work. Should the therapist report her client's violation to the authorities?*

This dilemma addresses one of the cornerstones of the psychologic profession: Maintaining Confidentiality (Standard 4.01; American Psychological Association, 2017; Section 3.1.1; BPS, 2018). This ethical standard clearly states that psychologists have an obligation to take reasonable precautions to protect their clients' information while acknowledging that confidentiality may be broken in conditions specified by law. Although it does not appear in the latest version of the APA's Code, it seems that the one and only exception to the confidentiality rule had never changed: "Information received in confidence is released only after most careful deliberation and when there is clear and imminent danger to an individual or to society" (American Psychological Association, 1959, p. 280; 1963, p. 57, 1968, p. 358, 1979, p. 4). However, this well-known phrase is far too general for some clinical situations, leaving a great deal of ambiguity concerning precisely when practitioners are required to breach confidentiality (Fisher, 2008), especially when the therapeutic alliance is on the line.

On the one hand, the *autonomy principle* clearly urges us to recognize the client as a "rational agent", respect his unique views, and refrain from paternalism and judgment. On the other hand, the *non-maleficence* principle stresses that even through acts of omission, it is possible to do great harm. In this case, intentionally refraining from breaching confidentiality could impose an extreme risk onto others – an infection with a serious and potentially deadly illness. Thus, and in accordance with the *beneficence principle*, the cost of infecting people may be considered greater than the benefit of, maintaining confidentiality.

At the same time, this dilemma reflects the issue of Potentially Competing Duties (Section 3.3.4.; PBS, 2018; Standard 1.02; American Psychological Association, 2017). This conflict arises when psychologists' ethical responsibilities run counter to edicts of the law. In this case, the therapist's duty to maintain confidentiality conflicts with her legal duty to report a dangerous violation of quarantine, as well as her "responsibilities to [the welfare of] society" (Principle B; American Psychological Association, 2017; Section 1.6; British Psychological Society, 2018). Indeed, the Georgetown framework as a whole, and the *justice* principle in particular, remind us that ethics always reside within context; a practitioner cannot fully weigh the benefits and costs of a certain scenario without taking into account the world in which they both live. Thus, it seems that the therapist in question is obligated to act upon the information at hand, by taking reasonable steps to protect the individuals threatened by her client's actions.

Notably, one might consider the means by which the therapist is about to carry out her decision as another, inseparable dilemma, as ethically informed decisions are often a continuous action. Thus, choosing the "best" available manner of breaching confidentiality, while minimizing the harm, is of the utmost importance. For example, the therapist should consider discussing the limits of confidentiality (Standard 4.02; American Psychological Association, 2017) with her client, and in light of the *autonomy principle*, might suggest him the opportunity of reporting his violation himself.

Dilemma #3

> *In order to provide care under emergency conditions, a young practitioner is asked to perform a trauma-focused cognitive-behavioral intervention (TF-CBT) – a form of therapy for which she does not have the necessary training for. This is also her first time working with the post-traumatic population. Should the practitioner provide such services, despite the possibility of doing harm?*

This dilemma addresses the concept of "Boundaries of Competence" (Standard 2.01; American Psychological Association, 2017; Section 3.2; British Psychological Society, 2018). The increased demand for mental health services during a crisis usually triggers an "all hands on deck" situation, in which many practitioners might be facing the need to get quickly acquainted with new techniques (e.g., group therapy, prolonged exposure, grief counseling), technologies (e.g., telemedicine), populations (e.g., play therapy with toddlers), and disorders (e.g., the new emerging diagnosis of COVID-19 anxiety; Ahorsu et al., 2020), for which they lack adequate training and familiarity. Therefore, they cannot ensure that they will be performing the therapy competently and appropriately, and risk doing harm to their clients by providing substandard treatment. This dilemma is particularly relevant to training psychologists who, in an emergency situation, may find themselves performing treatments they do not have any prior experience with.

In this case, applying the *nonmaleficence* and *beneficence* principles yields conflicting advice. On one hand, denying therapeutic care to someone who is suffering due to a limited number of appropriately trained mental-health stuff certainly disrupts beneficence. On the other, practicing without the proper training puts the client at risk of considerable harm, and thus could be regarded as negligent. A possible solution that would balance beneficence and nonmaleficence would prioritize offering treatment to the client in order to avoid the painful decision of denying care, while taking appropriate measures to ensure its quality, such as discontinuing the service as soon as the emergency has ended or alternative services become available.

The *autonomy* principle helps further clarify the actions a practitioner should take. By this principle, therapists should seek to respect their clients' wishes instead of assuming they know what will best suit their needs. Accordingly, the best course of action would be to make the limitations of the therapist's skills known to the client, and allow him or her to choose for himself or herself. This would also be in line with the requirement of Informed Consent to Therapy (Standard 10.01; American Psychological Association, 2017; Section 3.1; British Psychological Society, 2018), which states that practitioners must inform their clients of the potential risks involved in the therapeutic process, while presenting alternatives (if any).

Dilemma #4

> *"In order to meet the expected high load of new referrals who suffer from the psychological consequences of COVID-19, therapists working in public and community healthcare facilities are instructed by the directors of their institutions to cut short long-term therapeutic processes currently in place. Should they follow the orders or continue to serve their existing clients"?*

In this situation, the instructions issued by the directors of these mental-health institutions conflict with the professional Ethics Code (Standard 1.03; American Psychological Association, 2017; Section 1.10; British Psychological Society, 2018). Conflicting loyalties (sometimes called "dual agency") can be ethically thorny for therapists, as they must balance their duty to clients with their need to follow the rules of their home institution. This circumstance may result in adverse outcomes in client care (Pryor, 1989). In emergency situations, these challenges intensify, as organizational, political and financial demands may preclude or override clinical discretion.

Three of the Georgetown principles are relevant to this dilemma: *beneficence, non-maleficence*, and *justice*. However, beneficence and maleficence are insufficient by themselves, since an action taken out of beneficence for one client might indirectly be maleficent towards another. The new guidelines issued in the case above will ensure that distressed clients who have suffered a tragic loss during the pandemic can be seen quickly, but this will come at the expense of others whose therapy has been terminated prematurely. Alternatively, should therapists decline the new clients, they will be able to maintain the existing standard of care for those clients, but those who have experienced acute and major psychological trauma may experience delays of care or may not have access to care at all.

Justice, particularly *distributive justice*, is relevant in this case, as accessible mental health care can be considered a scarce resource. It provides another viewpoint on the problem. For example, from a distributive justice point of view, since far greater resources have already been allocated to existing clients, and since investing resources in the "newcomers" is expected to be of greater impact, resources should be reallocated to post-COVID-19 referrals.

Importantly, even after ethical decisions have been made, one must continue to ensure that the benefits have outweighed the costs. For example, with regards to the aforementioned conflict, treatment of at-risk clients (i.e., presenting an immediate danger to themselves or others) should not be interrupted, in accordance with the non-maleficence principle and the Code of Avoiding Harm (Standard 3.04; American Psychological Association, 2017; Section 3.3; British Psychological Society, 2018). Thus, by combining the three principles, therapists are able to navigate through their conflicting duties, and make informed, balanced, and justified decisions.

Discussion

The four Georgetown principles, which have been available as a useful ethical tool for medical professionals for over half a century, are suggested to provide urgently needed guidance for practicing psychologists at this time of crisis. Considering these principles in addition to our professional Ethical Code allows one to engage in more straight forward, ethically-informed decision-making processes, while taking appropriate actions. Notably, their strength does not stem from either one of the principles at hand, but from the *interactions* between them. The insights lie within the "layers" created by adding the principles one on top of the other, until a committed decision can be made and then followed. Despite the fact that some critics find this approach to be mainly reflective western values of ethics and thus in need of culturally sensitive adjustments (Holm, 1995), the Georgetown principles can point us towards ethical "blind spots", which are particularly common in situations of "double exposure", when both clients and therapists have been exposed to a shared traumatic reality (Baum, 2014).

Ethics, moral distress, and professional burnout

The current work calls attention to the unique challenges facing mental-health practitioners during and after the present pandemic. Experts are now warning about the potentially immense psychological impacts of COVID-19. Global increases in depression, anxiety and post-trauma rates are only a few of the expected adverse effects of this monumental crisis (Brooks et al., 2020), which are likely to spread just as widely as the virus that initiated them. In times of crisis, rational sober thought is often abandoned, and decisions are all too often made rashly and under the influence of feelings fear, guilt and confusion, which often cloud our judgment. This problem is especially critical, as new and unfamiliar ethical dilemmas are constantly arising, and calm consideration rather than emotional overreaction is all the more essential at these times. Thus, a pragmatic framework allowing practitioners to quickly weigh complex ethical issues, while effectively balancing between clinical and situational considerations, is vital.

When professionals cannot carry out what they believe to be ethically appropriate actions, moral distress occurs (Lamiani, Borghi, & Argentero, 2017). This is especially pervasive among practitioners facing ethically complex situations (McCarthy & Deady, 2008). Indeed, losing control of clinical decision-making processes in emergency care was found to be a leading factor in practitioners' distress, resulting in further trauma for clients (Van Heugten, 2014). Moreover, moral distress has a significant detrimental effect on therapists' job performance, health, and wellbeing (Mänttäri-van der Kuip, 2016). This issue is highly relevant during the present pandemic and will continue to be relevant in its aftermath. The tension between what is morally just and what is practically possible intensifies therapists' moral distress, which in turn, could result in burnout (Dzeng & Curtis, 2018).

Despite over three decades of research into the phenomenon of moral distress among healthcare professionals (e.g., nurses, surgeons, occupational therapists, pharmacists; Whitehead, Herbertson, Hamric, Epstein, & Fisher, 2015), not much attention has been given to this issue within the field of psychology. However, the extraordinary circumstances of the COVID-19 event suggest this issue requires our immediate attention, as we are soon to expect an unprecedented global demand for mental health services all around the world (Brooks et al., 2020). Moral distress threatens the ability of mental health services to provide appropriate care for those in need, and thus should be a priority of post-crisis public relief plans. Moreover, researchers and clinicians should join forces in order to develop appropriate scales for evaluating the unique characteristics of moral distress in psychologists, and explore the short- and long-term implications of this distress.

Resources for ethical guidance and support

In times of crisis, it is imperative that psychologists turn to one of the profession's most valuable resources – collaborative thinking. Bennett, Bryant, VandenBos, and Greenwood (1990) considered peer consultation as "one of the most important resources for maintaining and enlarging competence" (p. 26). While consultation is essential at any time, it is far better to ask questions in advance, not in the midst of an ethical crisis. Regarding topics as anxiety-provoking as confidentiality or professional competence, it is advised that psychologists develop safe places to obtain advice and support in a future crisis (Fisher, 2008). Ethical guidance can be obtained from official ethical boards and committees, senior supervisors, and respected colleagues. Not only that, but therapists might also consider their clients as another, very important, resource within the deliberation process. While psychologists tend to feel obliged to enter the session "fully prepared", the respect for autonomy principle reminds us that clients do know what is best for them, and thus, sometimes, could (and should) take an active part in the decision-making process. Some examples of such actions can be found in the dilemmas presented above.

Conclusions

At this moment, when novel ethical problems arise constantly and less and less time is available to properly address them, it is more important than ever for psychologists to be attuned to the potential pitfalls associated with making complex ethical decisions in the clinical setting. Furthermore, psychologists ought to be well-versed in the ethical standards of their profession, as well as the state and federal laws and regulations which govern their practice (Fisher, 2016). Going forward, training programs must be made aware of these concerns, and to include training in risk management, so that all psychologists are familiar with the concept of managing ethical dilemmas and are not caught unawares by the complex realities of clinical practice.

When faced with the need to make a split-second decision, the simple and pragmatic framework usually yields the best answer. We have made a case in this paper that the Georgetown principles, when coupled with other professional ethical guidelines, can constitute such a framework, and yield such answers. Furthermore, we have shown, how situations arising during the COVID-19 pandemic can be framed in terms of the Georgetown Principles, and can thereby be quickly comprehended and addressed. Some of the dilemmas psychologists face will be similar to the ones we have presented, while others will be radically different; but by keeping these ethical principles in mind, while recalling their professional guidelines and the laws that govern them, psychologists will be empowered to perform efficient and morally sound decision making that will benefit their clients, their colleagues, their nations, and our world.

Disclosure statement

No potential conflict of interest was reported by the authors.

References

Ahorsu, D. K., Lin, C.-Y., Imani, V., Saffari, M., Griffiths, M. D., & Pakpour, A. H. (2020). The fear of COVID-19 scale: Development and initial validation. *International Journal of Mental Health and Addiction*, 1. doi:10.1007/s11469-020-00270-8

American Psychological Association. (1979). *Ethical standards of psychologists*. Washington, DC: Author.

American Psychological Association. (2017). Ethical principles of psychologists and code of conduct. Retrieved from https://www.apa.org/ethics/code/

Association, A. P. (1959). Ethical standards of psychologists. *American Psychologist, 14*, 279–282.

Association, A. P. (1963). Ethical standards of psychologists. *American Psychologist, 18*, 56–60.

Association, A. P. (1968). Ethical standards of psychologists. *American Psychologist, 23*(5), 357–361.

Baum, N. (2014). Professionals' double exposure in the shared traumatic reality of wartime: Contributions to orofessional growth and stress. *The British Journal of Social Work, 44*(8), 2113–2134.

Beauchamp, T. L., & Childress, J. F. (1979/2001). *Principles of biomedical ethics* (5th ed.). New York: Oxford University Press.

Bennett, B. E., Bryant, B. K., VandenBos, G. R., & Greenwood, A. (1990). *Professional liability and risk management*. Washington, DC: American Psychological Association.

British Psychological Society. (2018). Code of ethics and conduct. Retrieved from https://www.bps.org.uk/news-and-policy/bps-code-ethics-and-conduct

Brooks, S. K., Webster, R. K., Smith, L. E., Woodland, L., Wessely, S., Greenberg, N., & Rubin, G. J. (2020). The psychological impact of quarantine and how to reduce it: Rapid review of the evidence. *The Lancet*, *395*(10227), 912–920.

Bush, S. S. (2019). Use of practice guidelines and position statements in ethical decision making. *American Psychologist*, *74*(9), 1151.

Calain, P., Fiore, N., Poncin, M., & Hurst, S. A. (2009). Research ethics and international epidemic response: The case of Ebola and Marburg Hemorrhagic fevers. *Public Health Ethics*, *2*(1), 7–29.

Centers for Disease Control & Prevention. (2020, February 29). Interim guidance for healthcare facilities: Preparing for community transmission of COVID-19 in the United States. Retrieved from https://www.cdc.gov/coronavirus/2019-ncov/hcp/guidance-hcf.html?CDC_AA_refVal=https%3A%2F%2Fwww.cdc.gov%2Fcoronavirus%2F2019-ncov%2Fhealthcare-facilities%2Fguidance-hcf.html

Centers for Medicare & Medicaid Services. (2020, March 30). Guidance for infection control and prevention of Coronavirus disease (COVID-19) in hospitals, psychiatric hospitals, and Critical Access Hospitals (CAHs). Retrieved from https://www.cms.gov/files/document/qso-20-13-hospitals-cahs-revised.pdf

Chinazzi, M., Davis, J. T., Ajelli, M., Gioannini, C., Litvinova, M., Merler, S., … Sun, K. (2020). The effect of travel restrictions on the spread of the 2019 novel Coronavirus (COVID-19) outbreak. *Science*. doi:10.1126/science.aba9757

Dzeng, E., & Curtis, J. R. (2018). Understanding ethical climate, moral distress, and burnout: A bovel tool and a conceptual framework, BMJ Publishing Group Ltd.

Fisher, M. A. (2008). Protecting confidentiality rights: The need for an ethical practice model. *American Psychologist*, *63*(1), 1.

Fisher, M. A. (2016). *Confidentiality limits in psychotherapy:Ethics checklists for mental health professionals*. Washington, DC: American Psychological Association.

Gillon, R. (2003). Four scenarios. *Journal of Medical Ethics*, *29*(5), 267–268.

Hain, R., & Saad, T. (2016). Foundations of practical ethics. *Medicine*, *44*(10), 578–582.

Hanson, S. L., Kerkhoff, T. R., & Bush, S. S. (2005). *Crisis and emergency care health care ethics for psychologists: A casebook* (pp. 9–37). Washington, DC: American Psychological Association.

Ho, C. S., Chee, C. Y., & Ho, R. C. (2020). Mental health strategies to combat the psychological impact of COVID-19 beyond paranoia and panic. *Annals of the Academy of Medicine of Singapore.*, *49*(3), 155–160.

Holm, S. (1995). Not just autonomy – The principles of American biomedical ethics. *Journal of Medical Ethics*, *21*(6), 332–338.

Hutchings, K. (2010). *Global ethics: An introduction*. Cambridge, UK: Polity.

Kächele, H., & Schachter, J. (2014). On side effects, destructive processes, and negative outcomes in psychoanalytic therapies: Why is it difficult for psychoanalysts to acknowledge and address treatment failures? *Contemporary Psychoanalysis*, *50*(1–2), 233–258.

Karabag, S. F. (2020). An unprecedented global crisis! The global, regional, national, political, economic and commercial impact of the Coronavirus pandemic. *Journal of Applied Economics and Business Research*, *10*(1), 1–6.

Lamiani, G., Borghi, L., & Argentero, P. (2017). When healthcare professionals cannot do the right thing: A systematic review of moral distress and its correlates. *Journal of Health Psychology*, *22*(1), 51–67.

Loewenberg, F., Dolgoff, R., & Harrington, D. (2000). *Ethical decisions for cocial work practice* (6th ed.). Itasca, IL: F. E. Peacock.

Lowman, R. L. (2006). *The ethical practice of psychology in organizations*. Washington, DC: American Psychological Association.

Macklin, R. (2003). Applying the Four Principles. *Journal of Medical Ethics*, *29*(5), 275–280.

Mänttäri-van der Kuip, M. (2016). Moral distress among social workers: The role of insufficient resources. *International Journal of Social Welfare*, *25*(1), 86–97.

McCarthy, J., & Deady, R. (2008). Moral distress reconsidered. *Nursing Ethics*, *15*(2), 254–262.

Phillips, S., Knebel, A., & Johnson, K. (2009). Mass medical care with scarce resources: The essentials. Agency for Healthcare Research and Quality, 2009 AHRQ Publication, 09–0016.

Platje, J., Harvey, J., & Rayman-Bacchus, L. (2020). COVID-19–Reflections on the surprise of both an expected and unexpected event. *The Central European Review of Economics and Management, 4* (1), 149–162.

Pryor, R. G. (1989). Conflicting responsibilities: A case study of an ethical dilemma for psychologists working in organisations. *Australian Psychologist, 24*(2), 293–305.

Ransing, R., Ramalho, R., Orsolini, L., Adiukwu, F., Gonzalez-Diaz, J. M., Larnaout, A., … Patil, I. (2020). Can COVID-19 related mental health issues be measured? Assessment options for mental health professionals. *Brain, Behavior, and Immunity*. doi:10.1016/j.bbi.2020.05.049

Sussman, M. B. (1995). *A perilous calling: The hazards of psychotherapy practice*. Hoboken, New Jersey: John Wiley & Sons.

Van Heugten, K. (2014). *Human service organizations in the disaster context*. New York: Springer.

Whitehead, P. B., Herbertson, R. K., Hamric, A. B., Epstein, E. G., & Fisher, J. M. (2015). Moral distress among healthcare professionals: Report of an institution-wide survey. *Journal of Nursing Scholarship, 47*(2), 117–125.

Wind, T. R., Rijkeboer, M., Andersson, G., & Riper, H. (2020). The COVID-19 pandemic: The 'black swan'for mental health care and a turning point for e-health. *Internet Interventions., 20*, 100317.

World Health Organization. (2020, March 11). WHO director-general's opening remarks at the media briefing on COVID-19—11 March 2020. Retrieved from https://www.who.int/dg/speeches/detail/who-director-general-s-opening-remarks-at-the-media-briefing-on-covid-19—11-march-2020#.Xoj7376UGsM.link

World Health Organization. (2020, January 20). Statement on the second meeting of the International health regulations 2005 emergency committee regarding the outbreak of novel coronavirus (2019-nCoV) [Press release]. Retrieved from https://www.who.int/news-room/detail/30-01-2020-statement-on-the-second-meeting-of-the-international-health-regulations-(2005)-emergency-committee-regarding-the-outbreak-of-novel-coronavirus-(2019-ncov)#.Xoj73VhXFwM.link

Psychotherapy at a public hospital in the time of COVID-19: telehealth and implications for practice

Zoe Silver, Mikaela Coger, Sebastian Barr and Rebecca Drill

ABSTRACT

As the crisis of global pandemic continues to unfold and alter the everyday workings of public life, early trends in the impact on mental healthcare treatment at a safety-net hospital illuminate implications for clinical work in the public sector under unprecedented conditions and beyond. While there are many important areas to consider and research to come, the current paper will explore the impact of the COVID-19 crisis on attendance of psychotherapy sessions. The authors point to early evidence from their caseloads in an outpatient psychodynamic psychotherapy training program showing a statistically significant decrease in missed appointments upon switching, in crisis, to a telehealth model. In this paper we explore possible reasons for this decrease in missed appointments, including psychological reasons (such as increased need for connection) and logistical reasons (such as eliminating barriers to attendance). Finally, we point to considerations and implications for practice during and after the crisis of the pandemic has subsided, and consider ways in which the changing approach may, in effect, increase access and remove barriers to care that pre-date our current crisis.

The COVID-19 pandemic has massively interrupted *status quo* parameters in mental healthcare at a public safety-net hospital in Cambridge, Massachusetts, where the mission is to provide care to traditionally underserved, vulnerable and diverse populations. In four short weeks, the large psychiatry department rolled out rapid and far-reaching changes to its service model in order to ensure access to psychiatric care during this period of working under stay-at-home orders and social distancing. The roll-out occurred in stages, beginning with a swift decision to change all outpatient visits to phone sessions within a 24-hour window when the call for social distancing became urgent. Over the following week, mechanisms to bill for these visits were implemented, which is an essential aspect in a hospital system already financially strained. This was followed by a procedure (2 weeks later) to conduct and bill for video sessions.

This paper offers a unique perspective of making this transition in a public safety-net hospital and specifically focuses on an unintended positive consequence of this transition, namely, a statistically significant decrease in missed appointments (i.e., when the patient cancels or does not show up). The first three authors of this paper are post-graduate fellows in a psychodynamic psychotherapy clinic/training program, and the last author is the clinical director. This program is a part of the larger Outpatient Psychiatry Department (OPD) of the only public acute care hospital in Massachusetts. The hospital has the highest concentration of Medicaid and low-income patient care (representing 51% of its payer mix) among hospitals in the state, and it has 2.6 times greater the proportion of Medicaid and low-income public payer care than the acute care hospital average (Center for Health Information and Analysis, 2018). Given the large majority of low-income patients, many cannot afford to be seen in private practice, or they have insurance that limits their options for obtaining private care. Patients pay little-to-no fee for psychotherapy and are not charged for missed appointments.

The following patient demographics are derived from a representative sample of patients in our clinic (*N* = 393) who participated in a research project that included self-reported demographic information. One hundred twenty-eight patients (33%) identified themselves as male, 260 (66%) female, and five (.01%) used another term (e.g., "fluid").[1] Sixty-one percent identified as White/Caucasian (not of Latina/Latino origin), 1.78% as Black, 4.32% as Black/African American, 6.87% as Latina/Latino, 1.78% as Asian, 0.025% as Pacific Islander, 11.45% as mixed racial/ethnic heritage (or endorsed more than one category), 4.58% as "other," and 7.63% left it blank.[2] Mean age was 35.38 (*SD* = 10.21), with a range from 18.3 to 69.9 years. Open-ended responses to a question about sexual-orientation yielded the following: 64.6% identified as heterosexual or straight, 3.8% as homosexual, gay or lesbian, 1.5% as queer, 5.3% as bisexual, 1.5% as fluid, 1.3% as pansexual, 0.5% as asexual, 1.5% used a term other than the ones just listed above (e.g., questioning), 5.3% as more than one category (e.g., bisexual/queer), 4.0% used a term or spelled the category in an ambiguous manner that could not be interpreted (e.g., "heterosexual," "yes," or "male"), and 9.9% left it blank, responded N/A, or declined to answer.

Yearly income levels were as follows: 27.7% under 12,000, USD 10.4% 12,000 USD to 15,999, USD 16.8% 16,000 USD to 24,999, USD 17.3% 25,000 USD to 34,999, USD 9.7% 35,000 USD to 49,999, USD and 5.9% 50,000 USD or above. Education levels were as follows: 28.0% of patients in the study had a high school diploma or equivalent, 44.0% had an associates or bachelor's degree, and 19.3% had either a graduate or professional degree.[3] Finally, from the same research project, a representative sample (*N* = 110) of diagnoses assessed by the treating clinician at the time of termination of treatment is as follows: 53% Depressive Disorders (e.g., Major Depressive Disorder, Dysthymia), 21% Anxiety-related Disorders (e.g., Generalized Anxiety Disorder, Panic Disorder, OCD), 8% PTSD, 7% Adjustment Disorders, 4% Bipolar Disorders/Cyclothymia, 4% ADHD/Impulse Control Disorders, 2% Premenstrual Disorder, 1% Psychological Factors Affecting a Pain Syndrome, and 1% Hypochondriasis.

The current scenario defined by COVID-19 is without precedent in our lifetimes and it is fraught with challenges and lessons to be learned. While we can take guidance from the experiences of clinicians in previous crises, the obstacles facing us now raise distinct challenges. There has been literature on conducting therapy after disasters and crises in recent decades, e.g., the AIDS crisis (M. Forstein, personal communication, March 17, 2020), 9/11 (Frawley-O'Dea, 2003; Saakvitne, 2002), Hurricane Katrina (Boulanger, 2013), the Boston Marathon bombing (J. Jenkins, personal communication, March 24, 2020) and these resources have helped therapists think about how to conduct therapy while managing their own internal states (e.g., feelings of vulnerability, anxiety, fear, etc.). However, in these earlier post-disaster situations, being together in the therapy room could offer a comforting and containing experience and, with few exceptions, was available immediately or nearly immediately after the crisis. What makes the COVID-19 pandemic crisis unique for the field of psychotherapy is that the personal, face-to-face contact that provides support is the very thing that people cannot access; social distancing and stay-at-home orders prevent it. The unclear timeline and absence of a visible endpoint sets this moment apart and poses additional challenges. While we as therapists can offer support and help our patients develop coping mechanisms, we are aware that the sequelae of such trauma (whether it be PTSD, bereavement, heightened anxiety, etc.) may not fully develop until sometime after.

Though there are many clinical and logistical aspects to the experience of transitioning from in-person psychotherapy to teletherapy (whether via phone or video conferencing) overall, as mentioned above, this paper will focus on one aspect in our experience working in a public safety-net hospital: the statistically significant reduction in the number of missed appointments that occurred in our caseloads upon switching to teletherapy. A survey of eight fellows in our clinic revealed that clinicians had a mean missed appointment rate of 14.25% ($SD = 9.42$) before the transition to telehealth and a mean missed appointment rate of 5.63% ($SD = 2.72$) after the transition to telehealth. A Wilcoxon Signed-Ranks Test indicated that this difference was statistically significant, $Z = -2.18$, $p = .03$. Thus, the rate of missed appointments in our clinic was statistically significantly lower in a four-week period following the transition to telehealth (March 30–24 April 2020) than in a four-week period before the transition (February 3–28, 2020).Note that the clinic began the transition to telehealth during the week of March 16.[4] These results are based on reports generated by each of the therapists in our clinic (except for one, who was on vacation for a significant portion of the time frame in which data were collected) including the number of missed/cancelled appointments and the total number of patients they would have seen for each of the 8 weeks. (See Figure 1).

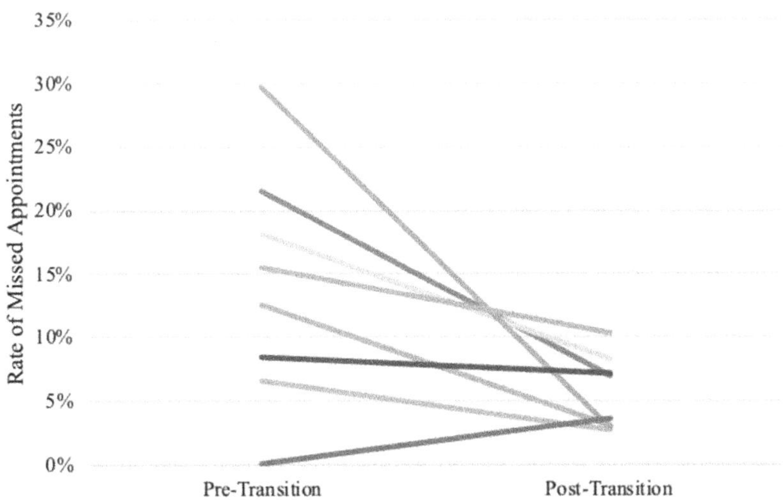

Figure 1. Rate of missed appointments before and after transitioning to telehealth. The graph above shows the changes in the average rate of missed appointments (cancellations and no-shows) for each of eight clinicians in the Program for Psychotherapy between the periods before and after the transition to telehealth.

While there are a number of limitations to consider regarding this data, which we will discuss below, the statistically significant reduction in missed appointments pre-and-post transition is striking, and we became curious as to why it was occurring. Authors have previously documented high no-show rates at public health facilities and have written about possible reasons for this, including clinical issues and logistical/practical challenges (DeFife, Conklin, Smith, & Poole, 2010; DeFife, Smith, & Conklin, 2013). For the sake of clarity, we have divided our ideas about contributors to this reduction in missed appointments into two categories: psychological and logistical factors.

We begin with a discussion about psychological factors that may have contributed to this phenomenon. One potential influence leading to higher attendance rates is an increased need for human connection during crises. As Judy Herman noted in her seminal book on trauma, "recovery can take place only within the context of relationships" (Herman, 2015, p. 133). Psychotherapists across all modalities know the importance of human connection regardless of whether or not they are using a trauma framework. Research has shown that the working alliance, as one aspect of the therapeutic relationship, is predictive of positive outcomes in psychotherapy (Flückiger, Del Re, Wampold, & Horvath, 2018; Horvath & Symonds, 1991; Jordan, 2003; Norcross, 2002; Uckelstam, Holmqvist, Philips, & Falkenström, 2020; Wampold & Imel, 2015; Xu & Tracey, 2015). In addition, in a study in our clinic which has been submitted for publication, in response to an open-ended prompt, "What do you find helpful about your treatment?," many patients either explicitly or implicitly referred to elements of the therapy relationship (Richardson et al., 2020). We speculate that attention to the relationship, which is an important component of psychodynamic psychotherapy, may contribute to a patient's greater commitment to maintaining a connection through this crisis and, therefore, lead to more consistency in attendance through the transition to teletherapy. Further, for patients who find the intimacy of therapy challenging, teletherapy provides an extra layer of insulation between patient and therapist that may help resolve resistances to connecting, and therefore increase their ability to tolerate attending sessions consistently (E. Silver, personal communication, May 28, 2020).

Given the importance of human connection, and the importance of the therapy relationship specifically, patients feeling socially isolated may be particularly craving connection with their therapists during this uncertain and frightening time. As mentioned above, therapists who specialize in working with trauma have established that human connection is healing (Herman, 2015; Saakvitne, Gamble, Pearlman, & Lev, 2000) and it is commonly accepted that social connection improves many aspects of both psychological and physical well-being (Murthy, 2020; Seppala, 2012). Even for those who are not fully isolated, maintaining ties to the "outside world" may be relieving; it may provide a break from new or expanded caregiving responsibilities and/or a connection to one's "pre-pandemic" life and psychological mind. For example, while some of our patients spent telehealth sessions focusing on the pandemic itself and the anxieties and fear aroused by it, others, while not ignoring the outbreak, continued to work on issues they had been addressing in therapy previously. While patients have always been able to use the clinical hour to meet their fluctuating needs, it seems that this might be particularly important during a pandemic and may contribute to the increased attendance that we have found in our caseloads.

The transition to teletherapy also necessitated some logistical changes that may have contributed to the increased attendance, and these logistical shifts may also have psychological meaning. For instance, in a standard therapy session, the meeting begins when the patient arrives, creating a dynamic in which the initiative lies with the patient. In the first week of our clinic's switch to teletherapy, all clinical interactions were administered through telephone. Suddenly, clinicians were required to take the initiative to call the patient at the start of the therapy hour. Once a HIPAA-compliant video platform was available, to initiate a session, therapists created a meeting and invited their patients via hospital email. Patients received the email invitation only after it was sent by clinicians, and they entered the virtual meeting at their convenience. This process allowed for some continuity of the in-person psychotherapy frame (i.e., the meeting started when the patient arrived); however, it was still ultimately clinicians' responsibility to set up the meeting and reach out to their patients. Additionally, text or email reminders were previously sent to patients 24–48 hours before the scheduled in-person appointment, but in the new system, patients no longer received those reminders, and instead received only the email invitation soon before the appointment was scheduled to begin. We wonder if some patients responded positively to the therapist's more active pursuit of them during this crisis, and interpreted it as a communication of the therapist's willingness to devote time and energy to maintaining the attachment. Particularly for patients who have been traumatized or marginalized (as is the case with many public hospital patients), this active pursuit may have been a relationally novel and thereby fortifying experience. Thus, the very shift in the frame whereby the therapist took more initiative in starting the session could have had the unintended but positive consequence of deepening the therapeutic relationship and increasing patients' motivation to attend therapy (J. Smith, personal communication, April 12, 2020).

It is possible that this shift in the frame increased convenience and decreased certain barriers to treatment, and therefore contributed to fewer missed appointments. For instance, logistical challenges that formerly contributed to missed appointments (such as commuting, scheduling, and arranging childcare) were, for some patients, eliminated or decreased under the new circumstances. Transportation was no longer necessary; late or missed buses or trains did not interfere with appointments. The majority of businesses and workplaces were closed, unfortunately leaving a significant number of our patients unemployed and with unstructured schedules. Patients who previously had to prioritize work by picking up extra shifts or working overtime no longer had this scheduling conflict. Patients who were still working during this time were likely working odd or different hours; at the same time, clinicians, also working from home, may have had more flexibility to accommodate shifting schedules. Family-related barriers such as childcare, daycare schedules, or elder care could have been less likely to interfere with therapy appointments for some. Notably, for others, who could not be relieved of these duties, the opposite may have been true.

It is important to acknowledge the limited scope of our experience as a singular clinic as well as limitations in our data collection. There are many situations in which the current crisis may in fact have made it *more* challenging for some clients to engage in teletherapy. For instance, some patients may not have been able to utilize the video platform because they did not have access to either a computer, internet, or a private space. These patients might have been required to continue with telephone therapy (rather than video therapy) regardless of their preference. Additionally, some who simply wanted to continue treatment by telephone could not choose to do so because certain insurance plans would not initially allow reimbursement for phone sessions (although this was resolved relatively early on). Furthermore, patients who lived with children, roommates, or family members may have struggled to find privacy, which could interfere with speaking candidly or continuing treatment at all. Patients who were homeless or had limited-to-no income may have had to use a pay-per-minute phone or may not even have had access to a phone or data plan at all. Elderly patients who were isolated and did not know how to utilize new technology may have been unable to engage.

Due to various social determinants of health (e.g., race, location, responsiveness of local government, discrimination in healthcare, living conditions, prevalence of pre-existing conditions, and poverty), certain populations (particularly the black community) have had a higher prevalence of deaths from the virus (Hawkins, 2020). For individuals in these communities, continued therapy may have been a significant challenge. In addition, barriers to mental healthcare in the United States pre-date COVID-19. The National Comorbidity Survey Replication (Mojtabai et al., 2011) illuminated such barriers, including lack of perceived need for treatment, attitudinal barriers (e.g., stigma), and structural barriers (e.g., financial, availability, transportation, and inconvenience), all of which are influenced by sociodemographic factors and severity of illness. These barriers in general, and the inequities that the pandemic crisis highlighted, underscore the structural issues of class and racism that exist in our society. While most of our patients found ways to continue their therapy, we are aware that differing levels of access and privilege have likely had an impact on continued attendance.

In addition, we acknowledge various limitations of our data that should be considered when drawing conclusions based on our findings. First, our data are representative only of our very small clinic; completing similar analyses with a larger sample size and across different types of clinical settings would help determine whether our findings are generalizable. Further, the lack of a centralized system for record-keeping of missed appointments meant that each clinician depended on their individual records and memories when reporting their data. Additionally, clinicians may have had different approaches to calculating the total number of missed and scheduled appointments per week. These limitations highlight the value of replication of this study on a larger scale with more uniform and rigorous data collection methodologies. Larger studies would also be able to determine whether there were patient factors (e.g., race, SES, length of current treatment) or clinic factors (e.g., type of therapy) that affected changes in attendance rates.

Although the limitations of our study should caution readers against generalizing these findings to settings that differ substantially from our clinic, we believe the results point to important implications and considerations for practice moving forward. For example, perhaps the reduction of missed appointments observed by these clinicians is reflective of a larger way in which the lowering of barriers during the crisis has improved service delivery. Perhaps we will learn from this experience how significant it is to our population to have the option for out-of-office care, later appointment reminders, and appointment flexibility. Once we are through the catastrophe and return to whatever the new normal will be, what lessons will we take with us?

Conversations have been emerging in various fields about how the pandemic is illuminating unnecessary red tape and bureaucratic processes that are being cut through to deal with this crisis. In this way, the crisis has revealed pre-existing inequities that are intrinsically woven into the fabric of American society, including social welfare, housing, healthcare, and education systems. Many Americans, particularly those who have been historically oppressed and marginalized, have long struggled to stay afloat as a result of these gaps and disparities in access and opportunity. Because the COVID-19 crisis is far-reaching and has also impacted individuals who are regularly privileged by such systems, various sectors have mobilized to rapidly respond to the needs of the public. For example, unemployment applications are being streamlined, and public health insurance companies are eliminating co-pays associated with certain medications and appointments. Various policies (e.g., those pertaining to health insurance, immigration, overcrowding in prisons) are shifting to deal with the current crisis, and areas of policy deficit are being exposed (e.g., public access to the internet, inequities in health and education, and barriers to care). For those who have long been in crisis, these responses were needed well before the pandemic. For the healthcare industry, this begets the question of how dire circumstances must get, and for whom, in order to implement widespread strategies that improve access.

Notes

1. We have since revised our demographic questionnaire so that the item asking patients to self-identify their gender is now an open-ended question with some examples as prompts to allow patients to respond to this item in whatever way they feel best reflects their gender identity (Drill et al., 2019).
2. Similarly, we have since revised our demographic questionnaire so that the item asking patients to self-identify their race/ethnicity is now an open-ended question with some examples as prompts to allow patients to respond to this item in whatever way they feel best reflects their racial/ethnic identity.
3. Not all participants answered every demographic question in the survey; therefore, some percentages do not add up to 100.
4. We purposefully did not choose the 2 weeks before or after the transition date to buffer against the immediate effects of the crisis and transition to telehealth.

Acknowledgments

The authors gratefully acknowledge the helpful comments of Janna Smith, MSW, LICSW.

Disclosure statement

No potential conflict of interest was reported by the authors.

References

Boulanger, G. (2013). Fearful symmetry: Shared trauma in New Orleans after hurricane Katrina. *Psychoanalytic Dialogues*, *23*(1), 31–44.

Center for Health information and analysis 2018 hospital cost report data access tool. (2018). https://www.chiamass.gov/hospital-cost-report-data-access-tool.

DeFife, J. A., Conklin, C. Z., Smith, J. A., & Poole, J. (2010). Psychotherapy appointment no-shows: Rates and reasons. *Psychotherapy Theory, Research, Practice, Training*, *47*(3), 317–413.

DeFife, J. A., Smith, J. A., & Conklin, C. (2013). Psychotherapy appointment no-shows: Clinicians' approaches. *Journal of Contemporary Psychotherapy*, *43*(2), 107–113.

Drill, R., Malone, J., Flouton-Barnes, M., Cotton, L., Keyes, S., Wasserman, R., . . . Beinashowitz, J. (2019). Inclusive language regarding gender, sexual orientation, and relationship status: The ongoing process and outcome of revising psychiatric materials. *Journal of Mental Health Training and Education*, *14*(6), 385–398.

Flückiger, C., Del Re, A. C., Wampold, B. E., & Horvath, A. O. (2018). The alliance in adult psychotherapy: A meta-analytic synthesis. *Psychotherapy, 55*(4), 316–340.
Frawley-O'Dea, M. G. (2003). When the trauma is terrorism and the therapist is traumatized too: Working as an analyst since 9/11. *Psychoanalytic Perspectives, 1*(1), 67–89.
Hawkins, D. (2020). The coronavirus burden is falling heavily on black Americans. Why? *The Guardian*. Retrieved April 18, 2020 from https://www.theguardian.com/commentisfree/2020/apr/16/black-workers-coronavirus-covid-19
Herman, J. L. (2015). *Trauma and Recovery*. New York: Basic Books.
Horvath, A. O., & Symonds, B. D. (1991). Relation between working alliance and outcome in psychotherapy: A meta-analysis. *Journal of Counseling Psychology, 38*(2), 139–149.
Jordan, K. (2003). Relating therapeutic working alliance to therapy outcome. *Family Therapy: The Journal of the California Graduate School of Family Psychology, 30*(2), 95-107.
Mojtabai, R., Olfson, M., Sampson, N., Jin, R., Druss, B., Wang, P., ... Kessler, R. (2011). Barriers to mental health treatment: Results from the National Comorbidity Survey Replication (NCS-R). *Psychological Medicine, 41*(8), 1751–1761.
Murthy, V. H. (2020). *Together: The healing power of human connection in a sometimes lonely world*. New York, NY: Harper Collins.
Norcross, J. C. (2002). *Psychotherapy relationships that work: Therapist contributions and responsiveness to patients*. New York, NY: Oxford University Press.
Richardson, H., Hunnicutt, P., Gill., A., Ernst, J., Drill, R., & Beinashowitz, J. (2020). *Qualitative study of psychodynamic psychotherapy*. Manuscript submitted for publication.
Saakvitne, K. (2002). Shared trauma: The therapist's increased vulnerability. *Psychoanalytic Dialogues, 12*(3), 443–449.
Saakvitne, K. W., Gamble, S. G., Pearlman, L. A., & Lev, L. (2000). *Risking Connection: A Training Curriculum for Working with Survivors of Childhood Abuse*. Lutherville, MD: Sidran Press.
Seppala, E. (2012, August 26). *Connect tothrive*. Psychology Today. https://www.psychologytoday.com/us/blog/feeling-it/201208/connect-thrive
Uckelstam, C. J., Holmqvist, R., Philips, B., & Falkenström, F. (2020). A relational perspective on the association between working alliance and treatment outcome. *Psychotherapy Research, 30*(1), 13–22.
Wampold, B., & Imel, Z. (2015). *The great psychotherapy debate: The evidence for what makes psychotherapy work* (Second ed.). New York: Routledge.
Xu, H., & Tracey, T. J. (2015). Reciprocal influence model of working alliance and therapeutic outcome over individual therapy course. *Journal of Counseling Psychology, 62*(3), 351.

A brief transdiagnostic pandemic mental health maintenance intervention

Trisha Arnold, Brooke G. Rogers, Alyssa L. Norris, Anna Schierberl Scherr, Kayla Haubrick, Megan E. Renna, Shufang Sun, Margaret M. Danforth, Christina T. Chu, Elizabeth S. Silva, Laura B. Whiteley and Megan Pinkston

ABSTRACT

The COVID-19 pandemic qualifies as a major national and global disaster. Behavioral health providers are poised to provide psychological crisis interventions to reduce the psychosocial effects. This paper presents a brief transdiagnostic mental health maintenance intervention tailored to treat adults and families with distress symptoms. The intervention components include evidence-based techniques which have been strategically selected to address distress related to the pandemic and to prevent the escalation of distress. The intervention aims to be flexibly incorporated into care based on the provider and needs of the presenting individuals. The intervention incorporates components of evidence-based treatments such as Cognitive Behavioral Therapy and associated "third wave" therapies (e.g. Dialectical Behavioral Therapy and Acceptance and Commitment Therapy). The intervention can be delivered via telehealth and includes the following modules: 1) Agenda Setting & Avoidance Identification; 2) Responding to Difficult News/ Normalizing Reactions; 3) Perspective Taking; 4) Situational Control/Acceptance; 5) Maintaining a Healthy Routine; 6) Coping with Stress; 7) Insomnia Preventions; and 8) Building Resiliency & Hope. The intervention includes a list of home based pleasurable activities, a list of technology modalities to maintain social interactions, and a handout for patients. Research is needed to further test this intervention and assess implementation strategies.

Background

The COVID-19 pandemic qualifies as a major national and global disaster. The pandemic not only affects individuals' physical health, but it also creates psychological distress for COVID-19 patients, family members, health service providers, and the general public. Despite the unifying effect of a sweeping global impact, the pandemic has simultaneously isolated, restricted, and altered our way of living. The Centers for Disease Control and Prevention recommend social distancing by limiting face-to-face contact with other people, maintaining at least six feet of physical separation, and avoiding social gatherings (Centers for Disease Control and Prevention, 2020a). Social isolation has also disrupted work, employment status, and daily routines with little-to-no advance notice for much of the population. While essential to promoting physical health, paradoxically, these dramatic changes to normal routine can negatively impact mental health for large portions of the population. The pandemic also presents individuals with uncertainty about timing and the toll the disease may take on individuals, families, and communities. Unpredictability across physical, social, and economic domains without ready access to typically used coping mechanisms could lead to widespread, significant, and long-lasting mental health effects. Given the restrictions of social distancing and the mental health effects, there is a need to develop mental health interventions that are both informed by empirical research but also responsive to the unique demands of this pandemic.

The COVID-19 pandemic presents an unprecedented challenge in its impact to our collective well-being. Although researchers are just beginning to assess the psychological impact of COVID-19, behavioral healthcare providers are already required to meet the needs of individuals as they seek services that will support them in making sense of and coping with this outbreak and its sequelae. Given the novel nature of COVID-19, research on infectious disease outbreaks in general can provide a framework for understanding the potential impact of this pandemic. Infectious disease outbreaks, such as the COVID-19 pandemic, can be associated with depression, anxiety, guilt, grief, stigma, and post-traumatic stress (Brooks et al., 2020; Chew, Wei, Vasoo, Chua, & Sim, 2020; Lau et al., 2005). Indeed, the limited research examining the mental health sequelae of COVID-19 in China suggests that the impact of this outbreak is similar to that of prior public health emergencies in that it is associated with significant increases in negative emotionality (e.g., anxiety and depressive symptoms) and reductions in positive emotionality (Lau et al., 2005; Li et al., 2020).

Although research is currently focusing on acute effects of this pandemic and isolation, research suggests that the impact of COVID-19 will be long-lasting (Brooks et al., 2020). Therefore, there is an urgent need for interventions that effectively mitigate the mental health impact to improve individual well-being, but also reduce burden to an already taxed healthcare system. Early research related to COVID-19 highlights the benefits of using technology to deliver mental health services (Dong & Bouey, 2020). Behavioral health care providers are poised to provide psychological crisis interventions to reduce the psychosocial effects of the COVID-19 outbreak. To our knowledge, there are no published brief transdiagnostic interventions in the United States tailored specifically toward coping with pandemic distress or mental health maintenance during the COVID-19 pandemic.

The proposed intervention

Existing models of transdiagnostic interventions emphasize eliciting stimuli (e.g., exposure to someone sick, unknown future) as causing distress rather than differences in the psychological, cognitive, emotional, interpersonal and behavioral processes as responsible for resulting distress and disorders (Barlow, Allen, & Choate, 2004; Norton & Paulus, 2017). A transdiagnostic approach identifies and targets the core processes that manifest psychological distress (Harvey, Watkins, Mansell, & Shafran, 2004). Consistent with the Research Domain Criteria (RDoC), put forth by the National Institute for Mental Health, transdiagnostic interventions apply the same treatment principals to address underlying processes (Cuthbert, 2014). Modular transdiagnostic interventions can be incorporated into other treatment approaches by utilizing only the relevant modules. Clinical practice advances highlight a paradigm shift towards a transdiagnostic conceptualization and treatment (Craske, 2012). In response to the public health emergency and urgent need for behavioral health interventions tailored to psychological symptoms specific to COVID-19, this paper presents a Brief Transdiagnostic Pandemic Mental Health Maintenance Intervention protocol. The purpose of this transdiagnostic intervention is to promote resilience in the face of COVID-19, which will be achieved through principles of Cognitive Behavioral Therapy (CBT) (Beck, 1997, 2011; Perlis, Benson-Jungquist, Smith, & Posner, 2005), Acceptance and Commitment Therapy (ACT) (Luoma, Hayes, & Walser, 2007), Dialectical Behavioral Therapy (DBT) (Linehan, 2015; Najavits, 2003), and Behavior Activation (BA) (Martell, Dimidjian, & Herman-Dunn, 2010). Given the prediction for increased demand for mental health services throughout and following the pandemic, behavioral health professionals need protocols that are sensitive to clients' presenting needs (Galea, Merchant, & Lurie, 2020). The proposed intervention can be provided alone or in conjunction with existing interventions for psychiatric conditions premorbid to the pandemic. The goal of this intervention is to provide skills that can help buffer the psychological impact of COVID-19 through increasing coping and promoting resilience.

Intervention development

The intervention includes a comprehensive set of evidence-based techniques to address mental health distress related to the pandemic and to prevent the escalation of distress throughout its duration. The intervention was created by clinical psychologists with a range of primary theoretical orientations which include CBT, ACT, DBT, and BA. The authors also include psychologists specializing in domains such as providing brief treatment for distress in primary care and outpatient psychiatric settings, treating sleep disorders, and developing brief interventions specific to infectious disease/chronic illness prevention, adjustment, and recovery. In developing this intervention, we gathered authors' clinical experiences from the current pandemic as well as in previously similar clinical situations (e.g., working with patients vulnerable to other types of infectious diseases) to identify key techniques and principles to inform this transdiagnostic intervention. After an initial draft of the intervention protocol, authors then provided further intensive feedback for refinement and improvement. Drawing on the authors' experiences providing care from a variety of theoretical orientations in a range of settings, the intervention aims to be flexibly incorporated based on the intervention setting, role of provider, and needs of the presenting individuals. Additionally, we include coping techniques that have been useful during other infectious disease outbreaks in the general population. These techniques include social support and assessing the positives of the situation (Chew et al., 2020).

This intervention is designed to be delivered flexibly via telehealth in line with social distancing and quarantine guidelines published by the World Health Organization (2020) and the Centers for Disease Control and Prevention (2020b). Researchers have emphasized the need for utilizing telehealth during the pandemic (Liu et al., 2020; Zhou et al., 2020). Fortunately, telemedicine has been documented to be feasible, acceptable to clients and clinicians, and effective more broadly (Kemp et al., 2020). For example, offering mental health services virtually has comparable efficacy to in-person care in treating depression, anxiety and trauma disorders (Andrews et al., 2018; Kuester, Niemeyer, & Knaevelsrud, 2016). As such, special considerations were given to telehealth/mHealth as pertains to the intervention's content and delivery. The intervention could also be delivered person-to-person when the context for delivery changes.

Intervention summary

This brief intervention is designed and tailored to treat adults with symptoms of distress caused by the ongoing COVID-19 pandemic, which may include intensified symptoms of anxiety, depression, sleep disturbance, and traumatic stress as a result of the COVID-19 specific events and policies (e.g., quarantine). In addition, due to stay at home recommendations and orders, people are home more than usual. Such transitions may require re-structuring one's life, such as changes from outdoor to indoor activities promoting one's health. This intervention will be most impactful when delivered by a mental health professional; however, it is possible to provide patients with the outlined guide that will support them in implementing the skills on their own. The intervention modules are in a strategic sequential order for clinicians to easily follow. Specific considerations for the delivery are provided throughout the modules to enhance successful delivery. Dialogues are provided not as an exact script that clinicians should use but as examples for clinicians to incorporate and adapt as needed. Consistent with APA's evidence-based treatment task force and multicultural guidelines (American Psychological Association, Presidential Task Force on Evidence-Based Practice, 2006), providers need to consider the patient's salient identities, demographic characteristics, specific regions, social statuses, disadvantages that may affect them in their presentation of COVID-19 stress and tailor the intervention to these features to enhance engagement with and effects of the intervention. Given that this intervention is designed to be brief, requiring few sessions, patients living with bipolar, schizophrenia, borderline personality, or other severe mental illnesses who may require more intensive care, may not be suitable candidates (Chong, 2020; Fonseca et al., 2020). However, it may be beneficial for clinicians to incorporate relevant modules into their current treatment approach.

Informed by literature on stages of change in psychotherapy and consistent with other transdiagnostic treatments, the intervention includes the following modules: 1) Agenda Setting & Avoidance Identification; 2) Responding to Difficult News/Normalizing Reactions; 3) Perspective Taking; 4) Situational Control/Acceptance; 5) Maintaining a Healthy Routine; 6) Coping with Stress; 7) Insomnia Preventions; and 8) Building Resiliency & Hope. Providers should only deliver the modules relevant to needs of the presenting individual. The Agenda Setting & Avoidance Identification Module focuses on naming, identifying, and validating how the pandemic is associated with a loss of control and increased uncertainty. The Responding to Difficult News/Normalizing

Reactions Module normalizes the patient's emotional response to the pandemic and describes the function of emotions. The Perspective Taking Module is designed to help the patient think flexibly and enhance alternative perspective taking about the pandemic. The Situational Control/Acceptance Module supports the patient in distinguishing between things they cannot control (pandemic itself; emotional reactions to pandemic) and things over which they can exercise control (e.g., own behavior), thereby promoting acceptance and agency. The Maintaining a Healthy Routine Module helps the patient develop routines that promote physical activity and other healthy lifestyle behaviors while practicing social distancing. The Coping with Stress Module provides psychoeducation on grounding techniques and describes a variety of mental, physical, and soothing grounding exercises. The Insomnia Preventions Module includes psychoeducation on the importance of sleep, the three facilitators of sleep (circadian clock, stimulus control, and sleep drive), and helps the patient develop a healthy sleep schedule. The last module Building Resiliency & Hope facilitates resilience and hope through reflection and taking a growth-oriented perspective related to the pandemic. Table 1 presents a brief summary of each intervention stage and Table 2 provides a list of pleasurable home activities as suggestions, and alternative ways to communicate with others through the pandemic. The intervention also includes the Pandemic Mental Health Maintenance Intervention handout to provide patients. See **Appendix A** for a copy of this handout.

Case example 1

Presenting patient

"Sarah" is a 44-year-old woman with a complaint of severe insomnia and increased stress that started in March/April in the context of COVID-19. Her husband has been furloughed and she is homeschooling her three children. Sarah works full-time remotely as a business office clerk and juggling work and home-school activities has been challenging. Many of her routines have been disrupted. For example, Sarah used to walk for exercise with a colleague during her workday. Since the transition to working from home, this routine has stopped. Sarah feels she is just "hanging on by a thread." Looking after her three kids, homeschooling, and worrying about her husband's lost income, takes all her energy. She feels stressed and tired all the time and has developed a new coffee habit – drinking three large cups of coffee per day to keep awake. Sarah tries to go to bed around 11:00 PM. She describes that it takes her hours to fall asleep. She often lies in bed until 3:00am. She states she feels panicked when she looks at the clock and sees the hours go by. She starts to worry about how long she will need to quarantine and the economic stressors her family is facing. Sometimes, she will start doing work on her laptop computer in bed until she feels tired at 3:00 am.

Primary reported symptoms

Insomnia, Anxiety, Stress

Selected modules

Module 2 Responding to Difficult News/Normalizing Reactions, Module 5 Maintaining a Healthy Routine, Module 6 Coping with Stress, and Module 7 Insomnia Prevention.

Table 1. Pandemic mental health maintenance intervention summary.

Intervention Module		Brief Description
Loss of Control	1.Agenda Setting and Avoidance Identification	This initial phase focuses on naming, identifying, and validating how the pandemic is associated with a loss of control and increased uncertainty. It should acknowledge the impact of the individual's named role transitions, which they likely did not choose. The clinician should use this opportunity to relate personally to this experience and humanize and normalize these feelings. This module also asks patients to describe strategies to get rid of this discomfort (e.g., to escape, avoid, opt-out, or excessively seeking information), and provides an explanation of how these strategies provide only short-term relief before discomfort or fear returns. The clinician should then lead the patient to question whether there might be another way. This perspective was drawn from Learning ACT (Luoma et al., 2007).
	2.Responding to Difficult News/ Normalizing Reactions	The clinician will further normalize the patient's emotional response to the pandemic by describing the function of emotions. This perspective was drawn from Learning ACT (Luoma et al., 2007) and Cognitive Behavioral Therapy (Beck, 1997; Beck, 2011; Perlis et al., 2005). The clinician can explain the origin of emotions in terms of fear and anxiety helping to guide us thousands of years ago when we were faced with a bear in the wilderness and how the function of that emotion was to keep us safe. The clinician should then discuss how in times like this it can feel like a threat just like a bear in the woods. The clinician should collaborate with the patient to question whether this type of anxiety is helpful or not. The clinician should bring awareness and understanding to the process of mourning the loss of what the patient thought the next period of time would be. If present, the clinician should address any feelings of guilt the expressed by the client (e.g., not doing enough to help end the pandemic; not appreciating job if they still have one; feelings of irritability toward family; survivor guilt for those recovered from COVID-19).
	3.Perspective Taking	The clinician help the patient think flexibly and enhance alternative perspective taking. Speciically, the clinician will guide the patient in describing past painful/uncertain situations in which the patient felt they had little or less control. The clinician will then support the patient's reflection on their coping thoughts and behaviors and any growth acquired from getting through the identified experiences. This perspective was drawn from Learning ACT (Luoma et al., 2007).
	4.Situational Control/Acceptance	The clinician will support the patient in distinguishing between things they cannot control (pandemic itself; emotional reactions to pandemic) and things over which they can exercise control (e.g., own behavior), thereby promoting acceptance and agency. The clinician will help the patient list things they have control over vs. what they do not have control over and help them develop acceptance of the current pandemic. Emphasis should be placed on all of the areas of life that the patient can control and should focus on how to prioritize these areas of life to improve psychosocial functioning. This perspective was drawn from Learning ACT (Luoma et al., 2007).

(*Continued*)

Table 1. (Continued).

Intervention Module		Brief Description
Coping Skill Development	5.Maintaining a Healthy Routine	The clinician will support the client in identifying active coping strategies, including developing routines that promote physical activity and other healthy lifestyle behaviors. Drawing from foundations of Behavior Activation Therapy (Martell et al., 2010), the clinician will guide the patient to develop understanding on how behaviors promote emotional changes. (Note: This is particularly important for patients affected by depression or experience a lack of interest in activities.) Additionally, the clinician will help the patient develop a daily or weekly schedule by first eliciting their own preferences, prior history of successful coping, and core values. The clinician will probe for targets in the following areas: physical activity and social relatedness/connection.
	6.Coping with Stress	The clinician will actively support the client in building self-compassion and self-soothing skills. The goal of this section is to provide psychoeducation on grounding techniques and describe a variety of mental, physical, and soothing grounding exercises (Linehan, 2015; Najavits, 2003). The clinician will then encourage the patient to pick five techniques to try at home.
	7.Insomnia Prevention	The clinician will help the patient develop a routine to promote healthy sleep. This includes psychoeducation on the importance of sleep and the three facilitators of sleep: circadian clock, stimulus control, and sleep drive, which are pulled form Cognitive Behavioral Therapy for Insomnia (Perlis et al., 2005).
	8.Building Resiliency and Hope	The clinician will facilitate resilience through reflection and taking a growth-oriented perspective. Additionally, the clinician will help the patient draw attention to reflect on potential positive aspects of the current situation. This perspective was drawn from Learning ACT (Luoma et al., 2007). The clinician provides a brief discussion on the importance of limiting exposure to news updates. The final goal of this section and one of the most important is to ensure the patient understands the importance of flexibility with the established schedule and grounding techniques.

Table 2. Suggestions for pleasurable/meaningful home activities and tools for social interaction.

Pleasurable/Meaningful Home Activities	Tools to Maintain Social Interaction
• Reading favorite or uplifting books, magazines, comics, newspapers, etc. • Make face masks to give to others • Watching "feel good" movies or shows • Listening to favorite podcasts or audiobooks • Cooking more involved, nutritious meals • Exercising (e.g., workout classes online or video) • Meditating or relaxing • Make encouraging cards for individuals living in quarantined assisted living facilities • Call a friend or family member to check in on them • Cleaning and organizing • Exploring creative pursuits (e.g., writing, blogging, drawing, painting, photography, dancing, practicing instruments, Karaoke-on YouTube) • Mail a small gift or handmade craft to a friend or family member • Developing new skills (e.g., DuoLingo, sewing, gardening) • Put up signs in your windows to provide encouraging messages to others	• Phone call/Text/Email • Write and mail a letter to a friend or family member and kindly request they write you a letter back • Video or audio conferencing (e.g., Facetime, Google Hangouts, Facebook video on messenger, Zoom, Jitsi, Cisco WebEx, Skype, Oovoo) • Social media applications (e.g., Snapchat, Instagram, Facebook, Twitter, Whatsapp, Pinterest, Tumblr, TikTok, Marco Polo) • Schedule quality time with individuals you live with • Chatrooms (e.g., Chatroulette, Zobe, Chat for Free, Second Life) • Live streaming platforms (e.g., Twitch, YouTube Live) • Forums (e.g., Reddit, Quora) • Online gaming (e.g., Xbox Live, PlayStation Plus, Chess) • Virtual (e-) book group • Wave and smile at neighbors as they walk or drive by • JQBX (shared music listening) • Netflix Party (chat over a movie) • Virtual spiritual or religious services

Tailoring of modules

Module 2 and Module 6 were tailored to address this patient's specific symptoms of anxiety and stress (i.e. loss of income). Module 5, Module 6, and Module 7 were tailored to address patient's lack of routine and enhance patient's quality of sleep.

Change process

By managing anxiety (Module 2; Module 6), reducing caffeine consumption and implementing sleep recommendations (Module 7), sleep started to improve. Her schedule started to normalize, and she was able to resume a healthy routine (Module 5). With the improvement in sleep and daily schedule, anxiety was more manageable, and patient was able to tackle some of the other stressors in her life more effectively including using problem solving to address the loss of income, homeschooling, and interpersonal relationships with her husband and children (Module 6).

Treatment considerations

The brief initial assessment and selected modules were completed in a 60-minute session with the patient. Patient returned for two 15-minute follow-up appointments to discuss improvements in sleep and adherence to her established routine schedule and selected coping techniques.

Case example 2

Presenting patient

"Bryman" is a 27-year-old man with a complaint of increased anxiety that started in March/April in the context of COVID-19. He works at a factory and fears that the company is not taking all necessary precautions to protect workers from contracting the virus. He reports having obsessive anxious thoughts about getting sick, getting his wife sick, and family members dying. He reports having thoughts that he "isn't doing enough" to help others get through the pandemic and worries he is not supporting his wife emotionally. Patient has a previous diagnoses of Generalized Anxiety Disorder, but reported that his anxiety has been well managed for 5 years by taking 20 mg of Zoloft daily. He reports that he has been taking his medication as prescribed, but still has elevated anxiety. He reports having a consistent routine because he is still working and is not experiencing difficulties sleeping at night. Patient reports feeling somewhat "hopeless" that the pandemic will never end.

Primary reported symptoms

Anxiety & Stress

Selected modules

Module 1 Agenda Setting and Avoidance Identification, Module 2 Responding to Difficult News/Normalizing Reactions, Module 3 Perspective Taking, Module 4 Situational Control/Acceptance, Module 6 Coping with Stress, and Module 8 Building Resiliency and Hope.

Tailoring of modules

Modules were tailored to address this patient's increased anxiety since the onset of COVID-19. Module 8 specifically addressed patient's feelings of hopelessness.

Change process

By identifying worries and avoidance thinking (Module 1) and acknowledging the reality of these fears (Module 2) patient felt heard and understood. The patient was then encouraged to recognize these worries in the context of the larger situation (Module 3), to take control of the things that were within his control (Module 4), and develop healthy coping skills to manage stress (Module 6). Therapist encouraged patient to recognize his efforts and strengths and utilize these to continue to do the best he could with his current situation (Module 8).

Treatment considerations

The brief initial assessment and selected modules were completed in a 60-minute session with the patient. Patient returned for one 30-minute follow-up appointment to briefly review modules discussed in session 1 and adherence to his selected coping techniques.

Discussion

Drawing upon cognitive behavioral models of psychotherapy, the primary objective of the Pandemic Mental Health Maintenance Intervention is to foster resilience and positive mental health during an unprecedented time. These aims are achieved through the provision of emotional validation, psychoeducation and guided learning to promote active coping skills rather than avoidance, and the development of an active schedule that promotes physical health, social connection, and sleep.

The Pandemic Mental Health Maintenance Intervention has many strengths which include transdiagnostic, brief, appropriate for a broad range of patients, and can be delivered via telehealth. Although the intervention is informed by evidence-based treatments and encouraged by clinical anecdotes, it has not been tested and proven to be efficacious in a sample population. Further, it is not designed to replace existing evidence-based treatments for psychological disorders. The intervention is designed to be brief; however, psychological consequences of COVID-19 could be long-term and thus more intensive treatment may be needed for those more affected by COVID-19 (i.e. patients who experienced death in the family, front-line medical workers). Future research should test this intervention in a randomized controlled trial and assess efficacious intervention implementation strategies.

The COVID-19 pandemic had a rapid onset and research examining the impact are still limited. Non-intervention research is needed to ascertain the specific psychosocial consequences of COVID to better inform tailored interventions. Given the potential positive impact of behavioral health professionals in addressing pandemic stress, mental health psychosocial interventions tailored for the pandemic are needed now. Thus, we encourage clinicians to utilize these modules with appropriate patients as needed. Drawing from experts with rich experiences in diverse settings, we present the first known intervention protocol for addressing COVID-19 pandemic stress. Future research should examine the overall effectiveness of this intervention as well as differences across patient populations.

Pandemic mental health maintenance intervention

Below, we provide a sequential overview of the intervention, its goals and key concepts in each module, as well as concreate examples. Modules should be selected and prioritized based on patients' presenting concerns. Dialogues are provided not as exact script that clinicians should use but as examples for clinicians to incorporate and adapt as needed. Length and number of sessions is dependent upon individual patient characteristics (i.e. ability to understand concepts, number of presenting concerns).

Note: Each first session should begin with 1) a brief intake to collect salient presenting symptoms, 2) rapport building, and 3) a description of this brief treatment.

1. **Agenda Setting and Avoidance Identification**:
   - Have them name and identify how the pandemic is associated with a loss of control and increased uncertainty. Specifically, have the patient acknowledge the real impact of the patient's named role transitions.
     - *"Welcome and thank you so much for agreeing to meet today for this pandemic-related mental health service."*
     - *"To begin, can you tell me how the pandemic has impacted your daily life? Specifically, how has it impacted work, and the way or frequency you interact with others? What kinds of emotional responses have you had to the pandemic?"* [Clinicians probe for anxiety and other feelings about uncertainty in social, financial, relational, health domains, e.g., anxiety about having COVID-19 or giving it to someone else, anxiety or sadness about losses.]
   - Explore how the patient has tried to get rid of discomfort (e.g., to escape, avoid, and opt-out) and begin to show the patient that those techniques only provide short-term relief.
     - *"Have you done anything to control the discomfort you are experiencing from the pandemic? How have those strategies worked for you? Were you able to permanently*

get rid of the discomfort? Have these techniques brought you closer to how you want your life to be during the pandemic?"
  - *"Many individuals try to avoid or escape uncomfortable emotions. Those techniques may be helpful in the short term; however, the feelings often return. Have you or others you care about experienced this? Do you think there are other ways one can cope with these responses?"*
- Help the patient see that trying to control their emotional response can be unhealthy and how acceptance of emotions provides an opportunity. Then review the steps toward emotional acceptance.
  - *"One alternative to trying to control emotions is inviting emotions to be present with you. Although we try, humans are not able to directly control emotions. For example, try not to feel anxious right now. If you feel anxious, [(imagine that I will start screaming at you/I am going to pinch you) every single time you feel anxious], okay? You can feel anything but anxiety. How are you feeling right this moment?"*
  - *"Instead of controlling our anxiety and other feelings about the pandemic, we can learn to acknowledge that it exists and is present. It takes less of our emotional energy to notice our emotional response to the pandemic than to fight with it."*
  - *"There are four steps to accept an emotional experience. The first step is to observe or bring awareness to the feelings in your body. The second step is to take a few deep breaths around those feelings in your body. The third step is to expand and make room for those feelings. The last step is to allow the feelings to be present and try to make peace with them. We will keep talking about this and how we might do this together today, okay?"*

2. Responding to Difficult News/Normalizing Reactions:
- Normalize the patient's emotional response to the pandemic.
  - *"This is a new experience, and everyone is responding in their own way. There is no right or wrong way to respond. How you feel may change frequently."*
  - *"When individuals are faced with a scary event, there are different ways in which they can respond. These responses include: fighting, freezing, or running from the event or emotional response to the event. These are all very normal responses to a new experience that is scary."*
- Briefly describe the function of emotions.
  - *"I know we might not always think about them this way, but emotions are sources of information that are neither good nor bad. Try to think about emotions like the air in the room. When it is cold, we get goosebumps; when it is hot, we sweat. Emotions are similar. Each emotion is a different source of information. Think about when you feel angry. Usually when we feel angry, it is information telling us that there has been an injustice done to ourselves or someone that we care about. Think about times when you felt sad. Usually we feel sad when we have lost something we care about or we are afraid we are going to lose something we care about. You see, we need emotions. They are not things to fear but rather information for us to consider. And, emotions tend to be tied to the things that are important to us."*
  - *"Let's talk about the emotion of fear or anxiety. This comes from the oldest part of our brain. This part of the brain doesn't think, it just reacts to situations as they arise. Our brains developed this way, in part, to protect us from danger. For example, let's say*

a tiger came running towards us, fear and anxiety would serve a purpose here. They would help our body react without having to think about it. What does our body do with fear and anxiety? What does your body do when it is anxious? [Get some examples] That's right. It speeds up our heart rate, our breathing, makes us jumpy (like we want to run), makes us sweat, etc. All of these body symptoms of fear/anxiety are purposeful – they make it easier for us to avoid that tiger. Now, the challenging thing, is that even if the things we fear or are anxious about today are less dangerous than a tiger, our body still reacts the same way … So now, we have reactions at inconvenient times or places, when it may not be helpful. The goal of this is to think about ways to deal with these reactions when they come up in ways that are helpful."

- [Optional Module] Exploring loss of someone close due to COVID-19.
  - *"Loss can be extremely difficult in general. In fact, it is probably one of the hardest emotional states that we as humans all have to go through at some point. Losing someone during this pandemic is extremely challenging because many of the ways we normally cope with grief include religious and cultural ceremonies, like funerals, that involve gathering with the community. It is normal to feel a range of emotions during loss. These can include anger, fear, loneliness, rage, sadness, and shock. Whatever you are thinking or feeling, it is important to acknowledge that emotion and know that there is no 'right' way to cope with loss. Instead, it is important you show yourself kindness and honor that emotional experience by allowing yourself to feel exactly what you are feeling when you need to feel it. I would encourage you to be fully aware of your grief and like an outside observer just notice what it brings up for you – we call this mindful grieving."*
- [Optional Module] Explain mourning the loss of an anticipated future. Note: consider omitting this section if the patient has recently lost a loved one.
  - *"Many of us had an idea of what the next few months would look like. We all had some sort of plans such as weddings, vacations, graduations, birthdays, and business related or work-related plans. Even our day-to-day activities and plans have been disrupted. Your plans have changed because of this pandemic. There is a part of us that has to mourn the loss of what we thought would be our future for the next couple of months and also what the months following may include. Just as if we were to lose something that we cared about, there is a similar mourning process for when our future is greatly altered. It is important to offer yourself kindness during this time while also acknowledging the grief."*
  - *"Our brains are designed to work by relative comparisons. That means, our brain is often comparing us to friends, neighbors, or colleagues. We compare what they own, how much money they have, and how they are doing. [Ask for examples.] Our brains can also compare us to ourselves. Do you ever do this? You may compare yourself to an earlier version of yourself, or even a future version that hasn't happened yet. The tricky thing about our brains is that no matter who we are comparing ourselves to – a neighbor, friend, colleague, former self, or future self – our brains always seem to tell us that we should be doing better. This can make us feel guilty and that we are 'not doing enough' even when we are doing the best we can."*
- [Optional Module] Address guilt related to the pandemic.
  - *"Some patients report feeling guilty because they are not out doing something about the pandemic. Have you felt this way?"* [If yes, continue. If not, skip to Unit 3]

- *This is a completely normal reaction. Many of us who are not nurses or doctors wish that we could do more. This is an okay reaction and means that you care about society as a whole. Remember, you have not done anything wrong by staying home; in fact, it will make a big difference if you stay at home as much as possible and support those around you the best that you can."*
- *"Some people might also feel guilty about things that used to be everyday parts of their lives – caring for a loved one like a parent, grandparent, or partner who relies on them, going to the grocery store or pharmacy for essential supplies like food and medicine. Although guidelines do recommend social distancing and staying home as much as possible, there are some things that are unavoidable. Remember that you do still need to keep yourself and your loved ones healthy and make sure that you have food to put on your table. You can only take care of yourself physically and emotionally if your basic needs are met."*
- *"Guilt may also come up in the context of the new normal. With many people working from home right now, shifting to a totally different work environment can be challenging. You may experience guilt about not being productive 'enough' while working from home, especially if you are also juggling caring for loved ones/children. If you have young children at home, you may feel guilty about how you are doing either keeping them entertained or helping them keep up with their online learning. It is important to remember that there are no rules or standards right now – we have never faced this type of situation before."*

3. Situational Control/Acceptance:

- Help the patient identify things over which they have control vs. things they cannot control.
  - *"I think it's important that we take a minute to reflect on the things that we do not have control over and the things that we do have control over. What are some things that you can control in the situation? What are things you cannot control?" For things you can control, go ahead and take action. For things you cannot control, it is important to recognize when you're encountering it and instead try to work toward accepting that there isn't anything you can do about it right now."*
- Help the patient develop acceptance.
  - *"Let's talk more about trying to accept what you cannot control. Recall a time you have been stuck in traffic. Remember how it is easy to get upset, weave lanes, honk your horn, all in attempt to change the traffic? How often do these strategies work in making you feel better? Often it is more helpful to recognize you're stuck, not that being stuck is OK, but there is likely nothing you can do to change the traffic jam at the present moment. This acceptance opens an opportunity to do what you can to make yourself feel better until the traffic clears, like opening a window, putting on your favorite music, or safely calling a loved one.*
  - *"Unfortunately, we cannot change some of the bigger things happening around us. What we can change, though, and what is in our control is how we respond to the situation. [To include if patient has a trauma history: when we have been through difficult times in the past, especially if we had those times as children, facing stressful life events like the pandemic can make us feel defeated or stuck again.] The important thing is to realize you have the ability to choose how you respond to these situations."*

4. Perspective Taking

- Have the patient describe past painful/uncertain situations in which they had no control. Then have the patient describe how they survived those experiences and any growth they acquired through the process.
- *"Tell me about a situation that you survived that was originally scary or out of your control. This could be something as simple as taking your driver's test for the first time, becoming a parent for the first time, or trying something new at work. These things are all scary and full of uncertainty; however, you can, and have, gotten through these situations. What did you do to get through these moments? Looking back on these situations, can you reflect on any growth that resulted because you persevered and got through? Not always, but often-times, these experiences tend to show people how strong they are and what they are capable of doing."*
- Have the patient reflect on any silver linings of their current situation.
  - *"Can you think of any benefits to having more time at home for the next couple of months?"* [More time with family, more time to clean/organize/fix things around the house, more time for leisure (watching TV shows, reading), having time to reflect on growth in the future]

5. Maintaining a Healthy Routine:

- Help the patient understand that you don't have to "feel" like doing something in order to engage in a behavior.
  - *"Sometimes we don't feel like doing activities that we know can make us feel better, or we think that we will do them when we feel the motivation to do them. It can be beneficial to schedule activities to make sure we are doing things to enhance our mood. For example, you can get up and get dressed each morning as if you were going somewhere, if that enhances your mood."*
- Help the patient develop a daily or weekly schedule based on their values while incorporating intentional body movement.
  - *"When we discuss things within our control, it can be helpful to maintain some sort of schedule to ensure you are doing behaviors that make you feel better. Let's take a few minutes to brainstorm how you would like your days to look during the pandemic. Are there things you usually do every day that you can continue doing? Are there specific meal times that work best? Are there things you can do to monitor your movement? Some people find it helpful to schedule in exercise or walks. Others find it helpful to set an alarm to get up and move every hour."*
- Help the patient brainstorm ways they can stay connected with others.
  - *"It is important that you do not feel alone throughout the pandemic. Even if you live with others, it can be helpful to maintain communication with other friends and family. Are there people you can call or video chat with throughout the week?"*
  - *"If you are living with someone, it is also healthy for you to schedule time apart from that person. This varies by individual, but some patients need alone time, which can be very helpful in mood maintenance."*
  - *"We also want to think about who we choose to become connected to and use for support. For example, now isn't a good time to call that negative family member of yours – the one who always puts you down and makes you feel worthless – now is the time to reach out to friends who support you and encourage you in your goals."*

- *"You may also find support from online support groups, 12-step recovery programs, or individuals who may have similar life circumstances, but do not personally know you. These can be great spaces for sharing your feelings and getting support from others who can be truly objective about your life circumstances. Have you thought about any of these?"*
- [Optional Module] If relevant, discuss medication (psychotropic and non-psychotropic) adherence with patients.
  - *"Many individuals often find it difficult to take their prescribed medications when not having a daily routine, going through difficult times, or experiencing more stress than normal. Has this been your experience?"* [If answer is yes, continue] *"Let's take a few minutes to discuss techniques other individuals have used to help them remember to take their medications during these difficult times. Some individuals find setting an alarm on their phone or asking a friend or family member to remind them as helpful. Would you be open to trying one of these techniques?"*

6. Coping with Stress:

- Begin the discussion of emotional grounding exercises.
  - *"Some days coping is a little bit harder. On these days it is okay to do things that you know will make you feel better. For example, on these occasions, wear your PJs all day or spend the day just watching TV if that makes you feel better. The important thing to remember is that this will end eventually and that this current schedule will not last forever.*

When emotions are particularly high, you can engage in emotionally grounding exercises."

- Provide psychoeducation on grounding techniques.
  - *"Grounding is a set of easy strategies that can help you create distance from emotional pain such as anxiety, fear, and sadness. It is a way to distract yourself by focusing on something else. Although grounding does not take the emotional pain away, it can be used to get through difficult emotional experiences and prevent things from getting worse. There are three types of grounding exercises which include mental, physical, and soothing. Just like running a marathon requires work and training, grounding techniques take practice. People benefit differently from different skills. Try out a variety of the techniques and make a list of the ones that work best for you."*
- Describe mental grounding exercises and provide examples.
  - *"Mental grounding exercises help the mind focus. Here are some mental grounding exercises for you to try."*

"Count to 10 over and over again."

"Describe your environment in detail, using all of your senses (smell, touch, taste, hear, see)."

- *"Play a Categories Game with yourself. For example, try to think of famous people that begin with each letter of the alphabet, types of cars, or TV shows."*

"Think of something funny to jolt yourself out of your mood."

- Describe physical grounding exercises and provide examples.

- *"Physical grounding exercises is the focusing on one's senses (touch, smell, taste, sight, feel). Here are a few physical grounding exercises for you to try."*

"Look at old family photos/videos."
"Run cold water over your hands for one minute or hold a piece of ice."
"Take a long hot bath or shower."

- *"Grab tightly onto a chair or hard surface as hard as you can (notice the sensations of the tight grip)."*
- *"Use a grounding object such as a ring, bracelet, piece of paper and touch it when you feel unpleasant emotions."*

"Play a calming song/sound."
"Jump up and down."
"Repeat a pleasant word to yourself over and over again."
"Light a scented candle."
"Eat a hard candy."
"Pet your cat/dog."

- Describe soothing grounding exercises and provide examples.

"Soothing is talking to oneself in a kind way. Here are a few soothing exercises for you to try."
"Say a coping statement over and over again. For example, you can say 'I will get through this.'"

- *"Offer yourself kind statements. Pretend you are talking to the child version of yourself. You can tell yourself – 'it's okay to be scared during this time.'"*

"Think of your favorite movie, color, animal, or season."
"Sing the words to an inspiring song, quotation, or poem."
"Plan a treat for yourself, such as making your favorite dinner to eat."
"Bring to mind things you are looking forward to in the future."
"Hug a pillow as if you were hugging yourself."

- Have the patient reflect on the discussed exercises and pick five techniques to try at home. [Have them write the chosen techniques down on a piece of paper]
  - *"We have talked about several different ways for you to ground yourself and cope with undesired emotions. Can you pick five of the exercises to try at home? Try to pick at least one from each category and write them down on a piece of paper."*
  - *"Also, it would be good if you could keep track of which ones are helpful and work and which ones do not. Everyone is different, so it takes some practice to figure out what works best for you. If you try something, and you hate it, or it doesn't work, then choose something else to try. Even if something doesn't work we are learning and collecting information about how to help cope in the future."*

7. Insomnia Prevention:

- Ask about sleep patterns and describe the importance of sleep.
  - *"Another important thing to consider is maintaining adequate sleep. Sleep not only impacts the amount of energy that you have, but it can also impact your mood, such as how sad or anxious you are. Some research suggests that healthy sleep can*

decrease anxiety and depression, which are commonly experienced in a pandemic." How has your sleep been affected so far? [Clinicians – pay attention to comments about them avoiding sleep/not wanting to go to sleep; staying in bed later; changes in other drivers of sleep (e.g., caffeine, lack of activity). Use these answers to guide focus in the next section]

- Describe the three facilitators of sleep: circadian clock, conditioning, and sleep drive.
  - *"There are three facilitators of sleep: circadian rhythms, conditioning, and sleep drive. Let me take a minute to explain each."*
  - *"Let's start with circadian rhythms. We tend to get up when the sun comes up and start to get sleepy when the sun goes down. We call these our circadian rhythms. During the pandemic, you want to make sure to maintain these rhythms. To do this, you want to maintain a consistent wake time, bed time, eating schedule, and exposure to sunlight. These are all cues to inform your body what time of day it is. Without these cues, some individuals develop what we call 'social jetlag', or an inability to sleep at preferred times. You don't need to necessarily sit in the sun to get exposure; however, you need to make sure that your eyes can see the sunlight coming in through a window."*
  - *"The next thing is what we call conditioning. Have you ever felt sleepy and then when you go to bed it's like a switch goes off and you are wide awake? This may be a sign that you have conditioned your brain to associate bed with wakefulness instead of sleep. You can strengthen the bed-sleep connection by only going to bed when sleepy, getting out of bed if you don't fall asleep quickly, and moving wakeful activities out of the bedroom (e.g., watching TV, playing on your phone, and even reading). Another behavior to limit is working while in bed. It can be helpful to set up a designated work station, so work is not coupled with sleep."*
  - *"The last thing that contributes to our sleep is what we call sleep drive. The more active you are throughout your day, the stronger your sleep drive is at night. When you are not physically active or if you nap, your sleep drive will lessen at night."*
- Help the patient develop a consistent sleep schedule.
  - *"It can be helpful to have a consistent sleep schedule. What would be a good sleep schedule for yourself? This is one of those things you can control!"*
- Discuss tools the patient can use to help get to sleep if they are having difficulties.
  - *"Some patients report having some difficulty sleeping because of elevated stress and anxiety. This is one helpful technique you can do to help yourself fall asleep. Schedule 20 minutes during the day, not close to your bedtime, to worry about things. Take the full 20 minutes to think about all the things that could come up for you to worry about at bedtime. Write down the full list of things you are worrying about. The next step is to go through each item you listed and write down what you can do about that worry or if you are unable to do anything about it write that down. Accomplish all the tasks you can do in service of fixing that worry. The last step is to fold the paper in half and put it on the table. Tell yourself you have finished worrying for the day."*

8. Building Resiliency and Hope:

- Help the patient gain resiliency by asking them how they want to reflect back on the pandemic. [Clinicians – spend a little time exploring this section and identifying values driven behaviors]

  - *"If we fast forward to the end of the pandemic, what do you want the days to look like? How would you like to spend your time?"*
- Discuss the importance of limiting the amount of news/pandemic related information consumed each day.
  - *"Being up-to-date and informed about the news is important, especially during a pandemic. However, if you are obsessively watching or reading the news it can exacerbate the stress and anxiety you are experiencing and may even make it more difficult for you to fall asleep or stay asleep at night. What have you noticed?"*

  - Discuss the importance of being flexible with the established schedule and coping techniques.
- *"We have spent a lot of time today creating a schedule for you and discussing coping techniques; however, it is important to remember that there will be good days and bad days. On the bad days, it is okay to be flexible with the schedule. If you don't adhere to the planned schedule, it is important to be nice to yourself and offer yourself kindness, because we are in the midst of a pandemic. This means that you are likely to experience more stress than normal. Practice the grounding exercises so that they can be more helpful to you on the bad days"*

9. Summary of Concepts Discussed:

Thank the patient for engaging in the session and review the concepts discussed.

- *"Thank you so much for your participation in the session today. I want to take a minute to summarize our session together:*

It is okay to feel whatever it is that you are experiencing right now.

- *It is important to recognize the possible heightened stress and anxiety levels and offer yourself some kindness.*

Focus on the things you can control and not on the things you are unable to control.

- *Maintain a schedule for eating, physical movement, social connection, and sleep can help you maintain healthy moods.*

Remember to practice the five grounding exercises.

- *Again, thank you so much for your time today. And, you should be proud that through all of this you took the time today to learn some new strategies to help manage your mental health and well-being."*

Disclosure statement

No potential conflict of interest was reported by the authors.

Funding

This work was supported by the National Institute of Mental Health [R25MH083620,T32MH078788, T32CA229114].

ORCID

Trisha Arnold http://orcid.org/0000-0003-3556-5717
Shufang Sun http://orcid.org/0000-0001-5215-128X

References

American Psychological Association, Presidential Task Force on Evidence-Based Practice. (2006). Evidence-based practice in psychology. *American Psychologist*, *61*(4), 271–285.

Andrews, G., Basu, A., Cuijpers, P., Craske, M. G., McEvoy, P., English, C. L., & Newby, J. M. (2018). Computer therapy for the anxiety and depression disorders is effective, acceptable and practical health care: An updated meta-analysis. *Journal of Anxiety Disorders*, *55*, 70–78.

Barlow, D. H., Allen, L. B., & Choate, M. L. (2004). Toward a unified treatment for emotional disorders. *Behavior Therapy*, *35*(2), 205–230.

Beck, A. T. (1997). The past and future of cognitive therapy. *The Journal of Psychotherapy Practice and Research*, *6*(4), 276–284.

Beck, J. S. (2011). *Cognitive behavior therapy: Basics and beyond* (2nd ed.). New York: Guilford Press. http://site.ebrary.com/id/10483589.

Brooks, S. K., Webster, R. K., Smith, L. E., Woodland, L., Wessely, S., Greenberg, N., & Rubin, G. J. (2020). The psychological impact of quarantine and how to reduce it: Rapid review of the evidence. *Lancet (London, England)*, *395*(10227), 912–920.

Centers for Disease Control and Prevention. (2020a, April 13). *How to Protect Yourself & Others*. https://www.cdc.gov/coronavirus/2019-ncov/prevent-getting-sick/prevention.html

Centers for Disease Control and Prevention. (2020b, April 4). *Social Distancing, Quarantine, and Isolation*. https://www.cdc.gov/coronavirus/2019-ncov/prevent-getting-sick/social-distancing.html

Chew, Q. H., Wei, K. C., Vasoo, S., Chua, H. C., & Sim, K. (2020). Narrative synthesis of psychological and coping responses towards emerging infectious disease outbreaks in the general population: Practical considerations for the COVID-19 pandemic. *Singapore Medical Journal*. doi:10.11622/smedj.2020046

Chong, S. C. (2020). Psychological impact of coronavirus outbreak on borderline personality disorder from the perspective of mentalizing model: A case report. *Asian Journal of Psychiatry*, *52*, 102130. Advance online publication.

Craske, M. G. (2012). Transdiagnostic treatment for anxiety and Depression. *Depression and Anxiety*, *29*(9), 749–753.

Cuthbert, B. N. (2014). The RDoC framework: Facilitating transition from ICD/DSM to dimensional approaches that integrate neuroscience and psychopathology. *World Psychiatry*, *13*(1), 28–35.

Dong, L., & Bouey, J. (2020). Public mental health crisis during COVID-19 pandemic, China. *Emerging Infectious Diseases*, *26*, 7.

Fonseca, L., Diniz, E., Mendonça, G., Malinowski, F., Mari, J., & Gadelha, A. (2020). Schizophrenia and COVID-19: Risks and recommendations. *Revista Brasileira De Psiquiatria (Sao Paulo, Brazil: 1999)*, S1516–44462020005009201. Advance online publication. doi:10.1590/1516-4446-2020-0010.

Galea, S., Merchant, R. M., & Lurie, N. (2020). The mental health consequences of COVID-19 and physical distancing: the need for prevention and early intervention. *JAMA Internal Medicine*. doi:10.1001/jamainternmed.2020.1562.

Harvey, A. G., Watkins, E., Mansell, W., & Shafran, R. (2004). *Cognitive behavioral processes across psychological disorders: A transdiagnostic approach to research and treatment*. Oxford: Oxford University Press.

Kemp, J., Zhang, T., Inglis, F., Wiljer, D., Sockalingam, S., Crawford, A., ... Strudwick, G. (2020). Delivery of compassionate mental health care in a digital technology-driven age: Scoping review. *Journal of Medical Internet Research*, *22*(3), e16263.

Kuester, A., Niemeyer, H., & Knaevelsrud, C. (2016). Internet-based interventions for posttraumatic stress: A meta-analysis of randomized controlled trials. *Clinical Psychology Review*, *43*, 1–16.

Lau, J., Yang, X., Pang, E., Tsui, H., Wong, E., & Wing, Y. (2005). SARS-related perceptions in Hong Kong. *Emerging Infectious Diseases*, *11*(3), 417–424.

Li, S., Wang, Y., Xue, J., Zhao, N., Zhu, T., Basile, G., ... Agodi, A. (2020). The impact of COVID-19 epidemic declaration on psychological consequences: A study on active weibo users. *International Journal of Environmental Research and Public Health*, *17*(9), 6.

Linehan, M. M. (2015). *DBT skills training manual* (2nd ed.). New York: Guilford Press. http://books.google.com/books?id=PLautAEACAAJ

Liu, S., Yang, L., Zhang, C., Xiang, Y.-T., Liu, Z., Hu, S., & Zhang, B. (2020). Online mental health services in China during the COVID-19 outbreak. *The Lancet Psychiatry*, *7*(4), e17–e18.

Luoma, J. B., Hayes, S. C., & Walser, R. D. (2007). *Learning ACT: an acceptance & commitment therapy skills-training manual for therapists*. Oakland, CA: New Harbinger & Reno, NV: Context Press.

Martell, C. R., Dimidjian, S., & Herman-Dunn, R. (2010). *Behavioral activation for depression: A clinician's guide*. New York: Guilford Press. https://doi.org/10.1176/appi.ps.2012p837a

Najavits, L. M. (2003). Seeking safety: A new psychotherapy for posttraumatic stress disorder and substance use disorder. In P. Ouimette & P. J. Brown (Eds.), *Trauma and substance abuse: Causes, consequences, and treatment of comorbid disorders* (pp. 147–169). American Psychological Association. https://doi.org/10.1037/10460-008

Norton, P. J., & Paulus, D. J. (2017). Transdiagnostic models of anxiety disorder: Theoretical and empirical underpinnings. *Clinical Psychology Review*, *56*, 122–137.

Perlis, M. L., Benson-Jungquist, C., Smith, M. T., & Posner, D. A. (2005). *Cognitive behavioral treatment of insomnia: A session-by-session guide*. Springer New York. https://doi.org/10.1007/0-387-29180-6

World Health Organization. (2020, March 31). *Coronavirus disease (COVID-19) advice for the public*. https://www.who.int/emergencies/diseases/novel-coronavirus-2019/advice-for-public

Zhou, X., Snoswell, C. L., Harding, L. E., Bambling, M., Edirippulige, S., Bai, X., & Smith, A. C. (2020). The role of telehealth in reducing the mental health burden from COVID-19. *Telemedicine and e-Health*, *26*(4), 377–379.

Part II

Therapeutic Relationship

Cultivating online therapeutic presence: strengthening therapeutic relationships in teletherapy sessions

Shari Geller

ABSTRACT

With the recent global pandemic, therapists have had to shift their psychotherapy practice online, as they have been unable to maintain a face to face relationship due to physical distancing measures. This has created an immediate need to understand how to build and maintain strong therapeutic relationships while navigating this new online therapeutic environment. With the removal of face to face therapy, there is a question of how the therapeutic relationship is to be maintained and fostered over the internet, through considering the necessity of cultivating and maintaining therapeutic presence. This article will discuss therapeutic presence as a precondition to effective therapeutic relationships and a positive therapeutic alliance. An exploration will follow of the challenges of cultivating therapeutic presence in online therapy ; followed by tips to encourage and support both the therapist and the client to remain present while engaging in telepsychotherapy. A final discussion will include implications for future research and clinical training for cultivating presence in telepsychotherapy as well as integrating what has been learned during the pandemic back into face to face sessions.

In a matter of days, psychotherapists across the globe had to shut down their in-person psychotherapy practice as the coronavirus pandemic escalated in early 2020. The need for social distancing required a quick shift to a virtual psychotherapy practice, with many therapists having minimal prior experience in developing online therapeutic relationships. Traditionally, psychological and emotional safety in the therapeutic relationship is generated by therapists and clients sitting together in the same room, in the same space, in a soundproof, private, and secure environment. During the pandemic, physical safety superseded this arrangement and to "flatten the curve" of coronavirus, we were all required to stay at home. Psychotherapy quickly transformed into being together yet at a physical distance, with two computer screens between therapists and clients.

We know from decades of psychotherapy research that the therapeutic relationship and the therapeutic alliance are the most consistent predictors of therapeutic change (Norcross & Lambert, 2011, 2019). Yet, relational factors that contribute to the development of strong therapeutic relationships and a positive alliance are less understood. Therapeutic presence is one common factor that has emerged in the literature and can be viewed as a necessary and preliminary step to creating safety, building a stronger therapeutic alliance, and increasing therapy effectiveness (Dunn, Callahan, Swift, & Ivanovic, 2013; Geller, 2017; Geller & Greenberg, 2012; Geller, Greenberg, & Watson, 2010; Geller & Porges, 2014; Hayes & Vinca, 2011, 2017; Pos, Geller, & Oghene, 2011). Presence strengthens the working relationship between therapists and clients, through the mechanism of evoking psychological and emotional safety (Geller & Porges, 2014).

Despite the recognition of therapeutic presence, foundational training in therapists' presence is just beginning to be developed in psychotherapy training programs as the inner work of the therapist is viewed as core to relating with presence (Geller, 2017; Geller & Greenberg, 2012). This training involves a focus on how to *be* with clients, which is foundational to what technique they *do* in their therapy session. It also helps therapists to stay grounded and attuned within themselves, which is key to attuning with clients (Siegel, 2007). This complex yet simple stance requires a commitment to self-growth and relational skill building. With this additional challenge of conducting therapy online, there are unique features to attend to when strengthening therapeutic relationships with presence. It is not the same as sitting in the room with a client and just transferring the therapeutic approach and relationship to the computer.

Some of the challenges of online presence are reflected in the actual setting of telepsychotherapy. Clients may be in their home environment with the very people they are having issues with. They can be distracted in an online environment. Therapists have technological challenges and report feeling more tired and experiencing professional self-doubt and loss of confidence working in this new way (Aafjes-van Doorn, Békés, & Prout, 2020). Many therapists have also had to cope with their own personal anxiety, grief, and trauma related to the pandemic while supporting their clients to do the same.

This article will expand on what therapeutic presence is as well as how it contributes to developing a strong therapeutic alliance. A discussion will follow on the unique challenges faced by therapists in cultivating presence in online therapy during the current pandemic, followed by concrete tips for cultivating presence in online therapy. The paper will conclude with implications of our learning about presence in therapy from the pandemic and a suggestion for future clinical training and research.

What is therapeutic presence?

Therapeutic presence is a way of *being* with a client that optimizes the *doing* and technique of therapy. It involves therapists bringing their whole self to the encounter with clients and being fully in the moment on a multitude of levels: physically, emotionally, cognitively, relationally and spiritually (Geller, 2017; Geller & Greenberg, 2002, 2012; Geller et al., 2010; Hayes & Vinca, 2011, 2017). This helps therapists to attune to their own moment-to-moment experience as well as the experience of their clients (Geller, 2017; Thompson, 2018). Therapists' presence involves being grounded in one's self, while receptively taking in the client's verbal and nonverbal experience and being responsive in the moment (Geller, 2019). Embodying and relating to clients with presence also helps therapists to stay grounded and centered amidst difficult emotions. Presence provides an invitation to clients to "feel felt" (Siegel, 2010), met, and understood, inviting a sense of safety and optimal engagement in the work of therapy (Geller, 2017; Ogden, 2018).

Therapeutic presence as a common factor

Therapeutic presence can be viewed as trans-theoretical, or a common factor, as it is valuable and recognized across various psychotherapeutic approaches (Geller, 2017; Geller, Pos, & Colosimo, 2012). Psychoanalysts such as Freud and Reik referred to maintaining an evenly suspended attention and listening to patients with a "third ear", maintaining an open, spacious, and attentive state of being (Epstein, 2007; Freud, 1930; Reik, 1948). Modern psychodynamic approaches highlight the present moment in the therapeutic relationship and invite therapists to approach clients with an open and authentic presence (Mitchell, 2000; Stern, 2004). Therapeutic presence was seen as an underlying condition to empathy, unconditional regard, and congruence by Carl Rogers' client-centered therapy (Baldwin, 2000), supported by later research suggesting presence as distinct and necessary for empathy to be felt and expressed (Geller et al., 2010; Hayes & Vinca, 2011; Pos et al., 2011). Presence is a key concept in Existential and Gestalt perspectives, which both focus on here and now contact and awareness through the senses, emotions, cognitions, and in a relationship (Perls, 1970; Yontef, 2005). Therapeutic presence is an essential stance in Emotion-Focused Therapy (EFT), to support and strengthen the therapeutic relationship and support clients to engage in the work of therapy and EFT tasks and modalities (Geller, 2019).

Recent interest in the therapeutic relationship in Cognitive Behavioral Therapy (CBT) has also highlighted the role of presence. Studies suggest that presence can be a significant clinical stance in CBT, as presence and attunement to the client in the moment can optimize the timing and effectiveness of therapeutic techniques (Geller et al., 2010; Kanter et al., 2009). Further support for presence as a common factor emerged from therapeutic research. Specifically, clients who rated their therapist as present were more likely to rate the therapeutic alliance and the session outcome positively, across Cognitive Behavioral Therapy, Emotion-Focused Therapy, and Person-Centered therapies (Geller et al., 2010).

Mindfulness and self-compassion approaches recommend therapists to have a personal practice of mindfulness and self-compassion to help cultivate therapeutic presence. Therapists' personal practices help to strengthen qualities of attention, awareness, warmth, compassion, and sensitivity which are the basis for attuning and understanding clients' experience, and in turn strengthen the therapeutic relationship (Geller & Greenberg, 2012; Germer, 2012; Segal, Williams, & Teasdale, 2002).

How does therapeutic presence help? Creating safety

Viewing therapeutic presence through the lens of Porges' (2011) polyvagal theory helps to explain the mechanisms of change that presence evokes. According to this theory, our nervous systems are constantly in bidirectional communication with other peoples' nervous systems (Geller, 2017, 2018; Geller & Porges, 2014; Porges, 1998, 2011, 2018; Thompson, 2018). When therapists are fully in the moment and attuned with their clients, their receptive and safe presence sends a neurophysiological message to clients that they are being heard, met, felt, and understood. This process elicits a reciprocal experience of safety between both therapist and client, and strengthens the therapeutic alliance (Badenach, 2018; Dana & Grant, 2018; Geller, 2017, 2018; Geller & Porges, 2014).

Research suggests that a safe therapeutic environment facilitates the development of new neural pathways for the client, which in turn contributes to the repair of attachment injuries and provides the positive social interactions that are essential for health and neural growth for the client (Allison & Rossouw, 2013; Rossouw, 2013). This sense of mutual safety and strong alliance also invites clients to be in their window of tolerance, a term coined by Daniel Siegel (1999), so they can open and engage in the necessary therapeutic work (Geller, 2017, 2018).

Therapists' presence serves as a co-regulator for clients' emotions (Geller, 2019). Attuned right brain to right brain communication to nonverbal communication (body posture, vocal expressions, facial expressions, gestures), a central part of attunement from a therapeutic presence perspective, is also a pathway to regulation in therapeutic relationships (Quillman, 2012; Schore, 2009, 2012; Siegel, 2010). When clients feel met and understood with their present-centered therapist, their brain likely establishes a "neuroception" of safety (Dana & Grant, 2018; Geller, 2018; Geller & Porges, 2014; Ogden, 2018; Porges, 1998, 2011). Clients who have experienced mis-attunement or trauma are often wired to perceive a situation, or person, as unsafe, even when the situation is safe (Geller & Porges, 2014; Gray, 2018). They relate to the world with a heightened state of fear and protection as their sympathetic nervous system (SNS) is aroused, or if it is over-aroused, the dorsal vagal wing of the parasympathetic nervous system (PNS) kicks in evoking a state of shut-down or freeze (Dana & Grant, 2018). When therapists relate with their clients as a calming presence, it activates their social engagement system and invites calm and connection in the ventral vagal wing of their clients' parasympathetic nervous system. Over time, this supports clients' felt sense of safety and regulation in the therapeutic relationship, which supports clients to feel safe to express their emotional vulnerabilities, pain, traumas, and fears and engage in the work of therapy (Geller, 2018; Geller & Porges, 2014; Ogden, 2018).

There are also intrapersonal aspects to the mechanisms of change from a presence perspective for therapists. With therapeutic presence, therapists use their selves and their attuned bodily awareness as tools for understanding their clients as well as for perceiving how their responses are facilitating the client's therapeutic process and the therapeutic relationship (Geller & Greenberg, 2012; Thompson, 2018). Their presence is like an antenna, reading the experience of the moment by resonating with clients' experience and attuning to their own felt experience of the moment. Therapists are looking for cues in the client's nonverbal expression. They are then listening internally for a combination of (a) their own resonance with their clients, (b) their understanding of the client's history and goals, and (c) clinical theory and wisdom (Geller, 2017; Geller & Greenberg, 2012).

The ongoing practice of presence in therapy demands much of a therapist's personal resources and active engagement. Therapists' self-care is also an integral part of the model of therapeutic presence (Geller, 2017; Geller & Greenberg, 2002, 2012). Practicing presence outside of session, in one's life and personal relationships, helps to build the neural pathways for presence to be able to be experienced in the session with clients. As well, the intentional aspect of self-care is a necessary part of lowering the risk of burnout and increasing the ability to sustain presence in session with clients.

The challenge of therapeutic presence in telepsychotherapy

Amidst the fears and challenges in navigating this global pandemic, therapists had the additional task of moving their therapy practice online. There are technological challenges, of course, in that transition – yet there was also the challenge of cultivating presence and building safe, helpful relationships with clients. Below are some common challenges of cultivating therapeutic presence and effective therapeutic relationships online, particularly in the time of the coronavirus pandemic.

Telepsychotherapy places physical distance between the therapist and client, which limits non-verbal communication (Oshni Alvandi, 2019; Sjöström & Alfonsson, 2012). A part of therapeutic presence is to use body to body non-verbal cues to communicate presence, which includes having a prosodic vocal tone, leaning forward, gesturing, having an open body posture, and soft facial features (Geller, 2017, 2018; Geller & Porges, 2014; Ogden & Goldstein, 2019). Through the bidirectional communication of the nervous system of therapists and clients, therapists' embodiment and expression of their calm and grounded presence can facilitate a sense of calm and safety for clients through the process of co-regulation, which allows for emotional stability and connection in the therapeutic relationship (Butler & Randall, 2013; Geller, 2017).

Similarly, trust is generated in the therapeutic relationship through the synchronization of physiological rhythms and bodily movements, expressed through mutual eye gaze and therapists' mirroring of gestures and expressions of the client (Geller, 2017; Marci, Ham, Moran, & Orr, 2007; Marci & Orr, 2006; Ramseyer & Tschacher, 2014). Research findings indicated that movement synchrony at the start of psychotherapy predicted client ratings of a positive therapeutic alliance and symptom reduction at the end of each session (Ramseyer & Tschacher, 2011). In online therapy, therapists have a reduced ability to express their presence with their full-body (prosody, open body posture, gestures, mirroring the movement of clients in real time), which limit their ability to attune and convey a sense of safety and build trust through presence. In a study exploring trust in mixed communication environments using social dilemma scenarios, it was found that trust can be delayed and more fragile in video and telephone conferencing (Bos, Olson, Gergle, Olson, & Wright, 2002).

Attuning to clients' non-verbal cues is also limited in online therapy. Reading facial expressions for markers of emotion or attuning to the gestures or posture to understand clients' emotional states are a part of the process of therapeutic presence. Therapists have reduced access to the physical cues of clients' emotions and experience (i.e. clients' gestures, posture, non-verbal expression) in virtual therapy (Oshni Alvandi, 2019; Sjöström & Alfonsson, 2012).

Another challenge in online therapy during the pandemic is the possible increased likelihood of therapists' countertransference. Clients express increased anxiety, trauma, and fear in relation to the pandemic, along with their ongoing longstanding issues and underlying pain. Therapists' anxiety and fear, as well as grief and loss in relation to the pandemic, can be activated by clients' shared distress, eliciting countertransference issues and interfering with the ability to be fully present and responsive to their clients' fears.

Increased fatigue can also occur for therapists working online (Aafjes-van Doorn et al., 2020). Being on a computer for excessive amounts of time can facilitate disconnection and exhaustion if not balanced with non-screen activities and connections (Dodgen-

Magee, 2018). Therapists' fatigue may be amplified by the stress they are experiencing in relation to the pandemic and the increased social isolation and lack of balance of outdoor time. Therapists may try to schedule themselves as they would in the office, yet more time may be required between sessions and after sessions to restore energy and wellbeing.

Technological challenges and glitches as well as lack of training in engaging in online therapy can also impact therapeutic presence and the alliance (Brahnam, 2014; Oshni Alvandi, 2019). Clients can attribute delays or glitches in the technology to a therapist's characteristics or lack of presence, rather than the actual technological issues (Schoenenberg, Raake, & Koeppe, 2014). While glitches are inevitable, technology challenges can be heightened for therapists who are not as familiar with the virtual platforms or technology, and who are lacking adequate training to conduct therapy online (Hafermalz & Riemer, 2016; Schoenenberg et al., 2014). Research shows that therapists are more likely to use the technology and strengthen therapeutic relationships when they are trained and supported in how to use telepsychology in their practice (Pierce, Perrin, & McDonald, 2020). Unfortunately, many therapists were not provided a training opportunity given the necessary response to the pandemic, with little time to develop skill in navigating this new environment.

A further challenge is that clients may not feel safe to express difficult emotions and vulnerabilities without the physical presence of their therapist. They also may be in the homes and environments with family or others that they have emotional challenges and complex relationships with. Finding ways for therapists to express presence so that clients can sense and feel their presence is critical. Also, helping clients find safe places within the home to express their emotional experience is important.

Can therapeutic presence and the therapeutic relationship be effective in online therapy?

Nascent research suggests that teletherapy is effective in working with clients who have various disorders (Varker, Brand, Ward, Terhaag, & Phelps, 2019). Research suggests that clients can both benefit from online therapy and develop a positive working alliance (Cook & Doyle, 2002; Reynolds, Stiles, & Grohol, 2006). Despite this research, therapists tend to have a negative view towards telehealth therapy and the possibility of developing a positive alliance online (Jerome & Zaylor, 2000; Rees & Stone, 2005; Wray & Rees, 2003). These negative views can impact how therapists rate the alliance in online therapy and may even impact how they approach online therapy with a bias that can inhibit the potential to generate a positive therapeutic alliance online (Rees & Stone, 2005). This bias could be based on limited resources (literature, training, and experience) around this approach and fear that therapists will not be able to attune to clients while in an online setting (Hafermalz & Riemer, 2016; Sjöström & Alfonsson, 2012).

The pandemic forced many therapists who may have been reluctant previously to offer virtual therapy to quickly move their therapy practice online. Hence, shifting their bias is imperative. The need for online therapy may remain for several months, even years, and there will likely be clients and therapists who want to stay with virtual therapy beyond the impact of the pandemic. While some studies suggest that clients favor face to face therapy over online therapy (i.e., Berle et al., 2014), a literature review suggests that clients generally do not have a preference between in-person or online therapy and it does not interfere with developing a therapeutic alliance (Simpson & Reid, 2014). Varker et al. (2019) suggest that there is great potential in telepsychology overcoming access barriers in rural communities and offering an effective method for various disorders. In fact, online therapy may offer novel ways to form strong therapeutic relationships with a variety of clients and may facilitate an even stronger therapeutic intimacy than in face to face therapy (Kocsis & Yellowlees, 2018). Not only is it a great option for rural communities and various populations, it is also time and cost efficient (Simpson, 2009).

With respect to therapeutic presence particularly in online therapy, there is minimal research. Nursing literature offers some examples where the presence can be felt by nurses in the nurse–patient interaction in telehealth interactions, which gives a suggestion that presence can be transferred online (Hafermalz & Riemer, 2016; Tuxbury, 2013). For example, Tuxbury (2013) interviewed 6 nurses about their experience of therapeutic presence in telehealth sessions with patients. Results of semi-structured interviews suggested that nurses who had previously engaged in the process to attain presence felt that it could also be accessed and experienced through non-video telephone and computer calls. This allowed nurses to offer care and develop presence in relationships with patients that they may not have the opportunity to meet in person.

Hafermalz and Riemer (2016) suggest presence can be generated in online therapy if nurses are trained and accustomed to the equipment and the technology. They can then focus on the relationship and engage aspects of presence such as expressing care, being present, and visualizing patients' difficulties through mirroring gestures and experience. The authors reference co-presence, a term used in information systems literature, which is the "illusion of having access to a remote or distant other that shares the same distant place, that is, being there with others" (Schultze, 2010, p.438). The adaptation of the concept of co-presence suggests that when nurses embody presence, they can adapt to the lack of physical distance and their mind and body perception can transcend time and space to provide the experience for both of really being together.

Similar suggestions come from psychotherapy research with CBT for the treatment of panic disorder with agoraphobia. Bouchard, Robillard, Marchand, and Riva (2007) demonstrate that in addition to empathy, warmth, understanding, and technique, clients are able to access a sense of presence that transcends the distance and helps them forget they are not actually physically with their therapist. Although telepsychotherapy does not allow individuals to be physically in the same room, it is possible to create the feeling that both people are in the same room even when they are not.

A conceptual understanding of how therapeutic presence can be expressed and received to optimize the effectiveness of cybertherapeutic engagement was proposed by Oshni Alvandi (2019). The author proposes three modules of counselling presence online – cognitive, counselling, and emotional. Cognitive presence includes the ability to empathize with clients. Counselling presence reflects the expression of qualities of presence such as listening, trust, compassion to ensure the client feels heard and understood. Emotional presence reflects feeling emotions with the client and helping clients to express and manage emotions. While the author discusses how missing nonverbal cues online can negatively impact therapists expressed presence, the expression of facial cues, gestures, and prosodic vocal tone can still be expressed online. This supports clients feeling safe, from a polyvagal perspective, in the online therapy environment

Tips for cultivating therapeutic presence online

Below are some tips to help therapists create an online environment to cultivate and communicate presence in online sessions, which can strengthen positive therapeutic relationships. Given the research of therapeutic presence in online psychotherapy is limited, the following discussion and suggestions are based on the few studies on online presence (i.e., Hafermalz and Riemer, 2016; Ogden & Goldstein, 2019; Oshni Alvandi, 2019; Tuxbury, 2013); and on the research, literature, and empirically validated model of therapeutic presence (Geller, 2017; Geller & Greenberg, 2002, 2012; Geller et al., 2010).

Creating safety

Online safety and security

- Ensure you are engaging with your clients on a telehealth system that has HIPPAA (PHIPA in Canada) compliance with the BAA agreement. This ensures a level of encryption that provides confidentiality and safety for all.
- Offering your embodied presence in session will further create psychological safety for your client and for yourself. Even if physical presence is not an option, therapists can deepen other aspects of presence when working online. Haddouk (2015) contends that physical distance should not be viewed as opposite to presence since research indicates psychological presence is also integral to the therapeutic alliance built online.

Consistency and set-up

- Set up a place in your home or office where you can see clients consistently and that mirrors your therapy room to the best that you are able. This can allow for a predictable environment for your clients.
- Consider using a larger screen to allow more visual contact and gestures with your full body versus from just the head up.
- Ensure privacy and remind your clients to ensure their own privacy by asking family members or people who share the home to be in a different room, with headphones on ideally.

Optimal distance

- Find a safe distance between you and the screen. Not too close that feels invasive to clients or not too far away that makes you look distant and small. You can ask clients to collaborate on finding an optimal distance that feels right to them, by asking them how they are experiencing the view of you (too close, too far, just right).
- Maintain your eye view at the level of the camera so clients experience you looking at them. If you are looking down at the camera, clients may experience you looming over them.
- Place the video box of your client as close to the camera as possible. This will help to maintain your eyes as close to the camera as possible to keep as direct eye contact as possible.

- Also have your notes, if you are referring to any notes in session, as close to the camera as possible (i.e. at the top of your computer screen) so you appear to be looking into the camera as you speak.

Lighting

- Experiment to find a place where the lighting is optimal – not too bright where there are reflections or too dark that you cannot be seen clearly. It is best to not have bright windows behind you, as this will cause your image to glare.
- Collaborate with your client to help them also find a place with optimal lighting so you can have a clearer view of their facial expressions and eye gaze.

Professional dress

- Dress professionally as you would in the office. It may be tempting to stay in comfortable bottoms assuming that clients cannot see your pants!

Optimizing clients presence

- Ensure clients have a private environment where they will not be disturbed and can feel safe to engage in therapy and express their emotions and experience. Empower clients on how to speak to members of their home to ask for what they need for this.
- Invite clients to intentionally minimize distractions – turning off phone, turning off background apps, such as email feeds, text alerts, or messages.
- Ask them to keep their camera on, so you can feel connected and read their visual and non-verbal cues. It also ensures confidentiality as it can support there are no other extraneous people present when the session is being conducted.
- Remind them to have Kleenex boxes on hand. I learned this in one of my first virtual sessions as I could not pass the box online!
- Invite them to prepare emotion regulation tools that they may be used to having accessible in the office, such as a weighted blanket, ice, or sensory balls, if that is part of your practice or items typically available in office with you.
- If you are engaging in therapeutic work that involves props, have clients prepare material they may need before the session. Some examples include EFT therapists guiding their clients to set up chairs beforehand or have empty chairs in reach for chair work. CBT therapists can ask clients to have their thought records accessible, and DBT therapists can remind clients to bring their diary cards or emotion regulation tools to session.
- Help clients to determine what they need in order to transition gently after sessions – given they do not have the time in the waiting room or travel home that they usually have, as they may want time to absorb the session before opening their door and re-entering their home environment.
- Provide written guidelines or a tip sheet to clients about the above preparation in advance of sessions, to optimize their ability to create a safe and supportive space to engage in online therapy. One study suggested that preparation and support offered to the client through the transition of the pandemic allowed

therapists to feel more positively about online therapy and supported the alliance to be sustained (Aafjes-van Doorn et al., 2020).

Pre-session/therapy day

- Take a walk or do something physically to shift to and from your "virtual office" – just as you would transition to your live therapy office.
- Take 5–10 minutes to center in yourself to help activate your embodied presence. Research suggests that a 5 minute practice prior to session contributes to a stronger therapeutic presence and positive therapeutic alliance (Dunn et al., 2013). Take some mindful breaths or execute a grounding yoga posture to prepare yourself to invite your client into the virtual therapy room. Then, intentionally invite clients into the virtual therapy room once you have prepared the ground within yourself. Simpson and Reid (2014) suggest the potentially greater inclination toward taking more time to prepare and settle into sessions would likely improve clinical outcomes in online therapy.
- Allow time for self-care outside of sessions – including moving your body or doing some gentle stretches. This is particularly important since your physical therapy space may be less comfortable than usual and being on screen can be more tiring than live person to person interaction. Self-care and cultivating presence outside of the therapy room is a part of the model of therapeutic presence. An increase in this kind of self-care is even more prominently needed during the pandemic.

During session

During the initial virtual session, discuss openly any feelings or concerns as you shift to this new virtual space.

Communicating presence, empathy and resonance

- Facial expression, prosody of voice (rhythm, timbre, volume, pace), eye gaze, non-verbal cues, gestures, are some of the ways we communicate our presence and attunement with clients. Ensure these are visible to clients so they can feel you with them in session. You may need to do more of this with online therapy, as the face is the main connection point between you and your clients.
- Stay attuned to your own experience as you connect with clients. This includes attention to your own affect tolerance and verbal and non-verbal cues of presence so clients can feel that you are present with them (Geller, 2017; Ogden & Goldstein, 2019).
- Maintain mutual eye gaze as the camera corrects for distance and you do not need to stare at the recording light. Ask your client if they feel your eye gaze is in contact with them given the limitations of direct knowledge of their experience online. Research suggests that mutual gaze results in clients feeling present and empathically attuned to (Marci et al., 2007).

Inviting synchronicity

- Allow yourself to co-regulate with clients by mirroring their expressions, eye gaze, vocal tone and pace, and entraining with their breathing rhythm. This can invite a felt sense of what their experience is and can allow clients to feel you present with them. This shared presence can evoke interpersonal synchrony and enhance a feeling of safety and connection (Geller, 2017; Koole & Tschacher, 2016; Imel et al., 2014; Ramseyer & Tschacher, 2014).
- Stay aware of matching the eye gaze of your clients. Clients' and therapists' physiological arousal has been shown to come into concordance when a therapist's eye gaze is in contact with their client's, and this can increase further a sense of interpersonal synchrony and connection (Marci & Orr, 2006).

Receptivity

- While starting the session with an open, centered place within yourself, continue through the session to let go of distraction or fixation on a certain insight in order to be present, open and receptive with clients' moment to moment experience. Tuxbury (2013) suggested that attaining online presence includes the ability of the nurse to be receptive and open to the patient and their experience.

Attuning to yourself

- Stay in contact with your own body and emotional state in a compassionate way – to recognize important states such as emotional resonance with clients' experience (awareness of how clients' emotions and experience are being felt in your own body) and countertransference responses (shutting down, triggers, etc.). Hafermalz and Riemer (2016) describe telenurses' experiences of presence and attunement through visualization and honouring their gut instincts during phone calls with patients.

Tracking clients' response

- Notice the nuances in clients' micro-expressions – noticing when they are open and in their window of tolerance or overwhelmed or shut down. To enhance a sense of co-regulation, adjust your posture or vocal tone as needed to meet your client with presence and empathy.
- Notice microexpressions of emotions in your clients' facial expressions. Emotions can be read most prominently in facial expressions (Ekman, 2004), and in online therapy, you have even more direct access to this point of contact.

Contact

- Keep confirming with the thumbnail image of yourself in online therapy that your camera is at eye level, so clients experience you looking directly at them.
- Pay attention to your responses so they are reflective of clients in the moment experience and larger therapy goals.

- Check-in with clients ongoingly about your distance and whether you or they need to adjust to allow for an optimal feeling of safety.

Managing countertransference and challenges to presence

- You and your clients are likely experiencing increased stress and trauma due to the coronavirus and staying indoors. If you find your resonance with clients' distress creating increased anxiety for you, then try a PNR (pause, notice, return) practice (see this and other practices in Geller, 2017), or a brief self-compassion or grounding practice to help you to re-center. This can help tap into a sense of common humanity, while also acting as a good modelling opportunity for clients.
- If the technology freezes or you fumble with how to use it, have compassion with yourself, acknowledge the trouble, and try again.
- If you find yourself in self-doubt as you cannot read clients' experience in the moment; then you can check in with them about their experience and acknowledge the shift in online therapy vs expecting yourself to attune to their experience with the same ease. You can also try a brief practice to help let go of self-doubt and re-center and bring your attention back to the moment (i.e. take three breaths with long exhalations and feel your feet on the ground or engage in a self-compassion practice).
- Overall, allow yourself to be authentic and be yourself in online therapy, acknowledging your humanness in moments of challenge can be helpful to you and your client.

Closing sessions/post work day

- Determine if you need more time than usual between sessions to transition, take notes, regroup, and do some physical stretching or moving.
- When finished with your therapy day, be intentional about closing your virtual therapy space as you would your live office – i.e. closing and putting away your computer, going on a walk, or some other ritual or gesture that lets you intentionally close your therapy day.
- Before engaging in the news and home life, ensure you have some time to transition and take care of yourself.

Conclusion

Telepsychotherapy is here to stay and therapists would benefit from understanding further how to cultivate therapeutic presence and effective therapeutic relationships online. While online therapy is necessary during this global pandemic, this modality will likely continue to grow long after the pandemic is over. The utilization of online therapy may have greater appeal to therapists and clients after having experience with it through this time of social isolation. Hence, a focus on cultivating therapeutic presence online in order to build and strengthen therapeutic relationships is essential. This would help clients to feel emotionally and psychologically safe with their therapists, even from a physical distance.

The ability to generate presence and cultivate positive therapeutic relationships is an important topic that this current pandemic is inviting us to learn more about. Therapists with a previous bias against telepsychotherapy need to bring a present state of mind, such as being open, flexible, curious, and non-judgmental to discovering how to cultivate presence and positive therapeutic relationships online. While there is still much to learn in this area, research exploring (a) whether presence can be cultivated and effectively communicated and felt in online therapy; (b) how therapeutic presence can contribute to creating a more positive therapeutic alliance in online therapy and (c) the development and evaluation of training programs in therapeutic presence, so that the cultivation of therapeutic presence could be integrated into future training programs in online therapy.

Training in cultivating therapeutic presence and effective therapeutic relationship would also increase the likelihood that therapists would use telehealth, which would allow access to therapy to a much broader community (such as those who live in rural communities, have physical, cognitive, or emotional limitations and cannot come into office, or want to access a particular therapist who is geographically distant). Training in both the logistics, technology equipment, and mode of therapy, including training in therapeutic presence, would increase this likelihood.

Training specifically in therapeutic presence in teletherapy would include preparing for presence – through intention prior to and in session as well as increasing self-care to offer balance and sustainability to do online therapy. It would also include helping therapists to embody presence through grounding and centering within themselves and activating a calming nervous system with exercises that enhance the ventral vagal nervous system. Helping therapists enhance the process of presence and relational engagement through attuning to their own experience when online would serve both as a tool to attune to clients and to recognize countertransference, therapeutic ruptures, or interpersonal responses so they can work with them in the moment. Not only would this training help therapists attune to their own experience, it would also highlight attuning to clients through mirroring or other related modalities.

Helping therapists to communicate their presence online is also an essential component of training. Even though nonverbal cues can be missed online and negatively impact presence, facial cues, gestures, and prosody can still be expressed over online therapy mediums (Oshni Alvandi, 2019; Ogden & Goldstein, 2019). Generating more understanding would be helpful on how technology-related issues (glitches, freezing, screen pixilation) and misunderstandings can negatively impact expressed presence (therapists' frustration showing through facial expression) and perceived presence (clients wondering if the therapist is angry with them) in online therapy. This can help therapists recognize when this is occurring and to soften their expression or communicate with clients to work through these potential ruptures. It will be important to address any ruptures and repair misunderstandings that are inherent to the use of technology and specifically, online therapy. With training and user-friendly technologies, therapists can learn how to exude presence to help clients to feel heard and understood. Clients therefore could feel emotionally and psychologically safe with their therapists, even from a physical distance.

In summary, despite its challenges, the coronavirus pandemic has taught us a great deal. The difficulty of cultivating and sustaining presence online and working through those challenges can hopefully benefit therapists to bring back to their face to face therapy. Since the challenges to presence mentioned in this article become heightened in online therapy, the experience of struggling and overcoming these obstacles can illuminate the resilience of therapists and their abilities to retune and refine their ability to be present and increase safety and intimacy in the therapeutic relationship. Therapists can hopefully carry forward their learning including the ability to remain humble and authentic to their strengths and weaknesses, to push through difficult times, and to grow themselves professionally when they are required to be creative in the provision of services. This will hopefully leave therapists more skilled in developing presence and therapeutic relationships, and to continue their work with increased self-care.

Disclosure statement

No potential conflict of interest was reported by the author.

References

Aafjes-van Doorn, K., Békés, V., & Prout, T. A. (2020). Grappling with our therapeutic relationship and professional self-doubt during COVID-19: Will we use video therapy again? *Counselling Psychology Quarterly*, 1–12. https://doi.10.1080/09515070.2020.1773404

Allison, K. L., & Rossouw, P. J. (2013). The therapeutic alliance: Exploring the concept of "safety" from a neuropsychotherapeutic perspective. *International Journal of Neuropsychotherapy*, *1*(1), 21–29.

Badenach, B. (2018). Safety is the treatment. In S. Porges & D. Dana (Eds.), *Clinical applications of the polyvagal theory: The emergence of polyvagal-informed therapies* (pp. 73–88). New York, NY: W.W. Norton & Company.

Baldwin, M. (2000). Interview with Carl Rogers on the use of the self in therapy. In M. Baldwin (Ed.), *The use of self in therapy* (2nd ed., pp. 29–38). New York, NY: The Haworth Press.

Berle, D., Starcevic, V., Milicevic, D., Hannan, A., Dale, E., Brakoulias, V., & Viswasam, K. (2014). Do patients prefer face-to-face or internet-based therapy? *Psychotherapy and Psychosomatics*, *84*(1), 61–62.

Bos, N., Olson, J., Gergle, D., Olson, G., & Wright, Z. (2002). Effects of four computer-mediated communications channels on trust development. Proceedings from SIGCHI *'02: Conference on Human Factors in Computing Systems*. New York, NY: ACM Digital Library. https://dl.acm.org/doi/10.1145/503376.503401

Bouchard, S., Robillard, G., Marchand, A., & Riva, P. R. (2007). Presence and the bond between patients and their psychotherapists in the cognitive-behavior therapy of panic disorder with agoraphobia delivered in videoconference. https://astro.temple.edu/~lombard/ISPR/Proceedings/2007/Bouchard,%20Robillard,%20Marchand,%20and%20Riva.pdf

Brahnam, S. (2014). Therapeutic presence in mediated psychotherapy: The uncanny stranger in the room. In G. Riva, J. Waterworth, & D. M. De Gruyter (Eds.), *Interacting with presence: HCI and the sense of presence in computer-mediated environments* (pp. 123–138). Berlin, Germany: De Gruyter.

Butler, E. A., & Randall, A. K. (2013). Emotional coregulation in close relationships. *Emotion Review*, *5*(2), 202–210.

Cook, J. E., & Doyle, C. (2002). Working alliance in online therapy as compared to face-to-face therapy: Preliminary results. *CyberPsychology & Behavior*, *5*(2), 95–105.

Dana, D., & Grant, D. (2018). The polyvagal playlab: Helping therapists bring polyvagal to their clients. In S. Porges & D. Dana (Eds.), *Clinical applications of the polyvagal theory: The emergence of polyvagal-informed therapies* (pp. 185–206). New York, NY: W.W. Norton & Company.
Dodgen-Magee, D. (2018). *Deviced!: Balancing life and technology in a digital world*. Lanham, MD: Rowman & Littlefield Publishers.
Dunn, R., Callahan, J. L., Swift, J. K., & Ivanovic, M. (2013). Effects of pre-session centering for therapists on session presence and effectiveness. *Psychotherapy Research*, *23*(1), 78–85.
Ekman, P. (2004). *Emotions revealed: Recognizing faces and feelings to improve communication and emotional life*. New York, NY: Henry Holt and Company.
Epstein, M. (2007). *Psychotherapy without the self: A Buddhist perspective*. London, United Kingdom: Yale University Press.
Freud, S. (1930). *Civilization and its discontent. Standard edition*. (J. Strachey, Trans.). New York, NY: Norton.
Geller, S. M. (2017). *A practical guide to cultivating therapeutic presence*. Washington, DC: American Psychological Association.
Geller, S. M. (2018). Therapeutic presence and polyvagal theory: Principles and practices for cultivating effective therapeutic relationships. In S. Porges & D. Dana (Eds.), *Clinical applications of the polyvagal theory: The emergence of polyvagal-informed therapies* (pp. 106–126). New York, NY: W.W. Norton & Company.
Geller, S. M. (2019). Therapeutic presence: The foundation for effective emotion-focused therapy. In L. S. Greenberg & R. N. Goldman (Eds.), *Clinical handbook of emotion-focused therapy* (pp. 129–145). Washington, DC: American Psychological Association.
Geller, S. M., & Greenberg, L. S. (2002). Therapeutic presence: Therapists' experience of presence in the psychotherapy encounter. *Person-Centered & Experiential Psychotherapies*, *1*(1–2), 71–86.
Geller, S. M., & Greenberg, L. S. (2012). *Therapeutic presence: A mindful approach to effective therapy*. Washington, DC: American Psychological Association.
Geller, S. M., Greenberg, L. S., & Watson, J. C. (2010). Therapist and client perceptions of therapeutic presence: The development of a measure. *Psychotherapy Research*, *20*(5), 599–610.
Geller, S. M., & Porges, S. W. (2014). Therapeutic presence: Neurophysiological mechanisms mediating feeling safe in therapeutic relationships. *Journal of Psychotherapy Integration*, *24*(3), 178.
Geller, S. M., Pos, A. W., & Colosimo, K. (2012). Therapeutic presence: A common factor in the provision of effective psychotherapy. *Society for Psychotherapy Integration*, *47*, 6–13. Psychotherapy Bulletin.
Germer, C. K. (2012). Cultivating compassion in psychotherapy. In C. K. Germer & R. D. Siegel (Eds.), *Wisdom and compassion in psychotherapy: Deepening mindfulness in clinical practice* (pp. 93–110). New York, NY: The Guilford Press.
Gray, A. (2018). Roots, rhythm, reciprocity: Polyvagal-informed dance movement therapy for survivors of trauma. In S. Porges & D. Dana (Eds.), *Clinical applications of the polyvagal theory: The emergence of polyvagal-informed therapies* (pp. 207–226). New York, NY: W.W. Norton & Company.
Haddouk, L. (2015). Presence at a distance. *Annual Review of Cybertherapy and Telemedicine*, *13*, 208–212.
Hafermalz, E., & Riemer, K. (2016). Negotiating distance: "presencing work" in a case of remote telenursing. Proceedings from ICIS '16: *The International Conference on Information Systems*. Dublin, Ireland: AIS Electronic Library. https://www.researchgate.net/publication/313794397_Negotiating_Distance_Presencing_Work_in_a_Case_of_Remote_Telenursing
Hayes, J., & Vinca, J. (2011). Therapist presence and its relationship to empathy, session, depth, and symptom reduction. Proceedings from SPR '11: The 42nd Annual Meeting for Society for Psychotherapy Research, Bern, Switzerland.
Hayes, J. A., & Vinca, M. (2017). Therapist presence, absence, and extraordinary presence. In L. G. Castonguay & C. E. Hill (Eds.), *How and why are some therapists better than others?: Understanding therapist effects* (pp. 85–99). Washington, DC: American Psychological Association.
Imel, Z. E., Barco, J. S., Brown, H. J., Baucom, B. R., Baer, J. S., Kircher, J. C., & Atkins, D. C. (2014). The association of therapist empathy and synchrony in vocally encoded arousal. *Journal of Counseling Psychology*, *61*(1), 146.

Jerome, L. W., & Zaylor, C. (2000). Cyberspace: Creating a therapeutic environment for telehealth applications. *Professional Psychology, Research and Practice, 31*(5), 478.

Kanter, J. W., Rusch, L. C., Landes, S. J., Holman, G. I., Whiteside, U., & Sedivy, S. K. (2009). The use and nature of present-focused interventions in cognitive and behavioral therapies for depression. *Psychotherapy: Theory, Research, Practice, Training, 46*(2), 220–232.

Kocsis, B. J., & Yellowlees, P. (2018). Telepsychotherapy and the therapeutic relationship: Principles, advantages, and case examples. *Telemedicine and e-Health, 24*(5), 329–334.

Koole, S. L., & Tschacher, W. (2016). Synchrony in psychotherapy: A review and an integrative framework for the therapeutic alliance. *Frontiers in Psychology, 7*(862), 1–17.

Marci, C. D., Ham, J., Moran, E., & Orr, S. P. (2007). Physiologic correlates of perceived therapist empathy and social-emotional process during psychotherapy. *The Journal of Nervous and Mental Disease, 195*(2), 103–111.

Marci, C. D., & Orr, S. P. (2006). The effect of emotional distance on psychophysiologic concordance and perceived empathy between patient and interviewer. *Applied Psychophysiology and Biofeedback, 31*(2), 115–128.

Mitchell, S. (2000). *Relationality: From attachment to intersubjectivity*. New Jersey: Hillsdale Analytic Press.

Norcross, J. C., & Lambert, M. J. (2011). *Psychotherapy relationships that work II* (Vol. 48, pp. 4). Washington, DC: Educational Publishing Foundation.

Norcross, J. C., & Lambert, M. J. (Eds.). (2019). *Psychotherapy relationships that work: Volume 1: Evidence-based therapist contributions*. Oxford, United Kingdom: Oxford University Press.

Ogden, P. (2018). Polyvagal theory and sensorimotor psychotherapy. In S. Porges & D. Dana (Eds.), *Clinical applications of the polyvagal theory: The emergence of polyvagal-informed therapies* (pp. 34–49). New York, NY: W.W. Norton & Company.

Ogden, P., & Goldstein, B. (2019). Sensorimotor psychotherapy from a distance: Engaging the body, creating presence, and building relationship in videoconferencing. In H. Weinberg & A. Rolnick (Eds.), *Theory and practice of online therapy* (pp. 47–65). New York, NY: Routledge.

Oshni Alvandi, A. (2019). Cybertherapogy: A conceptual architecting of presence for counselling via technology. *International Journal of Psychology and Educational Studies, 6*(1), 30–45.

Perls, F. S. (1970). Four lectures. In J. Fagan & I. L. Shepherd (Eds.), *Gestalt therapy now: Theory, techniques, and applications* (pp. 14–38). New York, NY: Harper Colophon Books.

Pierce, B. S., Perrin, P. B., & McDonald, S. D. (2020). Demographic, organizational, and clinical practice predictors of U.S. psychologists' use of telepsychology. *Professional Psychology, Research and Practice, 51*(2), 184–193.

Porges, S. W. (1998). Love: An emergent property of the mammalian autonomic nervous system. *Psychoneuroendocrinology, 23*(8), 837–861.

Porges, S. W. (2011). *The polyvagal theory: Neurophysiological foundations of emotions, attachment, communication, and self-regulation (Norton Series on Interpersonal Neurobiology)*. New York, NY: W.W. Norton & Company.

Porges, S. W. (2018). Polyvagal Theory: A primer. In S. Porges & D. Dana (Eds.), *Clinical applications of the polyvagal theory: The emergence of polyvagal-informed therapies* (pp. 50–69). New York, NY: W. W. Norton & Company.

Pos, A., Geller, S., & Oghene, J. (2011). Therapist presence, empathy, and the working alliance in experiential treatment for depression. Proceedings from SPR '11: *The 42nd Annual Meeting for Society for Psychotherapy Research*. Bern, Switzerland.

Quillman, T. (2012). Neuroscience and therapist self-disclosure: Deepening right brain to right brain communication between therapist and patient. *Clinical Social Work Journal, 40*(1), 1–9.

Ramseyer, F., & Tschacher, W. (2011). Nonverbal synchrony in psychotherapy: Coordinated body movement reflects relationship quality and outcome. *Journal of Consulting and Clinical Psychology, 79*(3), 284.

Ramseyer, F., & Tschacher, W. (2014). Nonverbal synchrony of head-and body-movement in psychotherapy: Different signals have different associations with outcome. *Frontiers in Psychology, 5*, 979.

Rees, C. S., & Stone, S. (2005). Therapeutic alliance in face-to-face versus videoconferenced psychotherapy. *Professional Psychology, Research and Practice, 36*(6), 649–653.

Reik, T. (1948). Listening with the third ear. New York, NY: Farrar Straus.

Reynolds, D. A. J., Stiles, W. B., & Grohol, J. M. (2006). An investigation of session impact and alliance in internet-based psychotherapy: Preliminary results. *Counselling and Psychotherapy Research*, *6* (3), 164–168.

Rossouw, P. J. (2013). The end of the medical model: Recent findings in neuroscience regarding antidepressant medication and the implications for neuropsychotherapy. [Departmental article]. *Applied Neuropsychotherapy*, Retrieved from http://www.neuropsychotherapist.com/the-end-of-the-medical-model/.

Schoenenberg, K., Raake, A., & Koeppe, J. (2014). Why are you so slow? — Misattribution of transmission delay to attributes of the conversation partner at the far-end. *International Journal of Human-computer Studies*, *72*(5), 477–487.

Schore, A. N. (2009). Right-brain affect regulation: An essential mechanism of development, trauma, dissociation, and psychotherapy. In D. Fosha, D. J. Siegal, & M. F. Solomon (Eds.), *The healing power of emotion: Affective neuroscience, development & clinical practice* (pp. 112–144). New York/ London: W W Norton & Company.

Schore, A. N. (2012). *The science of the art of psychotherapy (Norton series on interpersonal neurobiology)*. New York, NY: W.W. Norton & Company.

Schultze, U. (2010). Embodiment and presence in virtual worlds: A review. *Journal of Information Technology*, *25*(4), 434–449.

Segal, Z. V., Williams, J. M. G., & Teasdale, J. D. (2002). *Mindfulness–based cognitive therapy for depression*. New York, NY: Guilford Press.

Siegel, D. J. (1999). *The developing mind*. New York, NY: Guilford Press.

Siegel, D. J. (2007). *The mindful brain: Reflection and attunement in the cultivation of well-being*. New York, NY: W. W. Norton & Company, Inc.

Siegel, D. J. (2010). *The mindful therapist: A clinician's guide to mindsight and neural integration (Norton Series on Interpersonal Neurobiology)*. New York, NY: W.W. Norton & Company.

Simpson, S. (2009). Psychotherapy via videoconferencing: A review. *British Journal of Guidance & Counselling*, *37*(3), 271–286.

Simpson, S. G., & Reid, C. L. (2014). Therapeutic alliance in videoconferencing psychotherapy: A review. *The Australian Journal of Rural Health*, *22*(6), 280–299.

Sjöström, J., & Alfonsson, S. (2012). Supporting the therapist in online therapy. Proceedings from ECIS '12: The 20th European Conference on Information Systems. Barcelona, Spain: AIS Electronic Library. https://www.researchgate.net/publication/289165884_Supporting_the_therapist_n_online_therapy?enrichId=rgreq-71f42d9094fd1dd4ca7034c64b671e45-XXX&enrichSource=Y292ZXJQYWdlOzI4OTE2NTg4NDtBUzo0NDA3NTg5MTUzNDIzMzdAMTQ4MjA5NjUyMjkzNw%3D%3D&el=1_x_2&_esc=publicationCoverPdf

Stern, D. (2004). *The present moment in psychotherapy and every day life*. New York, NY: Norton.

Thompson, G. (2018). Brain-empowered collaborators: Polyvagal perspectives on the doctor-patient relationships. In S. Porges & D. Dana (Eds.), *Clinical applications of the polyvagal theory: The emergence of polyvagal-informed therapies* (pp. 127–148). New York, NY: W.W. Norton & Company.

Tuxbury, J. S. (2013). The experience of presence among telehealth nurses. *Journal of Nursing Research*, *21*(3), 155–161.

Varker, T., Brand, R., Ward, J., Terhaag, S., & Phelps, A. (2019). Efficacy of Synchronous telepsychology interventions for people with anxiety, depression, posttraumatic stress disorder, and adjustment disorder: A rapid evidence assessment. *Psychological Services*, *16*(4), 621–635.

Wray, B. T., & Rees, C. S. (2003). Is there a role for videoconferencing in cognitive–behavioural therapy. Proceedings from AACBT '03: *The 11th National Conference on Australian Association for Cognitive and Behaviour Therapy*. Perth, Australia.

Yontef, G. (2005). Gestalt therapy theory of change. In A. L. Woldt & S. M. Toman (Eds.), *Gestalt therapy: History, theory, and practice* (pp. 81–100). Thousand Oaks, CA: Sage.

Repairing alliance ruptures using supportive techniques in telepsychotherapy during the COVID-19 pandemic

Tohar Dolev-Amit, Liat Leibovich and Sigal Zilcha-Mano

ABSTRACT

The COVID-19 pandemic shifted many traditional face-to-face treatments to telepsychotherapy, forcing many therapists worldwide to adapt effective techniques developed in face-to-face treatment to telepsychotherapy. These include supportive techniques that may be particularly important at a time of rising anxiety, loneliness, helplessness, and depression. The present paper provides detailed guidelines for therapists on how supportive techniques developed in traditional face-to-face treatment can be effectively used in telepsychotherapy to resolve alliance ruptures. To this end, we used the conceptual framework of the core conflictual relationship theme (CCRT) formulation, making adjustments for identifying and resolving ruptures in the therapeutic alliance in telepsychotherapy. We demonstrated the proposed techniques for identifying and repairing ruptures with a case study of a patient participating in an ongoing RCT, whose treatment shifted in mid-therapy to telepsychotherapy because of the COVID-19 pandemic. The techniques presented and illustrated in this article may be used in the transition to remote therapy for a range of reasons, including patient or therapist relocation and more.

The present paper was written at the height of the COVID-19 pandemic, when many therapists worldwide were forced to shift from traditional face-to-face treatments to telepsychotherapy. Different remote therapy platforms, such as telephone, e-mail, and videoconferencing can be used in telepsychotherapy (e.g., Andersson et al., 2012; Backhaus et al., 2012; Kingsley & Henning, 2015). The sudden shift in treatment setting raises challenges, however, as therapists must work in an unknown environment without having all the knowledge needed for remote treatment.

Lack of knowledge or experience with telepsychotherapy may make it difficult for therapists to identify ruptures in the alliance (Safran & Muran, 2000; Safran, Muran, & Eubanks-Carter, 2011), including some ruptures that stem from the transition to the telepsychotherapy setting. The work of therapy regularly includes ruptures, and the transition to telepsychotherapy brings added challenges to their identification and resolution. Ruptures in the therapeutic alliance can be defined as tension or disagreement between patient and therapist on the goals of treatment, failure to collaborate on the tasks of treatment, or a strain in the emotional bond between them (Eubanks, Lubitz, Muran, & Safran, 2019). A rupture can manifest as a severe break or a subtle tension between patient and therapist. As alliance ruptures are an integral part of treatment, evident in over 91%of traditional face-to-face sessions (Muran, 2019), it is likely they will also be present in telepsychotherapy. Ruptures can be categorized into two main subtypes: withdrawal and confrontational (Eubanks, Muran, & Safran, 2015; Safran & Muran, 2000). In withdrawal ruptures, the patient moves away from the therapist or the work of therapy, whereas in confrontation ruptures the patient moves against the therapist or the work of therapy. When identified and successfully resolved, these events can lead to better treatment outcomes (Eubanks, Muran, & Safran, 2018; Safran & Muran, 2000). Given the significance of resolving ruptures, it is important to identify and successfully resolve them in telepsychotherapy.

Safran and Muran (1996, 2000) developed an empirically tested model of alliance ruptures and repair that emphasizes the importance of identification of ruptures and resolving them. They suggested that addressing and resolving ruptures properly can be a positive opportunity for therapeutic growth. Their model suggests that by systematically exploring, understanding, and resolving alliance ruptures, the therapist can provide patients with a new constructive interpersonal experience that has the potential to modify their maladaptive interpersonal schemas. This paper extends on Safran and Muran's conceptual and empirical writing to the specific difficulties rising from the transition to telepsychotherapy.

In the present paper, we introduce supportive techniques to repair ruptures in the alliance during telepsychotherapy based on the Core Conflictual Relationship Theme (CCRT; Luborsky, 1995) framework. The techniques described here are intended to help therapists during the current COVID-19 pandemic and in other situations in which patients and therapists are required to use telepsychotherapy, for example, patient or therapist relocation, illness, or vacation. Following a brief introduction to the concepts of alliance ruptures, supportive techniques, and the CCRT framework, we demonstrate the proposed techniques with a clinical illustration.

Identifying and repairing alliance ruptures using supportive techniques

The shift to telepsychotherapy can be a growth opportunity for therapists who wish to adopt new techniques and to adapt existing ones to online mode. These techniques include supportive ones, which are particularly important in times of heightened anxiety, loneliness, helplessness, and depression (Leibovich, Front, McCarthy, & Zilcha-Mano, 2019). Supportive techniques, in general, aim to strengthen the patient's ego, enhance self-esteem, and facilitate exploration of emotions, while encouraging higher-level defenses (Appelbaum, 2006; Pinsker, Rosenthal, & McCullough, 1991). In psychodynamic psychotherapy, supportive techniques were shown to improve depressive symptoms through the enhancement of the therapeutic alliance (Leibovich et al., 2019). Supportive techniques include, for example, the therapist demonstrating genuine interest and respect, while choosing to maintain the patient's vital defenses, such as repression or denial of certain emotions or thoughts that help patients in their current struggles; focusing on the here-and-now and on practical issues; noting the patient's gains, supporting the patient's aim to achieve the goals of treatment, and presenting realistically hopeful attitude regarding the attainability of these goals, and recognition of improvement toward the attainment of these goals. Therapists are advised to show their patients that they like them, believe in their strengths and ability to find solutions, and to work together with the patient as a team toward better self-understanding (Barber & Crits-Christoph, 1996; Book, 1998).

Supportive techniques may be implemented through the theoretical framework suggested by the supportive-expressive (SE) approach (Book, 1998; Leibovich, Nof, Auerbach-Barber, & Zilcha-Mano, 2018). SE psychotherapy is based on a formulation of the patients' CCRT, which includes three elements: a central wish from others (W), a perceived response from the other (RO), and a response of the self (RS) (Table 1). The CCRT is based on the fundamental assumption of psychodynamic theory that people internalize patterns in their early relationships and repeat them in later ones; thus, the purpose of psychodynamic therapy is to widen the repertoire of perceptions and responses. It has been demonstrated that alliance ruptures can be repaired by first identifying the patient's main conflictual interpersonal wish (W), then striving to actualize it in the therapeutic relationship using supportive techniques (Leibovich et al., 2018). Such implementation of supportive techniques has the potential to create a new corrective experience, enabling patients to practice new responses of their selves (RS), and can be instrumental in repairing ruptures in the alliance, both face-to-face and in telepsychotherapy.

Many therapists who are forced to switch to telepsychotherapy appear to assume that the need to use technology can interfere with the development of the alliance, and that they might be less effective in repairing ruptures when these occur (Monthuy-Blanc, Bouchard, Maïano, & Seguin, 2013; Rees & Stone, 2005). Similarly, patients may not be as inclined to attend remote sessions (Deen, Fortney, & Schroeder, 2013). Empirical evidence, however, suggests that patients' ratings of the alliance in telepsychotherapy are at least as strong as in traditional face-to-face treatment across a range of diagnostic groups (Backhaus et al., 2012; Germain, Marchand, Bouchard, Guay, & Drouin, 2010; Simpson & Reid, 2014). These findings suggest that also in telepsychotherapy, therapists can acquire skills that are effective in managing alliance ruptures. Today, when treatments are forced to move to telepsychotherapy, acquiring skills for repairing ruptures remotely is especially critical. The importance of knowledge of how repairing ruptures remotely can be acquired has been noted in the literature before (Beutel, Böhme, Banerjee, & Zwerenz, 2018; Simpson & Reid, 2014).

Table 1. The core conflictual relationship theme (CCRT; Luborsky, 1995) components and their manifestation in the present case study.

Components	Description	Manifestation in case study
Wish (W)	What the patient wanted in their relationship with another person.	Other people will show greater interest in her, care for her, and have faith in her.
Response other (RO)	How the patient believed this other person would respond if the patient were to articulate or act on his/her Wish.	Other people are all self-centered and care only for their own interests.
Response self (RS)	How the patient responded and felt in relation to/based upon the belief of the other person's response.	Sad, tired, hopeless about the future, and avoids interactions or behaviors that have the potential to hurt her.

Identifying and repairing alliance ruptures using supportive techniques in telepsychotherapy

Two steps are involved in repairing alliance ruptures: identifying the ruptures and repairing them (Safran & Muran, 2000). Previous research and clinical practice have shown that unnoticed and therefore unresolved ruptures can lead to deterioration of the alliance and dropout (Eubanks et al., 2019). Confrontation ruptures are easier to detect because they are characterized by overt expression of anger and dissatisfaction (Eubanks et al., 2015), and therefore may be easier to identify in telepsychotherapy. By contrast, withdrawal ruptures can go unnoticed by therapists in telepsychotherapy and face-to-face treatment alike (Eubanks et al., 2018). Withdrawal ruptures can manifest as the patient being laconic, silent, and giving short responses; showing flat, superficial, or detached emotions; changing or avoiding topics; or showing quick agreement. In the transition to telepsychotherapy, identifying ruptures, especially withdrawal ruptures, may be even more challenging. The therapists themselves might feel remote and frustrated for having to connect through a computer screen, and may confuse their feelings with an actual rupture.

Additionally, telepsychotherapy may result in technical difficulties that challenge the identification of ruptures, such as lack of body movement information, unclear facial nuances, lack of adequate sound quality, or video lags due to delay in the Internet connection, which may mask silence length. Ruptures may arise that are specific to telepsychotherapy, such as patients withdrawing because of having difficulty maintaining eye contact through the screen or reading text messages popping up on their computer. Patients can also avoid the work of therapy by doing housework, talking with other people in their surroundings, or attending to their pets during the session.

Despite the special difficulties in identifying ruptures in telepsychotherapy, therapists can use two techniques to enhance their ability to identify ruptures. The first is creating an appropriate setting and basic technical conditions, and the second is paying greater attention to the nuances of the patients' in-session behavior. Before starting telepsychotherapy, the therapist can prepare and make sure the setting and basic technical conditions are clear to the patient. The setting should be a quiet and private space, free from distractions. If this is difficult to achieve or it is not available to the patient, the therapist can help suggest a different setting, such as a car. Several basic technical solutions must be in place to help identify the ruptures in telepsychotherapy, making sure that the patient and therapist both have a stable Internet or phone connection, adequate lighting for the camera, and proper microphones.

The therapist must also attend to the nuances of the patients' in-session behavior, in the characteristics available to them, in order to identify ruptures, especially to identify withdrawal ruptures. For example, if the therapist is unable to see the patient's body movements or if the sound is unclear, greater attention must be paid to other characteristics, such as change in facial expressions or avoidance of eye contact. If the therapist is unable to see the patient or if there is a video delay, special consideration should be given to acoustic measures, such as becoming unresponsive, change in speech rate, unsteady or trembling voice quality, or longer silences (Dolev-Amit, Nof, Asaad, Tchizick, & Zilcha-Mano, in press). Therapists should also be aware of the contribution of the patient's new surroundings to the ruptures rising in treatment. If the patients are in their own home during the session while family members, romantic partners or roommates, are present, the therapist should pay more attention to topics the patients are reluctant or withdrawn from discussing. For example, this can be identified by more silences or shifting of topics. In addition, the therapists' awareness of their own feelings or reactions in the countertransference may also be a marker that a rupture has occurred (Safran & Muran, 2000). Ruptures can manifest as a feeling of detachment, a wish to avoid the situation or to be someplace else, boredom, pressure to find topics to talk about and to fill the session, or difficulty staying focused on the screen.

Once a rupture in the alliance has been detected in telepsychotherapy, the therapist should use the CCRT formulation to determine whether this is an enactment or a relational theme that is being reconstructed. It may be best to try to discover the patient's wish (W) that does not receive a satisfying response. The reason may be that the new situation and distance in remote treatment creates new opportunities for enactment and disappointment. In telepsychotherapy it is important for therapists to take more time to think about their countertransference feelings and reactions, and try to understand the patient's withdrawal as part of their dynamics and past experiences. The therapist can be inspired by Symington's (1983) concept of "act of freedom," which means that the therapist is looking for an act of freeing himself or herself from the "lasso" of the patient's relational enactment, and letting some new air and space into the therapy. This kind of "Act of Freedom" may be necessitated even more by the shift to telepsychotherapy.

With the transition to telepsychotherapy, the therapist may need to deal more directly with ruptures. To encourage talk about possible ruptures, therapists are advised to initiate a discussion about possible difficulties in the new setting right after the change to the online setting, and to end the first online session with a question about how the patient felt talking online. Actions of this type signal to the patient that the therapist expects difficulties and wants to talk about them. Another technique is to reflect the possible difficulty of the change in the conversation style as being connected to the online change, in a non-judgmental manner, such as "I think our conversation is less fluid today. Do you feel this too?" This technique extends an invitation to notice the changes and deal with possible ruptures (Safran & Muran, 2000).

During the transition to telepsychotherapy if the therapist feels that the patient was hurt by some of the therapist's actions, such as not agreeing to a face-to-face meeting, the therapist should talk about it directly, take responsibility, and allow the patient to express negative feelings, enabling overt negotiation of the alliance. This is particularly crucial because of the physical distance between the two. The therapist can also use supportive techniques that deal with alliance directly, such as discussing treatment goals and movement toward these goals, or admiring the patient's ability and willingness to move into an unfamiliar setting, which can enhance the alliance. Other supportive techniques, such as showing genuine interest and noticing gains, may enable the patient's specific CCRT wish to be better fulfilled in the therapeutic relationship, enhancing the alliance and repairing the rupture indirectly. In telepsychotherapy, the therapist must be more active than usual, taking charge of the session and showing greater interest, so that the patient feels the therapist's presence, to compensate for the missing therapeutic setting (quiet and comfortable room and reassuring physical presence).

In sum, we propose a four-step model for dealing with withdrawal ruptures in telepsychotherapy. In the first step, the therapist should make all the necessary preparations for the patient before switching to the online setting. In the second step, during first online meeting, the therapist should take time to comment about the change and initiate a conversation about possible ruptures. In the third step, during the remote sessions, the therapist should try to determine whether a rupture occurred. This will be based on cues in the elements of treatment that are available, such as facial expressions, eye contact, acoustic changes, and the therapist's own countertransference feelings.

In the fourth step, the therapist can choose to attend to the rupture directly, or indirectly. The therapist can address the rupture directly, by assuming responsibility or by initiating a talk about the goals and changing tasks of treatment due to the transition to telepsychotherapy. The therapist can also choose to attend to the rupture indirectly, by trying to better fulfill the patient's CCRT wish with indirect supportive techniques, which are adequate for telepsychotherapy, such as showing genuine interest in the patient or pointing out the patients' strengths and gains in dealing with their difficulties, especially during stressful times. The identification of a withdrawal rupture in telepsychotherapy and its resolution can be an opportunity for change and progress in the therapy process, as the following clinical illustration shows.

Clinical illustration

The following clinical illustration demonstrates the identification of ruptures and their resolution using supportive techniques.

Design

The clinical illustration below uses a case study from an ongoing randomized controlled trial (RCT) involving SE therapy for depression (Zilcha-Mano, Dolev, Leibovich, & Barber, 2018). Patients who met inclusion and exclusion criteria received 16 sessions of short-term psychodynamic treatment with either a supportive or an expressive focus. All patients provided informed consent before participating in the study, including agreeing to all treatment sessions being recorded. All background details are disguised to ensure the anonymity of the patient and therapist.

Measures

The following measures were used for the patient's description from the pretreatment assessment: Hamilton Rating Scale for Depression (HRSD; Hamilton, 1967), a 17-item clinical evaluation of depressive symptoms in which patients are assigned an overall score (e.g. depressed mood, feelings of guilt, insomnia); the Inventory of Interpersonal Problems – Circumplex (IIP-C; Alden, Wiggins, & Pincus, 1990; Horowitz, Rosenberg, Baer, Ureño, & Villaseñor, 1988), a 32-item self-report inventory assessing behaviors related to interpersonal problems, in which patients are assigned an overall score and a score for each of eight octants (domineering, vindictive, cold, socially avoidant, non-assertive, exploitable, overly nurturant, and intrusive); the Experience in Close Relationships (ECR; Brennan, Clark, & Shaver, 1998), a 36-item self-report measure assessing attachment orientation, in which patients are assigned a score for two primary dimensions (attachment anxiety, and attachment avoidance); the Working Alliance Inventory (WAI; Horvath & Greenberg, 1989; Tracey & Kokotovic, 1989), a 12-item self-report measure assessing the therapeutic alliance, in which patients are assigned an overall score and a score for three subscales (bond between patient and therapist, agreement on tasks and agreement on goals of treatment); and two items from the Post Session Questionnaire (PSQ; Muran, Safran, Samstag, & Winston, 2001, 2012), the first item indicates whether or not an alliance rupture occurred in the session ("Did you experience any tension or misunderstanding in your relationship with your (therapist/patient) during the session?") and the second refers to the extent to which the rupture was resolved ("To what degree do you feel the problem was resolved by the end of the session?").

Sessions were coded with the Rupture Resolution Rating System (3RS; Eubanks et al., 2015) to assess the ruptures. Coders watched recorded video sessions and detected events of tension or lack of collaboration between patient and therapist. Identified ruptures were coded as a confrontation or withdrawal. Each rupture was rated for clarity as a check minus (a weak or somewhat unclear example of the marker), a check (a solid example of the marker), or a check plus (a very clear, "textbook" example of the marker). All coders received six months of training from an experienced coder. During the coding phase, all coders received weekly supervision to maintain reliability. Inter-rater agreement reliability was .92 for withdrawal and .93 for confrontation.

Patient

Amy is a 21 years old Caucasian student, the youngest child in her family. She felt that her parents were already tired and "worn out" when she was born, and did not have much energy for her, so in her own description, "I kind of grew up by myself." Her immediate reason for coming to therapy was feeling lonely and frustrated for not being able to concentrate on her studies. Amy felt isolated from her friends and family after moving to a new city the year before, to begin her studies. She had just broken up with her boyfriend. She felt that no one in the faculty (teachers and students) knew her or cared about her. For some time, she had been feeling passive, hopeless, and lacking energy. The treatment goals seemed to be obvious to Amy: being less passive in her studies and being less lonely. She reported pretreatment that she was non-assertive and avoidant in her relationships (non-assertive IIP subscale = 14; avoidant ECR subscale = 4.54). Her pretreatment HRSD was 22, indicating severe depression.

Therapist

Terry is Caucasian and is in her 40 s. She holds more than 20 years of experience in psychodynamic therapy, and more specifically 5 years of experience in short-term SE therapy for depression.

Case formulation

Terry conceptualized Amy's CCRT after the first four sessions, as recommended in the treatment protocol (Book, 1998). The CCRT consisted of a wish that other people show greater interest in her, care for her, and have faith in her (W), but instead, it seemed to her that people were all self-centered and cared only for their own interests (RO). She felt sad and tired, hopeless about the future, and avoided interactions or behaviors that had the potential of further hurting her (RS) (Table 1).

Course of treatment

Amy started therapy face-to-face. At the first session she declared that she already felt better, that she decided not to let things affect her so much, began to allocate more time for her studies, started exercising, and signed up again on dating apps. It seemed that starting therapy for the first time encouraged and helped her feel that she was doing something for herself, without letting herself expect that the therapist will be caring or otherwise helpful, so as not to be disappointed once again. Nevertheless, during the therapy sessions Amy was emotionally withdrawn and laconic. In particular, at the start of therapy she denied the importance of interpersonal relationships and of events that were relevant to the work of therapy. An example of such a rupture occurred at session 2. Amy continued to talk about the recent breakup with her boyfriend, but when the therapist showed empathy, saying "You seem to be still upset about the breakup," Amy responded: "I don't really care about him. I'm fine," without adding anything and avoiding eye contact. This exchange was coded using the 3RS as a check plus for a denial and minimal response rupture (Eubanks et al., 2015). The therapist tried to show genuine interest in Amy. She noticed Amy's withdrawal style but did not confront her with a direct interpretation. Instead, she sought to attend to her wish by showing genuine interest, caring, and authentic admiration of her abilities to take care of herself. Amy seemed to respond to these efforts, but she remained laconic, showing evidence of withdrawal ruptures. These dynamics characterized the first half of the therapy (the first eight sessions).

After eight weeks in therapy, as a result of the COVID-19 pandemic, the government imposed social distancing, which ruled out face-to-face meetings. The therapist offered to change over to telepsychotherapy. In session 8 before the change, Amy rated the alliance as WAI = 5.58, and Terry as WAI = 4.41. The switch at session 9 went smoothly. Before the shift, Terry made sure that Amy had a private room, a stable Internet connection, and a working camera and microphone. Amy stayed in her dorm where she felt it was easier for her to continue studying, and since her roommates decided to leave the dorm, she had considerable privacy. She was comfortable using a computer in her everyday life and did not show any uneasiness or concern about the change. Terry conducted the sessions from a private room in her home, and was somewhat worried that her children, who were also home, would distract her, but they did not. Nevertheless, the dynamic of withdrawal evident in the face-to-face sessions was intensified after the transition to telepsychotherapy. Terry asked Amy at the beginning of the session to talk about any discomfort or other feelings related to the change to online therapy, but Amy dismissed her and said she had no problems. The interaction became even more laconic, and Terry found that she was bored and tired. She made an effort to select topics for conversation that would demonstrate her interest in Amy's life. Amy was overly accommodating toward the therapist, in an appeasing manner. She was smiling without a reason during the session, saying "yes" to everything Terry suggested. For example, Amy said "I started talking to a new guy this week. You're probably sick of hearing me talk about this every time." Terry answered "I'm not sick of it at all." Amy responded "I'm kidding, you're always so helpful." This was coded as a check for a deferential and appeasing rupture (Eubanks et al., 2015). Terry could not see whether Amy's body movements showed discomfort, but was able to hear Amy's voice changing as she talked, becoming more cynical, and noticed that she avoided eye contact.

Other types of ruptures that did not manifest in the face-to-face interaction started to evolve. Connecting to Amy through the computer screen made it even less lively for Terry, and new ruptures occurred. Amy started to withdraw even more, and during the session Terry was not sure whether or not Amy was looking at other messages that were popping up on her screen or on her cell phone. She did not maintain eye contact, and Terry could see her eyes were moving across the screen, and could not see her hands. Amy was disengaging from Terry and the work of treatment, which was coded as a check plus for minimal response rupture (Eubanks et al., 2015). Terry tried to attend to the rupture directly, by asking Amy whether she was looking at messages on the computer screen. She tried to sound inviting rather than accusing, but Amy dismissed this attempt by saying she was just taking a second answering her boss that she would get back to him later. After the transition, the alliance ratings did not meaningfully differ from before the transition for both Amy (WAI = 5.58) and Terry (4.58). However, both identified a rupture has occurred, as rated in the PSQ.

After the session, Terry reflected on these ruptures and her unsuccessful attempts to repair them. She thought about the reenactment of the CCRT dynamics and conflict, and was searching for an act of freedom from the enactment (Symington, 1983). Terry wished for something new that would enable her to resolve the recurring withdrawal ruptures as well as those that started to appear as the result of the transition to telepsychotherapy, to enhance the therapeutic alliance. Terry felt that it would not be beneficial to talk to Amy directly about the rupture because Amy might not be aware that something was wrong and feel accused or embarrassed. She was looking for an indirect path to better actualize Amy's wish to be cared for, and to feel others show interest and have faith in her.

The opportunity presented itself at session 10. The session began laconically, as usual, and Terry soon found herself tired, bored, looking at the clock on the computer screen, and feeling stressed that there will not be enough material to fill the session, and she would have to end it soon. Amy was continuing to withdraw. She was silent or minimal in her responses and kept saying that nothing was happening, since she did not go out of her apartment or meet anyone, so she had nothing to talk about. Amy began reporting on her last conversation on the dating app. A week earlier she started a conversation with a guy who seemed promising. But the day before he suggested that since they cannot meet because of the pandemic, although they lived close to each other, they should hold off their conversation until things get back to normal. Amy agreed, and Terry, rather tired and losing hope herself, also agreed that it was a reasonable step. Then Terry felt something rebelling inside her. She felt alive again, and she felt that she could do something different. The following conversation ensued, attesting to her identification of the ruptures and their resolutions using supportive techniques:

Terry: I hear you agree with him. You're probably worried you will get hurt again [validating, trying to explore together Amy's feelings].

Amy: Yes, maybe you're right, there's a right time for everything [withdrawal rupture of deference and appeasement].

Terry: Maybe (not interpreting the defense(. But I feel you might want something else. I feel like helping you go for it, don't just dismiss it by saying it's not so important. It's super important for you! It drags you down when you don't have it and lifts you up when you do have it [Terry is supporting the patient's treatment goal, and by being caring she also actualizes the CCRT wish].

Amy: Well that's true (smiling).

Terry: It's OK to say this is important for me. You're the kind of person who will go out of their way for her boyfriend, and will invest a lot into the relationship [Terry shows she believes in Amy's strengths].

Amy: I'm not sure he's the kind of guy who will appreciate this kind of investment.

Terry: I think most people appreciate it.

Amy: Well, he did write that he looks for someone caring (said in a livelier tone).

Terry: (smiling) So let yourself be that someone, and if he doesn't appreciate it, move on! You're allowed to want a relationship, it's OK to feel bad that you're alone. It's not natural for a person to be so alone. It's very difficult, and the restrictions now make it much worse [showing genuine respect and validating the difficulties to stress the strengths].

Amy: That's right (looks relieved).

Terry: You're a person who has a lot to give, and there's no reason for you to be on hold now. You're doing so much for this, for finding a relationship, your life is happening now, no reason to wait [recognition of improvement toward the attainment of the goals of the therapy].

Amy: Yes.

Terry: There are a million guys out there waiting for someone like you. Believe me, I personally know a few (smiling) [presenting a realistically hopeful attitude that these goals can be achieved, and humor always helps].

Amy: (laughing, and for the first time raising her head and looking directly at Terry) It's not that I got my expectations high with him [withdrawal rupture of denial].

Terry: I know, but with every promising message the expectation rises, it's just natural [explores emotions together, working as a team].

Amy: Yes, I suppose you're right. I'll get out of my room now and breathe some fresh air.

Terry: You need someone who likes your kind of creativity and caring. If he doesn't appreciate it, then you need someone else [stressing Amy's strengths and hopeful that her goals can be achieved].

Amy: That's right! And he made me more creative. I told you, the messages we sent to each other were not the usual stuff [Amy feels better and shows Terry she believes that Terry takes genuine interest in her].

Terry: That is right. You told me that. You have a chance here.

This exchange demonstrates how the ruptures were identified and repaired in an indirect way, using the CCRT framework and supportive techniques in an online session of telepsychotherapy. Terry noticed the recurring withdrawal ruptures based on the cues that were available to her. She felt the familiar countertransference of being tired, bored, and worried, and she could see Amy's denial and minimal response. She was able to identify the deferential and appeasing ruptures based on Amy's eye movements and acoustic change. Terry used her CCRT formulation to understand the reenactment, in particular the wish that did not receive an adequate response. Terry decided not to confront the rupture directly but work with it indirectly, using a variety of supportive techniques that can be deployed in telepsychotherapy. She was showing genuine interest and respect, without addressing Amy's vital defenses directly. She focused on the here-and-now and on practical issues, without going back to the patient's earlier dynamics and history. She noted the patient's gains, efforts, and improvement in moving to attain the goals of her therapy, supporting and being realistically hopeful about Amy achieving these goals. At this point in the therapy, Terry could genuinely show Amy that she liked her, and that she believed in her strengths and in her ability to cope with the difficult situation she was in. Although Terry was quite active and somewhat directive, and although Amy was far away and alone, Amy seems to have gotten the message that the two were working together as a team. Terry actualized Amy's wish of being cared for and not forgotten. She did so despite Amy's behavior, which rejected these efforts, as manifest in the withdrawal ruptures. Amy appears to have had a corrective emotional experience of being cared for. She became livelier as the interaction developed, and for the first time looked directly at Terry. The WAI improved for both Amy (WAI = 6.16) and Terry (WAI = 4.66) after the session and both identified that a positive resolution had occurred, as rated by the PSQ.

Concluding remarks

The transition to telepsychotherapy requires therapists to work in a new environment, outside their familiar setting, and to acquire new skills. Ruptures often occur in treatment and may be exacerbated during telepsychotherapy because of technical difficulties, dissatisfaction, or disappointment with the limited interaction. A model for rupture identification in remote treatment was demonstrated together with supportive techniques used to resolve the ruptures. This model extends on Safran and Muran's model (1996, 2000) of alliance rupture and repair, adjusting it for the specific difficulties rising in telepsychotherapy. The utility of the CCRT formulation as a basis for thinking about ruptures and about their possible resolutions was at the center of our suggested model. The identification of ruptures and their repair in telepsychotherapy is more difficult than in traditional face-to-face treatment. Our model showed techniques to enhance the ability to identify ruptures and supportive techniques aimed at resolving them. The model and techniques presented can help therapists in the transition to telepsychotherapy during the current COVID-19 pandemic as well as in other cases in which face-to-face treatment is not possible.

The model suggested in this article for identifying and repairing ruptures in telepsychotherapy is an addition to Safran and Muran's (1996, 2000)) classical model of identifying and repairing ruptures in the therapeutic alliance. It adds to the currently suggested models that address rupture identification and repair in given therapeutic situations or populations, such as the Identification Countertransference Empathy Freedom model (ICEF; Leibovich et al., 2018), which serves to enhance the alliance with depressed patients using supportive techniques, or the Child Alliance Focused Approach (CAFA; Nof, Dolev, Leibovich, & Zilcha-Mano, 2019), which is designed to enhance alliance and repair ruptures in children's therapy. These models, as well as the one suggested above, combine evidence-based principles with knowledge gathered from clinical practice, and bridge the gap between clinical practice and research. Ruptures in the alliance are problematic because they may lead to deterioration in the therapeutic process and to dropout, but they can also provide an opportunity for growth and development in the therapeutic process. As Leonard Cohen said, "There is a crack in everything. That's how the light gets in."

Disclosure statement

No potential conflict of interest was reported by the authors.

Funding

The research was supported by a grant from the Israel Science Foundation (Grant no. 186/15).

References

Alden, L. E., Wiggins, J. S., & Pincus, A. L. (1990). Construction of circumplex scales for the Inventory of Interpersonal Problems. *Journal of Personality Assessment, 55*, 521–536.

Andersson, G., Paxling, B., Roch-Norlund, P., Östman, G., Norgren, A., Almlöv, J., … Silverberg, F. (2012). Internetbased psychodynamic versus cognitive behavioral guided self-help for generalized anxiety disorder: A randomized controlled trial. *Psychotherapy and Psychosomatics, 81*(6), 344–355.

Appelbaum, A. H. (2006). Supportive psychoanalysis psychotherapy for borderline patients: An empirical approach. *The American Journal of Psychoanalysis, 66*(4), 317–332.

Backhaus, A., Agha, Z., Maglione, M. L., Repp, A., Ross, B., Zuest, D., … Thorp, S. R. (2012). Videoconferencing psychotherapy: A systematic review. *Psychological Services, 9*(2), 111–131.

Barber, J. P., & Crits-Christoph, P. (1996). Development of a therapist adherence/competence rating scale for supportive-expressive dynamic psychotherapy: A preliminary report. *Psychotherapy Research, 6*(2), 81–94.

Beutel, M. E., Böhme, K., Banerjee, M., & Zwerenz, R. (2018). Psychodynamic online treatment following supportive expressive therapy (SET) therapeutic rationale, interventions and treatment process. *Zeitschrift für Psychosomatische Medizin und Psychotherapie, 64*(2), 186–197.

Book, H. E. (1998). *How to practice brief psychodynamic therapy: The core conflictual relationship theme method.* Washington, DC: American Psychological Association Press.

Brennan, K. A., Clark, C. L., & Shaver, P. R. (1998). Self-report measurement of adult attachment: An integrative overview. In J. A. Simpson & W. S. Rholes (Eds.), *Attachment theory and close relationships* (pp. 46–76). New-York, NY: Guilford Press.

Deen, T. L., Fortney, J. C., & Schroeder, G. (2013). Patient acceptance of and initiation and engagement in telepsychotherapy in primary care. *Psychiatric Services, 64*(4), 380–384.

Dolev-Amit, T.*, Nof, A.*, Asaad, A., Tchizick, A., & Zilcha-Mano, S. (in press). *The melody of ruptures - identifying ruptures through acoustic markers.* Unpublished Manuscript.

Eubanks, C. F., Lubitz, J., Muran, J. C., & Safran, J. D. (2019). Rupture Resolution Rating System (3RS): Development and validation. *Psychotherapy Research, 29*(3), 306–319.

Eubanks, C. F., Muran, J. C., & Safran, J. D. (2015). *Rupture resolution rating system (3RS): Manual.* Unpublished Manuscript, Mount Sinai-Beth Israel Medical Center, New York.

Eubanks, C. F., Muran, J. C., & Safran, J. D. (2018). Alliance rupture repair: A meta-analysis. *Psychotherapy, 55*(4), 508–519.

Germain, V., Marchand, A., Bouchard, S., Guay, S., & Drouin, M. S. (2010). Assessment of the therapeutic alliance in face-to-face or videoconference treatment for posttraumatic stress disorder. *Cyberpsychology, Behavior, and Social Networking, 13*(1), 29–35.

Hamilton, M. A. X. (1967). Development of a rating scale for primary depressive illness. *British Journal of Social and Clinical Psychology, 6*(4), 278–296.

Horowitz, L. M., Rosenberg, S. E., Baer, B. A., Ureño, G., & Villaseñor, V. S. (1988). Inventory of interpersonal problems: Psychometric properties and clinical applications. *Journal of Consulting and Clinical Psychology, 56*(6), 885–892.

Horvath, A. O., & Greenberg, L. S. (1989). Development and validation of the working alliance inventory. *Journal of Counseling Psychology, 36*(2), 223–233.

Kingsley, A., & Henning, J. A. (2015). Online and phone therapy: Challenges and opportunities. *The Journal of Individual Psychology, 71*(2), 185–194.

Leibovich, L., Front, O., McCarthy, K. S., & Zilcha-Mano, S. (2019). How do supportive techniques bring about therapeutic change: The role of therapeutic alliance as a potential mediator. *Psychotherapy*. doi:10.1037/pst0000253.

Leibovich, L., Nof, A., Auerbach-Barber, S., & Zilcha-Mano, S. (2018). A practical clinical suggestion for strengthening the alliance based on a supportive–expressive framework. *Psychotherapy, 55*(3), 231–240.

Luborsky, L. (1995). Supportive-Expressive dynamic psychotherapy of depression: A time-limited version. In J. P. Barber & P. Crits-Christoph (Eds.), *Dynamic therapies for psychiatric disorders* (pp. 41–83). New-York, NY: Basic Books.

Monthuy-Blanc, J., Bouchard, S., Maïano, C., & Seguin, M. (2013). Factors influencing mental health providers' intention to use telepsychotherapy in first nations communities. *Transcultural Psychiatry, 50*(2), 323–343.

Muran, J. C. (2019). Confessions of a New York rupture researcher: An insider's guide and critique. *Psychotherapy Research, 29*(1), 1–14.

Muran, J. C., Safran, J. D., Samstag, L. W., & Winston, A. (2001). *Patient and therapist post-session questionnaires, version 2001*. New-York, NY: Beth Israel Medical Center.

Muran, J. C., Safran, J. D., Samstag, L. W., & Winston, A. (2012). *Patient and therapist post-session questionnaires, version 2012*. New-York, NY: Beth Israel Medical Center.

Nof, A., Dolev, T., Leibovich, L., & Zilcha-Mano, S. (2019). If you believe that breaking is possible, believe also that fixing is possible: A framework for rupture and repair in child psychotherapy. *Research in Psychotherapy: Psychopathology, Process and Outcome, 22*, 45–57.

Pinsker, H., Rosenthal, R., & McCullough, L. (1991). Dynamic supportive psychotherapy. In P. Crits-Christoph & J. Barber (Eds.), *Handbook of short-term dynamic psychotherapy* (pp. 220–247). New-York, NY: Basic Books.

Rees, C. S., & Stone, S. (2005). Therapeutic alliance in face-to-face versus videoconferenced psychotherapy. *Professional Psychology: Research and Practice, 36*(6), 649–653.

Safran, J. D., & Muran, J. C. (1996). The resolution of ruptures in the therapeutic alliance. *Journal of Consulting and Clinical Psychology, 64*(3), 447–458.

Safran, J. D., & Muran, J. C. (2000). *Negotiating the therapeutic alliance: A relational treatment guide*. New-York, NY: Guilford Press.

Safran, J. D., Muran, J. C., & Eubanks-Carter, C. (2011). Repairing alliance ruptures. *Psychotherapy: Theory, Research, Practice, Training, 48*(1), 80–87.

Simpson, S. G., & Reid, C. L. (2014). Therapeutic alliance in videoconferencing psychotherapy: A review. *Australian Journal of Rural Health, 22*(6), 280–299.

Symington, N. (1983). The analyst's act of freedom as agent of therapeutic change. *International Review of Psycho-Analysis, 10*, 283–291.

Tracey, T. J., & Kokotovic, A. M. (1989). Factor structure of the working alliance inventory. *Psychological Assessment: A Journal of Consulting and Clinical Psychology, 1*(3), 207–210.

Zilcha-Mano, S., Dolev, T., Leibovich, L., & Barber, J. P. (2018). Identifying the most suitable treatment for depression based on patients' attachment: Study protocol for a randomized controlled trial of supportive-expressive vs. supportive treatments. *BMC Psychiatry, 18*(1), 362–370.

Grappling with our therapeutic relationship and professional self-doubt during COVID-19: will we use video therapy again?

Katie Aafjes-van Doorn, Vera Békés and Tracy A. Prout

ABSTRACT

The social restrictions during the COVID-19 crisis led to many therapists providing therapy remotely, despite some therapists' concerns regarding its efficacy, technical challenges and their ability to build a strong therapeutic relationship online. This survey study reports on the experiences of 141 therapists who transitioned to providing video therapy during the pandemic. Aspects of the therapeutic relationship (e.g. working alliance, real relationship), experienced anxiety and professional self-doubt, attitudes towards and intention of video therapy use in the future were assessed. Although therapists reported some anxiety and self-doubt, most felt that online sessions had a sufficient working alliance and a strong real relationship. Therapists with more online therapy experience, lower levels of self-doubt and anxiety, and those who experienced a strong online real relationship during the pandemic, or thought their patients viewed it positively, tended to be more accepting of video therapy. Therapists were largely undecided as to whether they planned to use video therapy in the future; however, those with prior video therapy experience were more likely to endorse future utilization. Training is needed, especially for therapists with less online therapy experience, in order to foster a better experience and to support effective use of online therapy in the future.

In the world of telemental health interventions, video therapy (i.e. online therapy via a video conferencing) is one alternative to in-person therapy. Video therapy offers the benefits of telemental health (e.g., access in remote and rural areas, time and cost-savings; Simpson, 2009) while allowing for real-time synchronous interactions of speech and body movement. Most therapists have little training and experience in providing video therapy and many therapists believe that video therapies are less effective than sessions conducted in-person (e.g., Topooco et al., 2017). Commonly expressed concerns focus on the practicalities of conducting video therapy, such as the impact of technical glitches, insufficient internet literacy, or assuring confidentiality online (e.g., Topooco et al., 2017). Many therapists are also reluctant to use video therapy because of relational concerns, especially regarding difficulties with building a strong therapeutic relationship online (Connolly, Miller, Lindsay, & Bauer, 2020; Roesler, 2017; Sucala, Schnur, Brackman, Constantino, & Montgomery, 2013).

These concerns about the therapeutic relationship in video therapy are not necessarily based on empirical findings. Studies on the working alliance, one of the most researched aspects of the therapeutic relationship, suggest that patients benefit from video therapy and experience it positively. Although therapists tend to perceive a lower working alliance in video compared to in-person therapy (Rees & Stone, 2005), the working alliance in video therapies has shown to be high (see review by Norwood, Moghaddam, Malins, & Sabin-Farrell, 2018), and comparable to in-person therapies (e.g., Bouchard et al., 2000), especially when rated by patients (e.g., Ruwaard et al., 2009). It is thus possible that negative expectations of video therapy, rather than its actual relational deficits affect therapists' perceptions of the working alliance in video therapies (Rees & Stone, 2005). Another important aspect of the therapeutic relationship, the real relationship (i.e. the genuine and realistic personal relationship; Gelso, 2011), distinctly contributes to in-person treatment outcomes (Bhatia & Gelso, 2018), but has not yet been studied in video therapy.

During the COVID-19 pandemic, social distancing guidelines were instituted by health authorities in an effort to slow down the spread of the virus. Patients and therapists alike were advised to stay home, which meant that millions of in-person therapies transitioned to video at once. Consequently, many therapists began providing video therapy without much time to access training or support. Whereas using platforms allowed therapists and patients to continue ongoing treatments, it is unclear how these treatments are experienced by therapists. For many therapists, the experiences gained during the pandemic may shape their views and attitudes about video therapy and impact their attitudes towards future online work (Békés, Aafjes-van Doorn, Prout, & Hoffman, in press).

In the present cross-sectional survey study, we aimed to explore therapists' experiences of video therapy after switching from in-person to video sessions during the pandemic. More specifically, we examined: 1) Therapist perceptions of the therapeutic relationship (working alliance and real relationship) in video sessions compared to previous in-person therapy; 2) Therapist confidence in professional competence (professional self-doubt) and experienced anxiety related to providing video therapy; 3) Therapist attitudes towards video therapy technology in general, as well as intentions to continue using video therapy in the future.

Methods

Recruitment

An online therapist survey was advertised via professional listservs and social media. Due to the forced-choice logic of the online survey, no data were missing. Participants were eligible to take part if they were therapists (either licensed or in training) and if they had conducted at least one video therapy session since the start of the pandemic. The participants were first provided with an online information sheet and were asked for their consent before being directed to the online survey. The survey took approximately 15 minutes to complete and included several individual items as well as standardized measures in a set order. The study was reviewed by the Western Institutional Review Board. The present study reports on responses from 141 therapists collected between March 25 and 30 March 2020.

Measures

The survey included demographic questions, including age, gender, location, profession, and licensure. Several individual items inquired about previous in-person and video therapy experience, previous training and their experienced challenges with the transition to online therapy. Therapists were also asked to identify all the ways in which they prepared for the transition on a list of possible options, such as "I talked to colleagues", and "I read journal articles". Moreover, one item asked the therapists to rate their perception of patients' online experiences ("During the pandemic, how do your (previously in-person) patients tend to experience having therapy online?") on a 5-point Likert scale (1 = Extremely positive, 2 = Somewhat positive, 3 = Neither positive or negative, 4 = Somewhat negative, 5 = Extremely negative).

Standardized scales assessed the aspects of the therapeutic relationship (working alliance and real relationship), therapists' professional experience (self-doubt and anxiety), and attitudes towards acceptance and usage of video therapy more generally. In order to reflect therapists' overall experience of the working alliance, real relationship, and professional self-doubt in their online therapy, the instructions of the scales were slightly adapted to "In general, in your online sessions during the pandemic."

The **Working-Alliance Inventory-Short Form** (WAI-SF; Hatcher & GIllaspy, 2006) was adapted from the earlier versions of the WAI (Horvath & Greenberg, 1989) using extensive factor analyses. The WAI-SR assesses the level of agreement on the goals of treatment, agreement on the steps toward meeting the patient's goals, and the relationship between the patient and therapist. The ten items are rated on a Likert scale ranging from 1 (never) to 7 (always). A global working alliance rating of 4 (sometimes), the middle point of the scale, is interpreted as a neutral working alliance, with higher scores indicating a stronger working alliance (Horvath & Greenberg, 1989). The WAI-SF has shown adequate reliability and validity (Hatcher & Gillaspy, 2006).

In normal circumstances (not during an abrupt transition due to the pandemic), the therapist-rated alliance on the WAI-SF in video therapy is generally high (e.g., $M = 5.7$, $SD = .83$; Stubbings, Rees, Roberts, & Kane, 2013; $M = 5.4$, 95% CI = 4.72–6.07; Morland et al., 2015), similar to face-to-face therapy.

In the present study, total scores on the WAI-SF demonstrated good reliability (Cronbach's $\alpha = .87$). To examine the transition from in-person to video therapy specifically, the following item was administered: "Compared to in-person sessions, during my online sessions the therapeutic relationship felt … " to be responded on a three-point Likert scale (1 = more connected than in-person, 2 = the same, 3 = less connected than in-person).

The **Real Relationship Inventory–Therapist Form** (RRI; Gelso et al., 2005) assesses the real relationship in psychotherapy, defined as "the personal relationship existing between two or more persons as reflected in the degree to which each is genuine with the other and perceives the other in ways that befit the other" (Gelso, 2011, pp. 12). The RRI consists of 24 items on a Likert scale ranging from 1 (strongly disagree) to 5 (strongly agree), with higher overall scores reflecting a more genuine and authentic relationship. Reliability has shown to be high, with coefficient alphas ranging from .80 to .90 in various samples (e.g., Fuertes, Gelso, Owen, & Cheng, 2013; Fuertes, Moore, & Ganley, 2019; Marmarosh et al., 2009). Convergent and discriminant validity have been supported by the relation of the

RRI to ratings of working alliance, session quality, transference, patient insight, social desirability, and therapist and patient attachment (Fuertes et al., 2013, 2019; Marmarosh et al., 2009). Predictive validity has been supported by its relation with outcome (Fuertes et al., 2019; Marmarosh et al., 2009). As a point of reference, in studies on in-person treatments, the average real relationship has been reported as *M* = 3.81; *SD* = 1.01 (Bhatia & Gelso, 2018) and *M* = 2.94, *SD* = .12 (Gelso et al., 2012). The real relationship has not been previously assessed with regards to online therapies.

For the present sample, the internal consistency estimate was Cronbach's α = .86. To assess the experienced change in the real relationship since the switch to video therapy, the following item was added: "Compared to in-person sessions, during my online sessions the therapeutic relationship felt … " to be responded on a three-point Likert scale (1 = more authentic than in-person, 2 = the same, 3 = less authentic than in-person).

The **Professional Self-Doubt** scale (PSD; Nissen-Lie et al., 2017) assesses the level of uncertainty a therapist has in their ability to help a patient. The PSD includes nine items about how confident and competent the therapist feels, including phrases like; "Unsure how best to deal effectively with a patient," and "Afraid that you are doing more harm than good in treating a patient." Items are rated on a six-point Likert scale from 0 (never) to 5 (very often) and summed for a total score, with higher scores indicating more self-doubt. This 9-item PSD scale is derived from the larger 21-item scale on difficulties in psychotherapy practice, as part of the comprehensive self-reported DPCCQ questionnaire (Orlinsky et al., 1999) on professional training and development. Professional self-doubt predicts patient outcomes and may be used to surpass the inaccuracy of self-appraisal (Nissen-Lie, Monsen, Ulleberg, & Rønnestad, 2013; Nissen-Lie et al., 2017). Among licensed therapists, PSD, especially when coupled with self-compassion, has shown to be positively related to patient progress in treatment (Nissen-Lie et al., 2013); however, in trainees a decrease in professional doubt over treatment appears to be related to patient improvement (Odyniec, Probst, Margraf, & Willutzki, 2019). Research has shown that psychotherapy trainees and licensed therapists experience considerable professional self-doubt (e.g., trainees: *M* = 1.52, *SD* = .94; Odyniec et al., 2019; or licensed therapists; *M* = 1.24, *SD* = .70; Nissen-Lie et al., 2013).

The Cronbach's α in the present study was .84. To assess change in therapists' experienced competence and confidence we added the following two items: "Compared to in-person sessions, online sessions make me feel … " to be responded on a 3-point Likert scale (1 = more competent than in-person, 2 = the same, 3 = less competent than in-person) and "Compared to in-person sessions, online sessions make me feel … " to be responded on a 3-point Likert scale (1 = more confident than in-person, 2 = the same, 3 = less confident than in-person).

The **Unified Theory of Acceptance and Use of Technology** model (UTAUT, Venkatesh, Morris, Davis, & Davis, 2003) was used to assess attitudes towards acceptance and usage of video therapy. The UTAUT framework offers a comprehensive model of acceptance and subsequent utilization of technological innovations and has been adapted to various contexts, including occupational and physical therapy (Liu et al., 2015) and also for reviewing attitudes about video therapy (Connolly et al., 2020). The 21 items of the UTAUT are scored on a Likert Scale of 1 (Strongly disagree) to 5 (Strongly agree), with higher scores indicating a more positive attitude towards technology. The UTAUT has been validated in health care settings. The Cronbach's α for the subscales varies between .68 and .91. (Liu et al., 2015). The 13 items of the original UTAUT model have been used as determinant of technology-use (Venkatesh et al., 2003). Later researchers extended the UTAUT (e.g., Venkatesh, Thong, & Xu, 2012) including subscales on Anxiety (6 items) and Behavioral Intention (2 items). The UTAUT Anxiety scale refers to the feeling of apprehension or anxiety that one experiences when using technology (Compeau, Higgins, & Huff, 1999). The UTAUT Anxiety scale has been shown to have a direct negative effect on technology use and is thus seen as an important inhibitory variable (Cenfetelli & Schwarz, 2011). The UTAUT Behavioral intention subscale assesses explicitly declared intent and plan to use technology in the future (e.g., Wu, Tao, & Yang, 2007). In the present study the internal consistency of the UTAUT was $\alpha = .77$, the UTAUT Anxiety subscale had an $\alpha = .83$ and the UTAUT Behavioral Intention subscale an $\alpha = .94$. In this study the wording of the UTAUT items was adapted to reflect the video therapy context. Similar to the previous standardized measures, we added an item to assess changes in attitudes, inquiring about the therapists' views about video therapy before and during the pandemic.

Results

Therapists characteristics

The majority of the 141 therapists were female (N = 105; 74.5%) and identified as Caucasian (N = 120; 85.7%). Therapists ranged in age between 23 and 79, with an average age of 46 years (SD = 14.83). Most therapists were based in the United States of America (N = 96; 69.1%), Canada (N = 9; 6.5%), or European countries (N = 34, 24.5%) such as Hungary, Italy, United Kingdom, Germany, Norway, Sweden, Switzerland, Latvia, Ireland, Denmark, and Austria, in descending order. Most therapists were licensed (N – 107; 77.5%), in either clinical psychology (N = 91; 64.5%) or counseling (N = 14; 9.9%), or were clinical psychology trainees (N = 15, 10.6%). Most therapists had more than nine years of clinical experience (N = 94; 66.6%) of which 57 therapists had 17 years or more of clinical experience. Therapists worked with adult patients (N = 137; 94.5%), adolescents (N = 51; 36.2%), older adults (N = 45; 31.9%) or children (N = 31; 22.0%). Most worked in private practice (N = 101; 71.6%), outpatient clinics (N = 30; 21.3%) or hospitals (N = 12; 8.5%) and had an integrative therapy approach (N = 57; 40.4%) and identified with psychodynamic (N = 71; 50.4%), CBT (N = 50; 35.5%), humanistic (N = 28; 19.9%), and psychoanalytic (N = 23; 16.3%) orientations. The majority of therapists reported a caseload of 10–20 (N = 45; 31.9%), or 20–30 (N = 44; 31.2%) in-person patients per week. About half of all participating therapists had at least some experience with video therapy before the pandemic (N = 70; 49.6%).

Transition to video therapy during the COVID-19 pandemic

In order to prepare for the transition to video therapy most therapists spoke to colleagues (N = 94; 66.7%), followed posts on listservs (N = 86; 61.0%), read governmental guidelines (N = 69; 48.9%)), and/or prepared consent forms (N = 53; 37.6%). In addition, one-third of therapists also attended webinars on how to conduct video therapy (N = 47; 33.3%), read journal articles (N = 42; 29.9%) or spoke to a supervisor, (N = 42; 29.8%). Also, many therapists prepared their patients for the transition to video therapy by discussing it in person before ($N = 83$; 58.9%) and/or in the first session after the switch ($N = 92$; 65.2%). Many therapists provided their patients with technical support ($N = 58$; 41.1%), a consent form ($N = 62$; 44.0%) and/or an information sheet about the transition to video therapy ($N = 42$; 29.8%). Most therapists kept the same fees ($N = 133$; 94.3%) and the same cancellation policies ($N = 120$; 85.1%).

The most frequently reported challenges for the therapists during the transition to video therapy concerned technical difficulties with the online platform ($N = 86$; 61.0%). Other common challenges regarded patients' difficulty in finding a suitable space for therapy ($N = 68$; 48.2%) and the risk of the patient ($N = 59$; 41.8%) or the therapist ($N = 46$; 32.6%) getting distracted during session. Other reported concerns regarded the nature of the patient-therapist interaction, such as feeling less connected with the patient ($N = 58$; 41.1%), having difficulty reading the patients' emotions ($N = 52$; 36.9%) and difficulty feeling or expressing empathy ($N = 29$; 20.6%). Despite these challenges, very few therapists thought that their patients experienced video therapy negatively ($N = 10$; 7.1%), the vast majority perceived patient experience as either positive ($N = 88$; 63.8%) or neutral ($N = 40$; 28.4%).

Perceptions of the therapeutic relationship in video therapy

Even though therapists felt less connected to their patients during online sessions than in-person sessions ($M = 2.43$, $SD = .54$, range: 1.00–3.00), overall, they reported having a relatively good therapeutic relationship with their online patients, indicated by neutral ratings of the working alliance on the WAI-SF ($M = 4.09$, $SD = .48$, range: 2.70–5.00), albeit lower than therapist WAI-SF alliance ratings reported in the few available studies on video therapy treatment samples (Morland et al., 2015; Stubbings et al., 2013). For example, in comparing therapist working alliance ratings in the present study to those reported by therapists in the Morland et al. (2015) video therapy sample for women with posttraumatic stress-disorder, a one-sample t-test revealed a significant difference ($t(136) = 36.82$, $p < .0001$). Similarly, although therapists felt less authentic online than in-person ($M = 2.27$, $SD = .50$, range: 1.00–3.00), scores on the RRI indicated a good quality of the real relationship between patient and therapist during their online sessions ($M = 3.80$, $SD = .46$, range: 2.33–4.92), similar to the published in-person therapy samples (Bhatia & Gelso, 2018; Gelso et al., 2012).

Women reported higher working alliance in online sessions compared to men ($t(137) = 2.18$, $p < .05$), licensed practitioners reported higher alliance score than trainees ($t(136) = 2.33$, $p < .05$), and practitioners in North America (USA and Canada) compared to those in Europe ($t(137) = 2.08$, $p < .05$). Within the sample, higher online alliance was also reported by those who used a greater variety of methods (as opposed to fewer methods) to prepare patients for the transition ($r = .26$, $p < .01$), and those who perceived their patients' experience with video therapy more positively (as opposed to less positively) ($r = .32$, $p < .001$).

Similar to the working alliance, the perceived quality of the real relationship was related to using more methods to prepare the patients to the transition ($r = .18$, $p < .05$) and perceived positive patient experience ($r = .24$, $p < .01$). Age, years of clinical experience, number of patients seen weekly before the pandemic, previous video therapy experience, and views of video therapy before the pandemic were not associated with the perceived quality of alliance or the real relationship in online sessions.

Professional self-doubt and anxiety

On average, therapists experienced professional self-doubt sometimes or frequently ($M = 2.41$, $SD = .67$, range: 1.11–4.78) in video therapy during the pandemic, which is higher than the level of self-doubt experienced by therapists in a prior naturalistic study of PSD (Nissen-Lie et al., 2013; $t(136) = 20.45$, $p < .0001$), but still on the lower end of the 5-point Likert scale. Therapists felt less competent ($M = 2.28$, $SD = .52$, range: 1.00–3.00) and less confident ($M = 2.15$, $SD = .56$, range: 1.00–3.00) about their professional skills during online compared to in-person sessions. Higher levels of reported professional self-doubt were related to several demographic variables, such as younger age ($r = -.34$, $p < .001$), less clinical experience ($r = -.33$, $p < .001$), and worse perceived patient experience ($r = -.36$, $p < .001$).

Therapists' anxiety about using video therapy was moderate ($M = 2.87$, $S.D. = .86$, range: 1.00–4.83). Similar to professional self-doubt, higher anxiety was associated with female gender ($t(137) = 3.24$, $p < .05$), younger age ($r = -.30$, $p < .001$), less clinical experience ($r = -.36$, $p < .001$), smaller number of patients before the pandemic ($r = -.18$, $p < .05$), no previous experience with video therapy ($t(138) = 3.63$, $p < .001$), not being licensed yet ($t(136) = 3.28$, $p < .001$), perceiving patients as having a negative video therapy experience ($r = .27$, $p < .001$).

Attitudes towards using video therapy and intention to use it in the future

Overall in our sample, therapists reported somewhat positive attitudes towards video therapy ($M = 3.42$, $SD = 0.50$, range: 2.31–4.69). Although their views about video therapy had become more positive since the start of the pandemic ($t(140) = 2.06$, $p < .05$); they still thought that video therapy was somewhat less effective compared to in-person therapy ($M = 2.19$, $SD = 0.65$, range: 1.00–4.00).

Therapists who held more positive attitudes towards video therapy tended to have previous experience with video therapy ($t(142) = 3.53$, $p < .05$) and to have positive perceptions of their patients' online experience ($r = .30$, $p < .001$). Higher rated working alliance and real relationship were associated with more positive attitudes towards video therapy ($r = -.34$, $p < .001$ and $r = -.40$, $p < .001$, respectively) whereas professional self-doubt was associated with more negative attitudes ($r = -.34$, $p < .001$).

The sample of therapists as a whole was undecided as to whether they would like to continue using video therapy in the future (i.e. expressed a neutral response on the UTUAT Behavior Intention subscale), with large differences among therapists ($M = 3.14$, $SD = 1.23$, range: 1.00–5.00). Therapists who intended to use video therapy in the future were more likely to have prior experience with video therapy ($t(138) = 2.91$, $p < .01$), and tended to have positive perceptions of their patients' online experience ($r = .32$, $p < .001$).

See Table 1 for an overview of the correlations between the standardized measures. The relational, professional and technology-related scales were correlated in the expected direction. Specifically, scores on the real relationship and working alliance were positively correlated, and professional self-doubt and anxiety were positively related to each other

Table 1. Correlations among the measures of the therapeutic relationship, professional doubt and anxiety and attitudes towards video therapy technology.

	Measures	*M (SD)*	1	2	3	4	5	6
Therapeutic relationship	1. WAI	4.09 (.48)	-					
	2. RRI	3.80 (.46)	.52***	-				
Professional doubt	3. PSD	2.41 (.67)	.40***	−.42***	-			
& anxiety	4. UTAUT Anxiety	2.87 (.86)	−.19*	−.27**	.50***	-		
Attitude towards	5. UTAUT Acceptance	3.42 (.50)	.34***	.40***	−.34***	−.44***	-	
video technology	6. UTAUT Intention	3.14 (1.23)	.28***	.28**	−.28***	−.41***	.60***	-

WAI: Working Alliance Inventory. RRI = Real Relationship Inventory. PSD = Professional Self-Doubt. UTAUT = Unified Theory of Acceptance and Use of Technology Scale.
*p <.05; **p <.01, *** p <.001.

but negatively to the reported working alliance and real relationship, indicating that therapists with lower levels of professional self-doubt and anxiety reported a stronger working alliance and real relationship with their online patients during the pandemic. The attitudes towards and intention to use video therapy in the future were positively associated with ratings of the working alliance, and real relationship, and negatively related to professional self-doubt and anxiety (see Table 1).

Discussion

To our knowledge, this is the first study to explore certain aspects of the therapeutic relationship, including the real relationship, as well as professional self-doubt and anxiety in relation to attitudes towards the video therapy technology video therapy. The participants in this study indicated that they had made efforts to prepare themselves and their patients for the rapid transition from in-person to video therapy during the COVID-19 pandemic. Even though the therapists experienced challenges during the transition to video therapy, overall, they felt that their patients had a relatively good experience with the video therapy sessions.

In accordance with the literature on therapist concerns around video therapy (e.g., Topooco et al., 2017), therapists in this study reported technical and logistic concerns, but also about interpersonal and relational challenges of video therapy, such as difficulty communicating emotions and empathy online, and difficulty connecting with the patients. Despite these concerns, they reported a neutral working alliance online, albeit lower than those reported in previous studies on video therapy (Morland et al., 2015; Stubbings et al., 2013). Similarly, despite feeling that the patient-therapist relationship was less authentic than in-person therapy, results implicated a relatively strong real relationship online, similar to levels reported in studies of in-person therapy (Bhatia & Gelso, 2018; Gelso et al., 2012). This may indicate that this aspect of the therapeutic relationship remains intact on a video platform, or alternatively, that the current situation has a positive impact on the real relationship. It is possible that during the shared experience of the pandemic, therapists and patients feel more connected as human beings, possibly reflected in the relatively high real relationship scores.

Moreover, the surveyed therapists reported higher levels of professional self-doubt in their online sessions than previous levels reported in studies on in-person therapies (Nissen-Lie et al., 2013; Odyniec et al., 2019). Despite feeling less competent and less confident about their professional skills in video sessions, their scores only indicated a moderate level of self-doubt. Overall, therapists reported moderate levels of anxiety about using video therapy; however, professional self-doubt and anxiety were higher in younger and less experienced therapists in our sample. This is supported by prior research indicating that experience level is predictive of therapist self-efficacy (Mesrie, Diener, & Clark, 2018).

Furthermore, even though therapists thought that video therapy was somewhat less effective than in-person therapy, they still had relatively positive attitudes towards it, with a wide range of individual differences in their intention to use video therapy in the future. Specifically, therapists with positive relational experiences in their video sessions, with previous video therapy experience, and perceived positive patient experience had more positive attitudes and were more likely to use video therapy in the future, whereas therapists with high levels of self-doubt and anxiety, and with perceived negative patient experiences held more negative views and did not plan to utilize it after the pandemic.

Limitations

Several limitations of this study can be identified. First, given the cross-sectional observational study design, no pre and post pandemic scores were collected and the use of questions about the change may be informative but less valid. The threshold for participation – having conducted at least one video therapy session since the start of the pandemic – was low, which may have resulted in a high degree of variability among therapists in terms of their use of remote therapy platforms. Moreover, the validity of the standardized scales of working alliance, and real relationship could be questioned, given that these measures were used to assess the therapists' experiences with their typical online patient, rather than one patient in particular. Also, it is possible that these responses did not only reflect the transition to online therapy but also the context of the global pandemic, possibly increasing therapists' and patients' stress levels and thus indirectly relating to more professional doubt. Finally, there is also a possibility that the nature of the survey questions might have prompted the therapists to overstate their experiences (e.g., reporting more professional self-doubt than they might have reported if they would have been asked about their professional experience more generally).

Implications

This sudden uptake of remote therapies during COVID-19 sheds a unique light on telemental health and its challenges. The study results indicate that experiences during the pandemic might shape therapists' attitudes towards acceptance and usage of video therapy and their likelihood to continue using video therapy in the future. Therapists' views on video therapy tend to get more positive after trying it out and with usage, and therapists with more (online) experience tend to report fewer technical and relational challenges (Connolly et al., 2020). Thus, it is possible that during the first few weeks of a transition, video therapy experiences might appear more negative compared to in-person therapy, whereas with more experience therapists might adapt and be able to see more benefits of video therapy.

The relatively higher levels of professional self-doubt and anxiety in less experienced therapists might be unsurprising given the novelty of the treatment delivery method, and the lack of preparedness for this new situation. It would thus be important to provide more clinical training and support for (junior) therapists so that they can become more comfortable with providing video therapy. Besides traditional didactic training and supervision, telemental health platforms offer the opportunity to record, review and learn from therapy sessions.

Conclusion

Overall, our results show that, during the rapid transition to video therapy amidst the COVID-19 pandemic, therapists experienced some professional self-doubt and anxiety, and worried about technicalities and therapeutic relationship difficulties. However, despite this, they reported a relatively good working alliance and strong real relationship with their online patients, thought that their patients had a positive video therapy experience, and overall, they were moderately accepting of video therapy, but somewhat divided about intention to use it in the future. Moreover, factors that were related to more professional self-doubt and anxiety, such as lack of experience and worse in-session relational experience could be addressed in future professional trainings on how to best conduct video therapy. Since trying out video therapy is likely to lead to more positive attitudes towards it (Connolly et al., 2020), it is possible that once the initial stress subsides and therapists gain more experience and more training, they will feel more at ease using video therapy.

Disclosure statement

No potential conflict of interest was reported by the authors.

ORCID

Katie Aafjes-van Doorn http://orcid.org/0000-0003-2584-5897
Vera Békés http://orcid.org/0000-0003-3043-5155
Tracy A. Prout http://orcid.org/0000-0002-3650-5890

References

Békés, V., Aafjes-van Doorn, K., Prout, T. A., & Hoffman, L. (in press). Is it really that bad? Analytic therapists' experiences with remote therapy during COVID-19. *Journal of the American Psychoanalytic Association*.

Bhatia, A., & Gelso, C. J. (2018). Therapists' perspective on the therapeutic relationship: Examining a tripartite model. *Counselling Psychology Quarterly*, *31*(3), 271–293.

Bouchard, S., Payeur, R., Rivard, V., Allard, M., Paquin, B., Renaud, P., & Goyer, L. (2000). Cognitive behavior therapy for panic disorder with agoraphobia in videoconference: Preliminary results. *CyberPsychology & Behavior*, *3*(6), 999–1007.

Cenfetelli, R. T., & Schwarz, A. (2011). Identifying and testing the inhibitors of technology usage intentions. *Information Systems Research*, *22*(4), 808–823.

Compeau, D., Higgins, C. A., & Huff, S. (1999). Social cognitive theory and individual reactions to computing technology: A longitudinal study. *Management Information Systems Quarterly*, *23*(2), 145–158.

Connolly, S. L., Miller, C. J., Lindsay, J. A., & Bauer, M. S. (2020). A systematic review of providers' attitudes toward telemental health via videoconferencing. *Clinical Psychology: Science and Practice, Early View*, e12311. doi:10.1111/cpsp.12311

Fuertes, J. N., Gelso, C. J., Owen, J. J., & Cheng, D. (2013). Real relationship, working alliance, transference/countertransference and outcome in time-limited counseling and psychotherapy. *Counselling Psychology Quarterly*, *26*(3–4), 294–312.

Fuertes, J. N., Moore, M., & Ganley, J. (2019). Therapists' and clients' ratings of real relationship, attachment, therapist self-disclosure, and treatment progress. *Psychotherapy Research*, *29*(5), 594–606.

Gelso, C. J. (2011). *The real relationship in psychotherapy: The hidden foundation of change*. American Psychological Association.

Gelso, C. J., Kelley, F. A., Fuertes, J. N., Marmarosh, C., Holmes, S. E., Costa, C., & Hancock, G. R. (2005). Measuring the real relationship in psychotherapy: Initial validation of the therapist form. *Journal of Counseling Psychology*, *52*(4), 640–649.

Gelso, C. J., Kivlighan, D. M., Busa-Knepp, J., Spiegel, E. B., Ain, S., Hummel, A. M., … Markin, R. D. (2012). The unfolding of the real relationship and the outcome of brief psychotherapy. *Journal of Counseling Psychology*, *59*(4), 495–506.

Hatcher, R. L., & Gillaspy, J. A. (2006). Development and validation of a revised short version of the working alliance inventory. *Psychotherapy Research*, *16*(1), 12–25.

Horvath, A. O., & Greenberg, L. S. (1989). Development and validation of the working alliance inventory. *Journal of Counseling Psychology*, *36*(2), 223–233.

Liu, L., Miguel Cruz, A., Rios Rincon, A., Buttar, V., Ranson, Q., & Goertzen, D. (2015). What factors determine therapists' acceptance of new technologies for rehabilitation – A study using the Unified Theory of Acceptance and Use of Technology (UTAUT). *Disability and Rehabilitation*, *37*(5), 447–455.

Marmarosh, C. L., Gelso, C. J., Markin, R. D., Majors, R., Mallery, C., & Choi, J. (2009). The real relationship in psychotherapy: Relationships to adult attachments, working alliance, transference, and therapy outcome. *Journal of Counseling Psychology*, *56*(3), 337–350.

Mesrie, V., Diener, M. J., & Clark, A. (2018). Trainee attachment to supervisor and perceptions of novice psychotherapist counseling self-efficacy: The moderating role of level of experience. *Psychotherapy*, *55*(3), 216–221.

Morland, L. A., Mackintosh, M.-A., Rosen, C. S., Willis, E., Resick, P., Chard, K., & Frueh, B. C. (2015). Telemedicine versus in-person delivery of cognitive processing therapy for women with Posttraumatic Stress Disorder: A randomized noninferiority trial. *Depression and Anxiety*, *32*(11), 811–820.

Nissen-Lie, H. A., Monsen, J. T., Ulleberg, P., & Rønnestad, M. H. (2013). Psychotherapists' self-reports of their interpersonal functioning and difficulties in practice as predictors of patient outcome. *Psychotherapy Research*, *23*(1), 86–104.

Nissen-Lie, H. A., Rønnestad, M. H., Høglend, P. A., Havik, O. E., Solbakken, O. A., Stiles, T. C., & Monsen, J. T. (2017). Love yourself as a person, doubt yourself as a therapist?: Relationship of therapist professional and personal functioning to therapeutic outcome. *Clinical Psychology & Psychotherapy*, *24*(1), 48–60.

Norwood, C., Moghaddam, N. G., Malins, S., & Sabin-Farrell, R. (2018). Working alliance and outcome effectiveness in videoconferencing psychotherapy: A systematic review and noninferiority meta-analysis. *Clinical Psychology & Psychotherapy*, *25*(6), 797–808.

Odyniec, P., Probst, T., Margraf, J., & Willutzki, U. (2019). Psychotherapist trainees' professional self-doubt and negative personal reaction: Changes during cognitive behavioral therapy and association with patient progress. *Psychotherapy Research*, *29*(1), 123–138.

Orlinsky, D., Ambühl, H., Rønnestad, M., Davis, J., Gerin, P., Davis, M., … Northcut, T.; SPR Collaborative Research Network. (1999). Development of psychotherapists: Concepts, questions, and methods of a collaborative international study. *Psychotherapy Research*, *9*(2), 127–153.

Rees, C. S., & Stone, S. (2005). Therapeutic alliance in face-to-face versus videoconferenced psychotherapy. *Professional Psychology: Research and Practice*, *36*(6), 649–653.

Roesler, C. (2017). Tele-analysis: The use of media technology in psychotherapy and its impact on the therapeutic relationship. *Journal of Analytical Psychology*, *62*(3), 372–394.

Ruwaard, J., Schrieken, B., Schrijver, M., Broeksteeg, J., Dekker, J., Vermeulen, H., & Lange, A. (2009). Standardized web-based cognitive behavioural therapy of mild to moderate Depression: A randomized controlled trial with a long-term follow-up. *Cognitive Behaviour Therapy*, *38*(4), 206–221.

Simpson, S. (2009). Psychotherapy via videoconferencing: A review. *British Journal of Guidance & Counselling*, *37*(3), 271–286.

Stubbings, D. R., Rees, C. S., Roberts, L. D., & Kane, R. T. (2013). Comparing in-person to videoconference-based cognitive behavioral therapy for mood and anxiety disorders: Randomized controlled trial. *Journal of Medical Internet Research*, *15*(11), e258.

Sucala, M., Schnur, J. B., Brackman, E. H., Constantino, M. J., & Montgomery, G. H. (2013). Clinicians' attitudes toward therapeutic alliance in e-therapy. *The Journal of General Psychology*, *140*(4), 282–293.

Topooco, N., Riper, H., Araya, R., Berking, M., Brunn, M., Chevreul, K., … Andersson, G. (2017). Attitudes towards digital treatment for depression: A European stakeholder survey. *Internet Interventions*, *8*, 1–9.

Venkatesh, V., Morris, M. G., Davis, G. B., & Davis, F. D. (2003). User acceptance of information technology: Toward a unified view. *Management Information Systems Quarterly*, *27*(3), 425–478.

Venkatesh, V., Thong, J. Y. L., & Xu, X. (2012). Consumer acceptance and use of information technology: Extending the unified theory of acceptance and use of technology. *Management Information Systems Quarterly*, *36*(1), 157–178.

Wu, Y.-L., Tao, Y.-H., & Yang, P.-C. (2007). Using UTAUT to explore the behavior of 3G mobile communication users. *2007 IEEE International Conference on Industrial Engineering and Engineering Management*, 199–203. doi:10.1109/IEEM.2007.4419179.

When distance brings us closer: leveraging tele-psychotherapy to build deeper connection

Cory K. Chen, Nicole Nehrig, Lauren Wash, Jennifer A. Schneider, Sagiv Ashkenazi, Elana Cairo, Angel F. Guyton and Amy Palfrey

ABSTRACT

In this paper, the authors describe how patients and therapists may, paradoxically, perceive a greater sense of closeness as a result of the physical distance inherent in conducting psychotherapy over synchronous video telehealth. Case material is used to illustrate ways in which tele-psychotherapy facilitated engagement, strengthened the alliance, and created unique therapeutic opportunities that may not be possible when therapy is conducted in person. This paper aims to challenge preconceived notions about the ability to develop a strong therapeutic relationship with patients and implement lasting change through tele-psychotherapy. Implications for future clinical work are discussed, with particular consideration of the recent COVID-19 outbreak's influence on psychotherapy.

Over the last 20 years, there has been a steady increase in the use of telemental health (TMH) technologies to provide tele-psychotherapy (Frueh et al., 2000; Gros et al., 2013; Hollis et al., 2015; Monnier, Knapp, & Frueh, 2003; Richardson, Frueh, Grubaugh, Egede, & Elhai, 2009). While data is not yet available, it is likely that with the COVID-19 pandemic, the use of remote technologies to deliver psychotherapy is skyrocketing. This has been facilitated by many state boards having relaxed requirements in order to ensure that patients receive needed care during this stressful time. At the time of writing, therapists across the world are utilizing technology to maintain connection and deliver critical mental health services in the face of a global public health crisis that forces therapists and patients to remain physically apart. For many, this represents a first exposure to TMH treatment. However, some institutions, like the Veteran's Health Administration (VHA), have been increasingly utilizing TMH for the last 15 years (Deen, Godleski, & Fortney, 2012; Godleski, Darkins, & Peters, 2012; Wallace, Weeks, Wang, Lee, & Kazis, 2006; Weeks et al., 2004). In 2016, the VHA began a TMH initiative to provide treatment for Veterans in areas that did not have access to specialty mental health services (U.S. Department of Veterans Affairs [VA], 2018). Over time, the VHA significantly increased its use of TMH. During the 2019 fiscal year, more than 99,000 Veterans nationwide attended telehealth sessions at home using the VA Video Connect app, 200,000 of which were TMH appointments. (U.S. VA, 2019). VHA telemental health providers deliver a range of services including individual, couples, and group psychotherapy, psychological evaluations, and neuropsychological assessment (Chen et al., 2019; Shreck et al., 2020). There is strong evidence to suggest that TMH is an effective mode of treatment delivery for a variety of mental health conditions including post-traumatic stress disorder (PTSD), depression, anxiety, insomnia, alcohol abuse, and eating disorders with outcomes comparable to treatments delivered in person (Egede et al., 2015; Frueh, Henderson, & Myrick, 2005; Germain, Marchand, Bouchard, Drouin, & Guay, 2009; Holmqvist, Vincent, & Walsh, 2014; Luxton et al., 2016; Mitchell et al., 2008; Theberge-Lapointe et al., 2015; Wierwille, Pukay-Martin, Chard, & Klump, 2016; Yuen et al., 2013).

Despite its increasing utilization, there has been reluctance among therapists to deliver treatment via TMH. Many therapists have been deterred by the onerous process of navigating the complexities of licensure, state mandated telehealth training requirements, uncertain insurance reimbursement, risk management, and other logistical issues associated with TMH (Brooks, Turvey, & Augusterfer, 2013; Kruse et al., 2018). It is often considered an option of last resort with the assumption that in-person treatment is more effective, meaningful, or helpful to patients. Even the words used to describe TMH as "virtual" or "remote" can connote a falseness or coldness that understandably evokes hesitation and skepticism among therapists who pride themselves on their authenticity and warmth.

Critics of TMH have suggested that the physical distance between patient and therapist might contribute to a loss of perceived emotional safety for the patient. They worry that the lack of a stable containing environment, in the form of the therapist's office, can affect how patients are able to explore painful material during therapy (Argentieri & Mehler, 2003; Leffert, 2003; Russell, 2018; Scharff, 2012). Additionally, some worry that the ability to convey warmth and empathy through video technology might be curtailed (Germain, Marchand, Bouchard, Guay, & Drouin, 2010; Rees & Stone, 2005). Critics have also voiced concern that TMH may limit access to patients' verbal, non-verbal, and unconscious communications during therapy (Brahnam, 2017). Disruption in video and sound quality, coupled with the restricted view of the patient's body language, can make dynamic and introspective therapeutic work more difficult and may impede lasting change (Bayles, 2012; Essig & Russell, 2017; Gutiérrez, 2016). However, few systematic empirical studies have been done to study these concerns.

While these concerns are important to address when providing tele-psychotherapy, there has been little written about the unique ways that TMH may enhance the depth, connection, and intimacy between therapist and patient (Ehrlich, 2019). The authors serve as psychotherapists at one of the VHA's Telemental Health programs and have been providing a range of psychological services from a variety of theoretical orientations to Veterans across the country for years prior to the COVID-19 pandemic. In this paper, it is argued that, not only is the characterization of TMH as a poor substitute for in-person treatment patently false, but that for some patients TMH may open new avenues for connection and exciting possibilities for treatment not available in person. Case material is presented to illustrate these ideas for patients that have engaged in TMH. Cases have been de-identified and disguised to protect patient identities and some represent amalgamations of multiple patients seen across therapists in our program.

Significant variability exists across patients' reactions to TMH. Some of that variability may even occur within the course of a single patient's treatment. Thus, some of the ideas presented in this paper may seem contradictory, but in fact reflect the reality that aspects of TMH may foster closeness for some and create distance for others. While other papers have described the potential pitfalls of "virtual treatment," the authors focus on ways that tele-psychotherapy has deepened clinical work, broadened the range of areas explored, and facilitated the intimacy of the therapeutic relationship.

Meeting patients where they are

Tele-psychotherapy has the potential to reach patients by reducing barriers to treatment engagement. The issues that bring some patients to treatment may also interfere with their capacity to obtain the help they need. For example, a patient who has agoraphobia may be unable to leave their home to reach the therapist's office. A severely depressed patient may be overwhelmed by the effort to prepare for and travel to sessions but have the capacity to engage in a session that does not require them to leave their home. TMH may help these isolated patients ease into engaging more fully with their lives and potentially gain the skills to transition into in-person treatment, if indicated. TMH allows therapists to reach and be present for patients at moments when they feel most alone, both literally and figuratively – to "meet" patients where they are.

> "Brian," a 55-year-old, Asian American, male was seen in short-term psychodynamic treatment for severe depression that made it difficult to leave him home and regularly attend therapy. At the start of treatment, Brian tearfully expressed ambivalence about fully opening up to others, describing a fear of rejection, despite a deep longing for connection. The therapist noted the contrast between this statement and the vulnerability that the patient displayed with this disclosure. Upon reflection, Brian described being unable to imagine being as vulnerable had the treatment been in-person. As therapist and patient explored this feeling, Brian articulated fears that true closeness would expose his imagined defects and ultimately lead to rejection. Thus, for Brian, connection represented both hope and danger. The therapist's physical absence buffered that threat while maintaining the potential for new possibilities of connection. As treatment progressed, Brian experienced telehealth as a way to titrate his fears of failing to meet others' expectations. He was able to increase his ability to tolerate fears of disappointing others in the service of greater connection. He also began to translate these changes into deeper and fuller relationships outside of treatment. As termination approached, Brian reported pride in his growing ability to desire, rather than fear, closeness. As the treatment ended, he was able to describe and enjoy fantasies of meeting the therapist in person.

Similarly, some patients with severe PTSD may be triggered by travelling to the therapist's office. The intensity of their avoidance interferes with their ability to obtain the help they need. While careful not to collude with this avoidance, TMH therapists may have unique opportunities to scaffold exposures or provide skills training in ways that can help the patient better tolerate treatment. In addition to helping therapists meet patients where they are, TMH offers the opportunity for patients to take their therapists where they need to go.

> "Jen" was a 40-year-old, African American, female Veteran who presented with severe PTSD following Military Sexual Trauma (MST), as well as depression, anxiety and chronic pain. She had been socially isolated for a number of years and felt extremely triggered when travelling to the VA for appointments. Jen reported that she would never have engaged in treatment if not for telehealth. The treatment began with in-vivo exposures to decrease her social isolation. Using a tablet, Jen's therapist was able to travel with her as she engaged in these

exposures to different areas of her neighborhood. Jen's confidence and sense of self-efficacy increased such that she reported being willing to begin trauma-focused psychotherapy and a course of Cognitive Processing Therapy was initiated.

Finally, travel time, inflexible work schedules, travel costs, caregiving responsibilities, health issues, and physical disabilities may represent significant barriers to obtaining treatment, particularly for patients with fewer resources. TMH, while associated with an initial cost for the technology necessary (e.g. smart phone, computer, tablet, stable high-speed wifi, etc.), may lessen sociocultural barriers to accessing treatment as patients do not incur the repeated costs associated with traveling for in-person treatment sessions or have to navigate environments that are not accessible or perceived to be unwelcoming due to aspects of the patient's identity (e.g. gender identity, sexual orientation, race/ethnicity, etc.). These features of TMH may present both exciting opportunities and new challenges associated with engaging a population of patients that had not previously sought treatment and are underrepresented in our research literature.

Safe distances

The freedom patients experience in speaking to a therapist can be facilitated by the relative anonymity of both parties. Embarrassment, shame, and anxiety around disclosing sensitive material can be eased by the patient's trust that their words will be safely contained within the therapy space. Knowing that what they disclose will not intrude into their daily life can, for some patients, be a prerequisite for engagement. However, for patients who reside in small communities, that sense of anonymity can be severely compromised.

The stigma associated with seeing a therapist and the possibility that they may be observed entering the therapist's office by someone they know may deter some individuals from seeking help. For some patients, acquaintances, friends, or even family may work in the clinics where the patient would receive psychotherapy. Patients themselves may be medical providers or mental health professionals. The fantasy (or sometimes real possibility) that their sessions could be overheard by others serves as a significant inhibitor of the safety and trust necessary to fully engage in treatment. In these small communities, the likelihood of social circles overlapping and creating complicated dual relationships serves as an additional barrier to treatment; it may be uncomfortable for a patient to know that they will see their therapist later that day at their child's soccer game or religious services. Even those who do seek treatment in these situations may be inhibited from fully disclosing more sensitive aspects of their feelings or lives. This process can occur unconsciously as the patient's mind closes off access to these more threatening aspects of themselves. The embarrassing thought, shameful memory, or conflicted impulse never reaches the patient's awareness, thus foreclosing its exploration in the therapy room.

TMH provides access to a pool of therapists that may be hundreds of miles away thus providing a sense of anonymity and safety that would not otherwise be available. In some communities, where most people know one another, TMH may offer a relatively novel experience to feel free of the fear that what is spoken to one person will be shared with the broader community. That sense of the therapist being an "outsider" may allow patients to play with new ways of being in the treatment that would be too threatening with someone "inside" the community.

> "Andrew," a 35-year-old, White, male who worked as a lawyer in a small rural community presented with a vague sense of dissatisfaction in his relationships. He had been reluctant to seek treatment as he noted that the size of his community would make it impossible to maintain a sense of confidentiality as many of his family, friends, co-workers, and even his own clients, used the same firm for a range of services. Andrew was concerned about the stigma associated with seeing a therapist and concerned about the negative impact it might have on his reputation and livelihood.
>
> TMH to his home allowed Andrew to maintain the confidentiality he needed to engage in treatment. Once therapy began, Andrew described the impossibility of sharing all of his feelings, particularly the parts of himself that he viewed as vulnerable and weak, with his colleagues, friends, or family because of a need to maintain a professional image. Andrew's rigid investment in this image left him feeling inauthentic and alienated. His ability to be open and vulnerable with the therapist came, in part, because the therapist was viewed as distinctly outside of his world. This separation made Andrew feel safer, as the therapist could hold parts of him that did not conform to the image he presented to those around him. Having the therapist accept and hold these parts of him helped Andrew to explore and begin to integrate them into a fuller and more complete sense of self. This became a launching point from which to experiment with sharing those parts of himself with others.

Dangers of proximity

The co-location of therapist and patient in the same physical space can evoke or inhibit a range of reactions and can vary across patient and moment. As previously mentioned, one critique of tele-psychotherapy is that the absence of two physical bodies in the same space can result in a sense of alienation within the therapeutic relationship (Germain et al., 2010). For some patients, however, the proximity of another's physical body may evoke anxieties that inhibit a patient's capacities to make contact with aspects of their internal experience.

Patients who have suffered trauma may perceive themselves to be tainted or toxic in ways they worry will infect others (Boulanger, 2007). Often such patients describe fears that sharing their traumatic memories will traumatize the listener. The physical proximity of the therapist can evoke a patient's sense of themselves as a potential contagion, compelling them to quarantine damaging, shameful material contained within themselves. For these patients, the screen can serve as a psychic filter, protecting the therapist from the full brunt of the patient's imagined toxicity. One therapist described working with a Veteran with PTSD, whose index trauma involved his role as the perpetrator of domestic violence in a past relationship. The Veteran described significant shame and guilt and noted that he avoided discussing this history in past in-person treatments. The Veteran specifically described concerns about the therapist's wellbeing and noted that the distance created by the screen allowed him to feel less anxious about the impact of his words on the therapist. This allowed him to show increased vulnerability and examine his complex feelings about his history of violence and its impact. Alternatively, for some patients with trauma, proximity to the therapist can evoke fears of harm and result in an additional barrier to developing the trust and alliance necessary to engage fully in treatment (Herman, 1997). For these patients, the absence of the therapist from the physical space can add to a sense of safety, as the possibility of physical harm is reduced, allowing trust in the therapy relationship to develop more rapidly.

TMH may also increase the therapist and patient's willingness to explore intense feelings of rage. Physical distance from patients may allow therapists greater safety and freedom to explore aspects of the patient's experience that might otherwise be frightening, for the therapist, to invite into the room. One therapist noted an example of seeing a couple with a history of severe intimate partner violence. The husband made efforts to unnerve the therapist with threats regarding what would happen to the therapist and his wife if his wife decided to leave the marriage as a result of couples' therapy. Knowing that he could not physically harm her, the therapist was better able to manage her own fear which helped her set firm limits in treatment. Other patients fear that their rage will become overwhelming and dangerous. These patients are inhibited by fears of harming the therapist. The physical absence of the therapist may allow some patients to access these feelings knowing that the distance serves as protection from the patient's perceived destructiveness.

> "Mike," a 55-year-old, Latino, male Veteran was referred for long-standing depression and anxiety. He had a tendency to largely avoid his own affect and described feeling fearful of allowing himself to fully connect to the depth of his emotions. While he described feeling "numb" much of the time, he occasionally had powerful anger outbursts that frightened him.
>
> After several sessions over telehealth, Mike began describing his relationships with his family, from whom he was estranged. During one session, he began sweating and turned red when talking about his father. When he was asked to share his in vivo emotional experience, he broke down in tears and shared the rage he felt towards his parents for their estrangement from him. He was encouraged to stay with his emotions, and despite obvious discomfort, he was able to verbalize his feelings. A similar pattern happened throughout the treatment course, and over time, he became better able to identify, tolerate, and share his affect.
>
> As termination neared, Mike was asked to reflect on the treatment. He described it as his "first truly successful course of therapy" despite many previous courses of in-person treatment, and he relayed feeling a greater acceptance of himself and his emotions. He specifically attributed this to telehealth. He had previously been fearful that he would fly into a fit of rage if he let himself fully feel his emotions. In prior therapies, this worry about scaring his therapists inhibited him from showing anger. The physical distance offered by TMH allowed Mike to fully experience his rage as he worried less about the harm he might cause the therapist. The therapist also noted that the physical distance allowed her to feel safer as well, making room for greater curiosity that may have been otherwise taken up by anxiety. As a result, Mike was able to see that both he and his therapist could tolerate and survive the full depth of his affect, which facilitated decreased numbness outside of session. Over time, Mike was also able to express these feelings in more skillful ways and, during stressful times could access support from others rather than detaching and isolating himself.

The exploration of erotic feelings in the therapy can also be facilitated by TMH. While for some, the absence of the therapist's physical body in the room results in a deadening of impulses and fantasies; for others, the physical presence of the therapist may be overstimulating or dangerous as the "real" possibility of physical touch results in panic and a disconnection from these overwhelming feelings. The therapist's physical distance from the patient may allow the patient permission to explore aspects of their inner life and fantasies that they would not otherwise dare touch.

"Jonathan," a 27-year-old, White, male sought treatment for depression and longstanding social isolation. During the treatment, Jonathan disclosed details of sexual abuse by his mother during childhood as well as violence that he himself perpetrated. In the face of the shame he described experiencing, the therapist was able to retain her capacity to be supportive and warm rather than react with the judgment and criticism he feared. As the treatment progressed, Jonathan began to express feelings of warmth, affection, and desire towards the therapist – feelings that he rarely allowed himself to acknowledge. When asked about what allowed him to express these feelings, Jonathan reported that the distance created by TMH made him feel safer and more willing to both experience and share these feelings. The physical distance of TMH created a transitional space where his fears of being violated by the therapist as well as fears of rejection or criticism could be better managed. Speaking about his feelings of love towards the therapist and describing his fantasies about the relationship he wished he could have with her led to the Veteran's increasing contact with these desires that had long been too dangerous to allow into his awareness. This exploration became a starting point for deepening his connection to his desire to be cared for and challenged core beliefs that he was undeserving of this care. Over time the Veteran was able to generalize these experiences with the therapist to other relationships in his life.

Intimate spaces

The location of psychotherapy sessions can impact therapeutic intimacy. While telepsychotherapy is sometimes provided between medical institutions, it can also be delivered from the therapist's home to a patient's home. Particularly during the COVID-19 pandemic, for therapists and patients following shelter-in-place orders, this became one of the few options for continuing treatment. For both parties, video sessions provide a window into the other's private space.

What therapists see in the patient's background sometimes reveals new aspects of the patient's life. Therapists can catch glimpses (or be deliberately shown) bookshelves, artwork, family photos, or other aspects of the spaces within which our patients reside. The features of the patient's space (e.g. how disorganized, cramped, clean, etc.) provide new information about the patient's daily life in ways that patients themselves may struggle to convey or believe are insignificant. Explicit discussion of what is seen and being shown and its impact on the therapist's understanding of the patient or the therapy relationship can be critical for using this information to further the treatment and to navigate complex issues that may arise around unintended "visual disclosures." Additionally, the patient's capacity to set clear boundaries and keep others (e.g. children, older parents whom they provide care for, etc.) from intruding into the private space of the session also provides therapists with information and opportunities to empathize in ways that might not otherwise be available in the controlled environment of the therapist's office. Pets sometimes make unexpected appearances during sessions and have been observed helping patients to regulate their distress and tolerate sitting with emotions, thoughts, and memories that would otherwise have been overwhelming. Family members have also made unanticipated "intrusions" into the session. One male patient, who presented with panic disorder and complex trauma from childhood and military combat, lit up with joy when he heard his young daughter returning home a few minutes early from school. Seeing how dramatically his mood shifted in her presence opened up exploration of the meaning and significance of this relationship and furthered exploration of his childhood trauma and the ways he strove to differentiate his own parenting from what he endured.

Patients can also peek into the therapist's private space. Despite their best efforts, patients may catch unplanned glimpses of unruly pets or children in ways that, for some patients, can create a greater sense of closeness to the therapist as a real person or open up unexpected avenues of exploration. While sometimes disruptive, there are instances when these serendipitous moments precipitate responses from patients that catalyze the therapeutic work.

> "Linda," a 75-year-old, African American, woman came to treatment for longstanding PTSD symptoms connected to extensive childhood trauma. During one of her sessions, the patient could hear the therapist's daughter crying in the background. As Linda observed the therapist becoming distracted and concerned about the noises his daughter was making, Linda's eyes welled up with tears. The therapist inquired into her experience and Linda began to describe her fantasies of what she believed the therapist was like as a father, how that contrasted with her own history as a child, and how she wished to be cared for in the ways she imagined the therapist cared for his daughter. Greater access to these feelings helped Linda to connect to, reflect on, and mourn her own painful childhood and explore new possibilities for herself and her relationships in her present life.

What is possible for patients and therapists to think, feel, and do is context dependent. The characteristics of the session setting will both evoke and inhibit certain associations, memories, feelings, and actions. While some authors have expressed concerns regarding the potential "informality" that may result from tele-psychotherapy (Fleuty & Almond, 2020; Russell, 2018), the "informality" does not necessarily result in superficial or frivolous engagement. The "formality" of meeting in a professional setting, such as a medical center, may inhibit some patients' capacity for creativity and play. The less formal environment of the patient's home may open up possibilities to engage in the serious work of playing with difficult material. Furthermore, a patient speaking about the argument they had with their partner from the room where the argument occurred may allow closer connection to a range of feelings that may not be as accessible in the therapist's office. Additionally, for couples therapists delivering treatment through TMH, observing who gets up to let out the dog, subtle ways members of the couple may care for one another (e.g., getting the other a glass of water), or who handles intrusions from children can provide greater clarity around patterns of interaction that may not be easily observable in the therapist's office.

Finally, for both therapist and patient, inviting the other into a space that can be associated with intimacy and safety may help facilitate similar feelings within the therapy relationship. For some patients, travelling to the therapist's office may include enduring a range of stressors (e.g., harassment, an unsafe neighborhood, lengthy commutes, environmental triggers for those with PTSD, etc.) that cause the patient to arrive to session with defenses activated. While exploring those defenses and aspects of the patient's lived experience can be helpful, TMH may offer a method of gaining more rapid access to vulnerable or sensitive aspects of the patient's inner life that may have been closed off otherwise.

The space created by absence

Patients can react differently to the physical presence of an other. For some patients, the therapist's physical presence can help regulate the patient's emotional reactions and evoke a sense of calm and safety (Beebee & Lachman, 1988; Geller & Porges, 2014).

However, for other patients, the therapist's physical presence can be overstimulating or implicitly demanding. The physical and psychological distance created by meeting a therapist on a screen can mitigate some of these barriers to accessing the patient's feelings. For these patients, distance reduces awareness of the therapist's presence in ways that can facilitate the treatment. For example, one patient seen via TMH for eating disorder treatment spoke of her envy, rage, and shame in the presence of women whom she perceived as thin and described her pattern of immediately discontinuing treatment with providers who evoked those feelings. This patient noted that it was difficult to clearly see the therapist's body on the screen and admitted that because of that ambiguity, she was able to tolerate engaging with the therapist in treatment. Decisions around what of the therapist's body is shown and what remains ambiguous are not available in the same way for patients seen in person. If these choices are made in deliberate, thoughtful ways, they have the potential to facilitate patients' engagement.

Similarly, patients who are hyper-attuned to others and become distracted from their inner life can experience a greater sense of freedom to direct their attention to and explore themselves when not "needing to" attend to an other in the room. The utilization of TMH can serve to remove some of the therapist generated cues that inhibit free association. Additionally, for some patients who tend to make negative attributions for other's behavior, TMH may mitigate these tendencies. For example, "Mike" (described above), noted that he had been hyperaware of the body language of his prior in-person therapists, vigilantly scanning for signs that therapists were judging him. This caused Mike to prematurely end multiple treatments due to his belief that the therapist was critical and did not empathize with him. In contrast, in TMH Mike described assuming that any misunderstanding or miscommunication was a result of technical issues with sound or visual quality. This unanticipated effect of TMH contributed to Mike's ability to engage in the treatment and begin to explore the assumptions that had caused him to abruptly end other therapies.

Staying safe by connecting on video

The shared global experience of the COVID-19 pandemic serves to both isolate us and bring us together. Individuals across the world end conversations with the send-off "stay safe." Across co-workers, friends, lovers, and family, we are attempting to bridge physical distance with technology. While social distancing helps to both individually and collectively keep us safe, the virtual world has become a primary method for maintaining real connection. Therapists and patients are "in it together" in ways that make it clear that we are all "more human than otherwise." In the context of these world events, many therapists self-disclose aspects of their own fears, frustrations, and uncertainties in ways that can help to validate the patient's reality. Therapists are also forced to share (intentionally or unintentionally) aspects of their life circumstances or situation as the voices (or crying) of children can be heard in the background or school closures require navigation of childcare responsibilities that impact session scheduling. These disclosures allow some patients to see therapists more clearly and fully. For some, this can manifest in a recognition of the therapist's vulnerability and expressions of concern and care towards them. For others, this can induce rage and envy as the patient's fantasies of being the most important person to the therapist are challenged. Ultimately, this increased authenticity through awareness of a shared humanity has the potential to lead to deeper work and is only possible through the virtual connections that allow us to maintain our relationships despite the isolation imposed by the pandemic.

Conclusion and future directions

New technologies often elicit mixed reactions across people. There are those who enthusiastically adopt and excitedly tout the advantages of the novel. Some are indifferent. And there are others who express skepticism and concern about the technology's potential unforeseen implications and effects. Tele-psychotherapy certainly provokes this range of responses. Some focus entirely on its convenience and capacity to provide access to patients who desperately need help. Some observe its increasing use with apathy – unthreatened and secure in the continued need and utility of in-person treatment and largely unchanged in how they practice. Others see tele-psychotherapy as a threat to the core values of the profession, a reflection of broader problems of alienation and disconnection in society, and a harbinger of a world where technology replaces "real" human connection. Perhaps, like most tools, tele-psychotherapy contains within it a range of possibilities – the potential to be either weaponized or curative.

The therapist's mindset in approaching tele-psychotherapy has a significant impact on the experience of the dyad in the room. The therapist's apathy or fear may have a concordant impact on the treatment, deadening or paralyzing the work as tele-psychotherapy's anticipated dangers preoccupy the therapist's consciousness. While it can be easy to say that its differences from in-person treatment represent "grist for the mill," without recognition of the grains that can be productively harvested the therapist may mistake the newly nourishing for the dangerously indigestible. This paper attempts to provide therapists with a "field guide" to assist in recognizing various possibilities for how tele-psychotherapy can be used to nurture connection. It is hoped that future work will elaborate on the details of the therapeutic process, specific implications for technique, or provide a nuanced discussion of the artistry critical to the work of this mode of psychotherapy.

COVID-19 is presenting a range of new challenges for tele-psychotherapy. Many therapists have been forced to transition from in-person treatment to tele-psychotherapy and greater exploration and reflection on how therapists navigate these transitions amid the chaos would be valuable. Additionally, COVID-19 has brought with it a range of health and economic anxieties that have had significant interpersonal implications – potentially leading to greater loneliness, isolation, and/or interpersonal conflict. The too frequent experiences of loss, bereavement, and mourning, absent the typical rituals and processes used to help navigate those experiences, has been a challenge for many and must be addressed by therapists who are themselves providing support at a distance. Furthermore, while we previously discussed the shared experience of the pandemic having the potential for creating a sense of shared humanity, the impact of the pandemic varies based on ones' relative resources and privilege. While we are all attempting to weather the "same storm," we are also not in the "same boat." Those with more resources may weather the pandemic in beach homes while those who were barely making ends meet further struggle to remain afloat. These discrepancies in experience have been brought into stark relief and must also be navigated by therapists who themselves may experience a range of reactions and feelings about their greater or less degree of privilege compared to their patients. Future work that specifically attempts to examine the range of ways that tele-psychotherapy has been deployed, navigated, and leveraged to address these issues is critical. Finally, empirical research that goes beyond the question of "does it work" and moves towards examining questions of "how it impacts the treatment process," "for whom," "under what circumstances," "at what moment" have the potential to refine our ability to deploy these new approaches most effectively and with greater nuance.

Adversity demands creativity and innovation. If, as Freud suggested, helping our patients to "work and love" represent key goals of psychotherapy, the immense global economic and relational impact of the COVID-19 pandemic makes our work critical for navigating the suffering of this moment (Erikson, 1950). As therapists, we are called upon to adapt to changing needs and evolving barriers to our work and relationships with our patients. While tele-psychotherapy represents one way of bridging the gap that separates therapists and patients during this crisis, it also offers a range of new possibilities and opportunities for connection. It is critical for therapists to remain open to the frustration and mourning associated with losing our routine modes of relating. And we must also remain flexible, hopeful, and open to the potential for creative surprise and growth that comes with holding the tension between the safely familiar work our field has been engaged in for over a century with the unknown possibilities for closeness that greater space and distance may evoke.

Acknowledgments

Acknowledgement to Adam Wolkin and Seena Mathew, for their involvement in the VA NY Harbor Health Care System Telemental Health Hub implementation and ongoing support.

Disclosure statement

The authors have no conflicts of interest or financial disclosures to report.

Funding

This work was supported by funding provided by U.S. Department of Veterans Affairs (VA) Office of Rural Health (ORH). Visit www.ruralhealth.va.gov to learn more.

ORCID

Cory K. Chen http://orcid.org/0000-0002-9283-8913
Nicole Nehrig http://orcid.org/0000-0002-9495-8126
Lauren Wash http://orcid.org/0000-0002-9279-6602
Sagiv Ashkenazi http://orcid.org/0000-0003-3744-7132
Angel F. Guyton http://orcid.org/0000-0002-9759-353X

References

Argentieri, S., & Mehler, J. A. (2003). Telephone 'analysis':'Hello, who's speaking?'. *Insight, 12*(1), 17–19.

Bayles, M. (2012). Is physical proximity essential to the psychoanalytic process? An exploration through the lens of Skype. *Psychoanalytic Dialogues, 22*(5), 569–585.

Beebee, B., & Lachmann, F. (1988). The contribution of mother-infant mutual influence to the origins of self- and object representation. *Psychoanalytic Psychology, 5*(4), 305–337.

Boulanger, G. (2007). *Psychoanalysis in a New York book series. Wounded by reality: Understanding and treating adult onset trauma.* Hillsdale, NJ: Routledge.

Brahnam, S. (2017). Comparison of in-person and screen-based analysis using communication models: A first step toward the psychoanalysis of telecommunications and its noise. *Psychoanalytic Perspectives, 14*(2), 138–158.

Brooks, E., Turvey, C., & Augusterfer, E. F. (2013). Provider barriers to telemental health: Obstacles overcome, obstacles remaining. *Telemedicine and e-Health, 19*(6), 433–437.

Chen, C. K., Palfrey, A., Shreck, E., Silvestri, B., Wash, L., Nehrig, N., … Chodosh, J. (2019). Implementation of Telemental Health (TMH) psychological services for rural veterans at the VA New York Harbor Healthcare System. *Psychological Services.* doi:10.1037/ser0000323

Deen, T. L., Godleski, L., & Fortney, J. C. (2012). A description of telemental health services provided by the veteran's health administration in 2006–2010. *Psychiatric Services, 63*(11), 1131–1133.

Egede, L. E., Acierno, R., Knapp, R. G., Lejuez, C., Hernandez-Tejada, M., Payne, E. H., & Frueh, B. C. (2015). Psychotherapy for depression in older veterans via telemedicine: A randomised, open-label, non-inferiority trial. *The Lancet Psychiatry, 2*(8), 693–701.

Ehrlich, L. T. (2019). Teleanalysis: Slippery slope or rich opportunity? *Journal of the American Psychoanalytic Association, 67*(2), 249–279.

Erikson, E. (1950). *Childhood and society.* New York, NY: Norton.

Essig, T., & Russell, G. I. (2017). A note from the guest editors. *Psychoanalytic Perspectives, 14*(2), 131–137.

Fleuty, K., & Almond, M. K. (2020). Remote access therapy for veterans with psychological problems: Current state of the art. *Military Medicine.* doi:10.1093/milmed/usaa020

Frueh, B. C., Deltsch, S. E., Santos, A. B., Gold, P. B., Johnson, M. R., Meisler, N., … Ballenger, J. C. (2000). Procedural and methodological issues in telepsychiatry research and program development. *Psychiatric Services, 51*, 1522–1527.

Frueh, B. C., Henderson, S., & Myrick, H. (2005). Telehealth service delivery for persons with alcoholism. *Journal of Telemedicine and Telecare, 11*(7), 372–375.

Geller, S. M., & Porges, S. W. (2014). Therapeutic presence: Neurophysiological mechanisms mediating feeling safe in therapeutic relationships. *Journal of Psychotherapy Integration, 24*(3), 178.

Germain, V., Marchand, A., Bouchard, S., Drouin, M. S., & Guay, S. (2009). Effectiveness of cognitive behavioural therapy administered by videoconference for posttraumatic stress disorder. *Cognitive Behaviour Therapy, 38*(1), 42–53.

Germain, V., Marchand, A., Bouchard, S., Guay, S., & Drouin, M. S. (2010). Assessment of the therapeutic alliance in face-to-face or videoconference treatment for posttraumatic stress disorder. *Cyberpsychology, Behavior, and Social Networking, 13*(1), 29–35.

Godleski, L., Darkins, A., & Peters, J. (2012). Outcomes of 98,609 US department of veteran's affairs patients enrolled in telemental health services, 2006–2010. *Psychiatric Services, 63*(4), 383–385.

Gros, D. F., Morland, L. A., Greene, C. J., Acierno, R., Strachan, M., Egede, L. E., … Frueh, B. C. (2013). Delivery of evidence-based psychotherapy via video telehealth. *Journal of Psychopathology Behavioral Assessment, 35*, 506–521.

Gutiérrez, L. (2016). Silicon in "pure gold"? Theoretical contributions and observations on teleanalysis by videoconference. *The International Journal of Psychoanalysis, 98*(4). doi:10.1111/1745-8315.12612

Herman, J. L. (1997). *Trauma and recovery: The aftermath of violence—From domestic abuse to political terror.* New York, NY: Basic Books.

Hollis, C., Morriss, R., Martin, J., Amani, S., Cotton, R., Denis, M., & Lewis, S. (2015). Technological innovations in mental healthcare: Harnessing the digital revolution. *The British Journal of Psychiatry*, *206*(4), 263–265.

Holmqvist, M., Vincent, N., & Walsh, K. (2014). Web-vs telehealth-based delivery of cognitive behavioral therapy for insomnia: A randomized controlled trial. *Sleep Medicine*, *15*(2), 187–195.

Kruse, C. S., Atkins, J. M., Baker, T. D., Gonzales, E. N., Paul, J. L., & Brooks, M. (2018). Factors influencing the adoption of telemedicine for treatment of military veterans with post-traumatic stress disorder. *Journal of Rehabilitation Medicine*, *50*(5), 385–392.

Leffert, M. (2003). Analysis and psychotherapy by telephone: Twenty years of clinical experience. *Journal of the American Psychoanalytic Association*, *51*(1), 101–130.

Luxton, D. D., Pruitt, L. D., Wagner, A., Smolenski, D. J., Jenkins-Guarnieri, M. A., & Gahm, G. (2016). Home-based telebehavioral health for US military personnel and veterans with depression: A randomized controlled trial. *Journal of Consulting and Clinical Psychology*, *84*(11), 923.

Mitchell, J. E., Crosby, R. D., Wonderlich, S. A., Crow, S., Lancaster, K., Simonich, H., ... Myers, T. C. (2008). A randomized trial comparing the efficacy of cognitive–behavioral therapy for bulimia nervosa delivered via telemedicine versus face-to-face. *Behaviour Research and Therapy*, *46*(5), 581–592.

Monnier, J., Knapp, R. G., & Frueh, B. C. (2003). Recent advances in telepsychiatry: A update review. *Psychiatric Services*, *51*, 1604–1609.

Rees, C. S., & Stone, S. (2005). Therapeutic alliance in face-to-face versus videoconferenced psychotherapy. *Professional Psychology: Research and Practice*, *36*(6), 649.

Richardson, L. K., Frueh, B. C., Grubaugh, A. L., Egede, L., & Elhai, J. D. (2009). Current directions in videoconferencing tele-mental health research. *Clinical Psychology: Science and Practice*, *16*, 323–338.

Russell, G. I. (2018). *Screen relations: The limits of computer-mediated psychoanalysis and psychotherapy*. Abingdon, United Kingdom: Routledge.

Scharff, J. S. (2012). Clinical issues in analyses over the telephone and the internet. *The International Journal of Psychoanalysis*, *93*(1), 81–95.

Shreck, E., Nehrig, N., Schneider, J. A., Palfrey, A., Buckley, J., Jordan, B., ... Chen, C. K. (2020). Barriers and facilitators to implementing a US Department of Veterans Affairs Telemental Health (TMH) program for rural veterans. *Journal of Rural Mental Health*, *44*(1), 1.

Théberge-Lapointe, N., Marchand, A., Langlois, F., Gosselin, P., & Watts, S. (2015). Efficacy of a cognitive-behavioural therapy administered by videoconference for generalized anxiety disorder. *European Review of Applied Psychology*, *65*(1), 9–17.

U.S. Department of Veterans Affairs. (2018). *Telemental health in the department of veterans affairs*. Retrieved from https://www.va.gov/anywheretoanywhere/docs/TeleMental_Health_factsheet.PDF

U.S. Department of Veterans Affairs. (2019). *VA reports significant increase in Veteran use of telehealth services* [Press release]. Retrieved from https://www.va.gov/opa/pressrel/includes/viewPDF.cfm?id=5365

Wallace, A. E., Weeks, W. B., Wang, S., Lee, A. F., & Kazis, L. E. (2006). Rural and urban disparities in health-related quality of life among veterans with psychiatric disorders. *Psychiatric Services*, *57*(6), 851–856.

Weeks, W. B., Kazis, L. E., Shen, Y., Cong, Z., Ren, X. S., Miller, D., ... Perlin, J. B. (2004). Differences in health-related quality of life in rural and urban veterans. *American Journal of Public Health*, *94*(10), 1762–1767.

Wierwille, J. L., Pukay-Martin, N. D., Chard, K. M., & Klump, M. C. (2016). Effectiveness of PTSD telehealth treatment in a VA clinical sample. *Psychological Services*, *13*(4), 373.

Yuen, E. K., Herbert, J. D., Forman, E. M., Goetter, E. M., Juarascio, A. S., Rabin, S., ... Bouchard, S. (2013). Acceptance based behavior therapy for social anxiety disorder through videoconferencing. *Journal of Anxiety Disorders*, *27*(4), 389–397.

A methodology to improve eye contact in telepsychotherapy via videoconferencing with considerations for psychological distance

F. Grondin, A. M. Lomanowska, V. Békés and P. L. Jackson

ABSTRACT

Telepsychotherapy by videoconference (VC) is an effective way to treat clients over the Internet, yet therapists often report concerns that VC could affect the therapeutic relationship by hindering the perception of nonverbal behaviors such as eye contact. To date, no simple procedure describes the technical adjustments needed to compensate for the unnatural angle between the eye gaze of the participants and the webcam that is pervasive to most commercial VC systems. This article describes the steps towards a practical and inexpensive VC setup that enables eye contact between therapists and clients. Moreover, this setup allows users to choose between two camera framing conditions: a zoomed-out, head-to-waist framing or a zoomed-in, head-to-chest framing. These two setups were tested by four therapist-client dyads in simulated telepsychotherapy sessions. Participants indicated that they preferred the framing condition congruent with their desire to be "closer" or "farther" from their partner, highlighting how their perception of psychological distance was related to the degree of camera zooming in VC. The article provides recommendations for different adaptations that therapists and clients can implement to maximize their experience of telepsychotherapy by VC.

Introduction

Telepsychotherapy, also referred to as telepsychology, teletherapy, e-therapy, cybertherapy, online therapy, or e-mental health, is rapidly gaining in popularity. Using information technologies such as videoconferencing (VC), practitioners can meet clients over the Internet and provide mental health services to those in remote areas, or in areas with fewer mental health practitioners, as well as to those with reduced mobility or other physical constraints. Additionally, therapy provided through VC saves time, travel and other costs for clients, such as childcare or taking time off work, and it also permits individuals to seek help without the potential stigma of visiting a mental health facility. Providing remote therapy also lowers associated time and costs for practitioners.

Under exceptional circumstances such as the global COVID-19 pandemic, telepsychotherapy can also represent the only means of continuing therapy while complying with the public health recommendation of social distancing. Accordingly, therapists quickly recognized the necessity of using VC to provide mental health services during the pandemic and switched to using this medium with clients.

Although the benefits of continued access to therapy during a pandemic are self-evident, psychotherapists have previously expressed concerns about the efficacy of VC as a therapeutic medium (e.g., Topooco et al., 2017) and about its impersonal quality. In a recent systematic review, Connolly, Miller, Lindsay, and Bauer (2020) found that therapists often reported concerns that VC could interfere with the therapeutic relationship due to difficulties in detecting nonverbal cues, such as crying or fidgeting, signs of intoxication, as well as maintaining eye contact.

Addressing these concerns, systematic reviews and meta-analyses of telepsychotherapy by VC have shown that this modality produces similar therapeutic outcomes as comparable in-person treatment for depression, anxiety, and posttraumatic stress disorder (Backhaus et al., 2012; Hilty et al., 2013). Other systematic reviews have found that therapeutic alliance is generally as strong in VC as it is in-person (e.g., Simpson & Reid, 2014). These empirical accounts emphasize that telepsychotherapy by VC offers the possibility of effectively providing services online, while also acknowledging that many aspects of telepsychotherapy can still be optimized or enhanced to maximize therapeutic gains. These aspects include the expression and perception of emotionality in VC sessions, particularly the communication of nonverbal cues.

Nonverbal cues are a very important source of information for therapists and clients across therapeutic orientations (e.g., Foley & Gentile, 2010). Videoconferencing systems typically transmit auditory (vocal inflexions and intonations) and visual nonverbal cues (gestures, body posture, facial expressions, and eye contact) with high fidelity; however, visual cues can be altered or filtered out of VC sessions. This filtering effect can occur due to limitations in transmission quality that prevents the instantaneous communication of relevant cues as well as the framing of the video that limits how much of the body is visible (Grondin, Lomanowska, & Jackson, 2019). The filtering effect is important to consider because numerous studies show an association between these visual cues and empathy (Hall, Harrigan, & Rosenthal, 1995), the latter being a crucial factor in therapeutic success (Elliott, Bohart, Watson, & Murphy, 2018). In a study on nonverbal behaviors, eye contact has been linked to increased levels of perceived empathy, alliance and treatment credibility (Dowell & Berman, 2013). However, eye-contact is especially difficult to establish in VC as most VC systems include a deviation in the angle between the gaze target (i.e., the other person's eyes on the screen) and the webcam used to transmit one's own image (see Figure 1). The resulting "gaze angle" often creates the mutual impression of looking at each other's chin instead of each other's eyes. Users can rapidly learn to interpret this altered gaze as intended eye contact (Grayson & Monk, 2003), yet the possibility of experiencing mutual gaze is lost. This alteration in eye contact could have an impact on the unfolding of VC sessions, since eye contact can be interpreted as an indicator of the therapist's attention towards the client which is important in facilitating rapport (Leach, 2005) and client's self-awareness (Baltazar et al., 2014). Therapists and clients can elect to look directly at the webcam when they speak, but this approach does not enable the synchronous dyadic exchange of eye contact that occurs in face-to-face

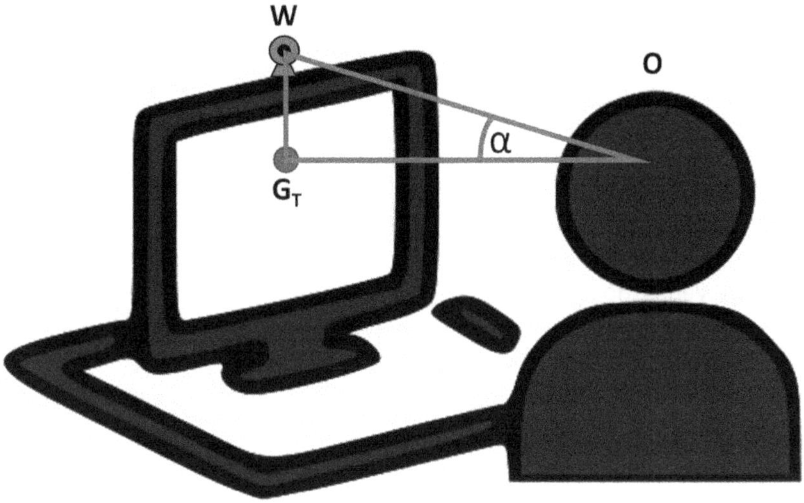

Figure 1. Schematic representation of the gaze angle, adapted from.Grondin et al. (2019)

interactions. If the therapist looks at the webcam, they cannot see the client well at the same time and can easily miss the momentary reactions of the client during the intervention (and similarly for the client). In addition, remembering to look at the webcam when speaking can incur a certain cognitive load for therapists and clients and impact the naturalness of the interaction. These challenges highlight the importance of developing technical solutions to automatically enable eye contact in VC sessions as opposed to relying on conscious behaviors such as looking directly into the webcam.

Numerous technological adaptations have been proposed to address the effect of the gaze angle on eye contact perception, particularly in the field of life-sized videoconferencing (i.e., VC systems that respect the actual physical dimensions of body parts as a function of their distance from the observer; for a review, see Regenbrecht & Langlotz, 2015). However, most of the solutions designed to this day require the use of specialized equipment (like a half-silvered glass) or advanced computational skills and software. In order to be practical and accessible for clinical practice, the solution should be simple to implement and inexpensive for both therapists and clients. It should also preserve the flow of the interaction, since using algorithms or video interpolation could increase the delay in video or sound transmission between interactants and potentially hamper the experience of therapists and clients.

To address the need for a practical and accessible solution, we devised a method that satisfies these criteria and can be quickly and effectively implemented in clinical practice. The method involves minimizing the gaze angle using commonly available webcam mounting equipment. This approach is derived from previous experimental reports that estimate that the illusion of eye contact is preserved when the gaze angle (the angle featured in Figure 1) is smaller than 7° (Chen, 2002). Deviations larger than this angle in any direction (e.g., over or beside the area of the eyes) are quickly detected. Sensitivity to a few degrees difference in the gaze angle is also supported by an experiment in telemedicine showing that 87% of participant responses attributed better eye contact to pictures taken at a 7° gaze angle compared to pictures taken at a 15° gaze angle (Tam, Cafazzo, Seto, Salenieks, & Rossos, 2007). In that study, 49 of the 53 participants (92.5%) also indicated that the difference in eye contact between the two pictures "mattered to them" as patients, with the four remaining participants indicating that they were more interested in what the clinician had to say than in achieving eye contact. In summary, despite the central importance of eye-contact to empathy (Dowell & Berman, 2013) and alliance (Duff & Bedi, 2010), no study to date has tested whether specific manipulations of eye contact had a significant impact on telepsychotherapy sessions. Moreover, although guidelines have been published by professional associations to meet with certain ethical standards associated with telepsychotherapy (American Psychological Association, 2013), the scientific literature about telepsychotherapy has yet to produce general, clinically-sound procedures for practitioners to adopt when aiming at optimizing VC sessions.

In the following sections, we elaborate on our methodology aimed at preserving eye contact in VC sessions in the context of an experimental investigation of perceptions of empathy and telepresence in simulated telepsychotherapy sessions. The methodological section describes the numerous adjustments required to sufficiently lower the gaze angle to enable eye contact. These adjustments produced two variations of setups: a zoomed-in, head-to-chest framing and a zoomed-out, head-to-waist framing. In a second phase, four therapist-client dyads completed 10-min segments under each condition of framing as part of the piloting phase of the research project. Brief interviews were conducted with both therapists and clients to determine their preferred eye contact setup. We report on their experience of these two setups and detail specific adjustments that therapists and clients can take to minimize the gaze angle beneath the documented 7° threshold while also facilitating the perception of other visual nonverbal behaviors such as posture and gestures. We end with suggestions of therapeutic practices to optimize the experience of VC sessions with clients.

Methodology

Participants

Therapists were four graduate students (one male; aged 24, 25, 26, and 29 years old) who had completed at least two years of and had invested 600 hours and above into clinical practica as part of their doctoral degree in clinical psychology. Therapists adhered to either cognitive-behavioral, psychodynamic, or an integrative approach to treatment. Because the larger research project involved meeting clients in simulated clinical interactions, therapists were instructed to explore the theme of discussion chosen by clients with attention, warmth, and openness, but refrain from doing an actual clinical intake or psychotherapy session. Therapists were compensated for their time with a research assistant contract.

Clients were four university students (one male; aged 21, 24, 25, and 25 years old) who discussed a personal theme chosen from a list (Hill, 2014, p. 19) for 20 min. For ethical purposes, clients who reported acute personal distress such as suicidal ideations were redirected towards professional mental health resources. Clients received 15 Canadian dollars to compensate for the travel costs associated with the study.

Therapists and clients did not have extensive prior experience using videoconferencing, which they all reported using casually (one call or less per week). However, they all reported frequent usage of a computer (nearly everyday, 3–5 hours a day). Ethics approval was granted by the Université Laval Ethics Committee (project number: 2017–007 phase II).

Materials

VC sessions were conducted using the software Zoom v.4.6.0 (Zoom Video Communications, Inc.) and commercial high-definition webcams (Logitech C920 S model, Logitech). The video feeds were displayed on 24″ high-definition LCD monitors. The webcams were mounted on commercial 25″ goosenecks mounts (Acetaken brand) to allow for flexibility in the adjustment of webcam positioning. Two pairs of noise-cancelling headsets were employed to limit extraneous distractions. Both rooms used for testing were well lit by fluorescent tubes and devoid of windows.

Initial setup

Based on the available literature on gaze angle and eye contact tolerance (i.e., the extent of incremental variations in gaze angle before the perception of an alteration of eye contact, which is 7° in videoconferencing interactions; Chen, 2002; Tam et al., 2007), a first setup featuring a gaze angle of around 6° was produced and tested by experimenters (Figure 2). This testing was done with the purpose of confirming firsthand the extent of

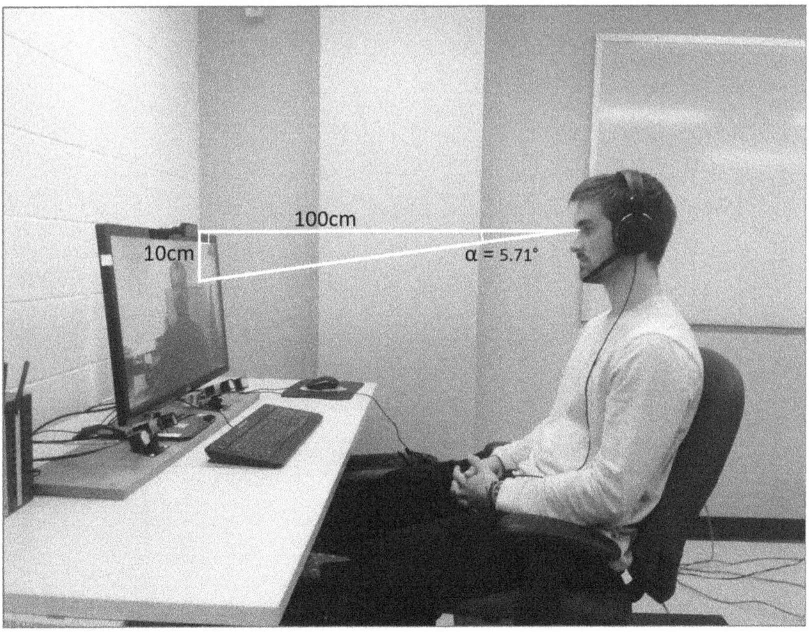

Figure 2. Initial setup to enable eye contact. Although the gaze angle (approximatively 5.71°) is within the tolerance of 7°, this setup was found to alter eye contact perception.

eye contact tolerance in VC. Experimenters on each side of the videoconferencing call sat 1 meter away from the computer monitor on top of which the webcam was mounted and centered. The distance between the webcam lens and the gaze target (the other individual's eyes on the screen) was approximatively 10 cm. Contrary to the available literature, this initial setup did not enable eye contact between individuals. The alteration of eye contact could be clearly observed when one individual was asked to gaze directly at the webcam and then back at the other individual's eyes on the monitor.

Final setup

To minimize the gaze angle, multiple steps were taken on both sides of the videoconferencing call to narrow the distance between the webcam lens and the gaze target. First, a gooseneck webcam mount was used to position the webcam upside down (Figure 3).

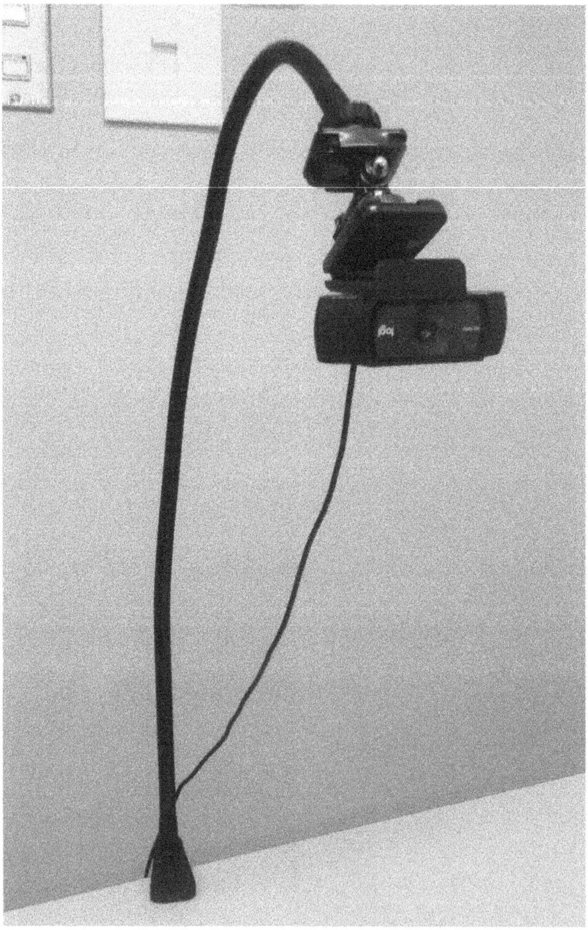

Figure 3. The gooseneck webcam mount used to lower the webcam over the edge of the monitor screen. The mount is inexpensive, easy to use, and can be locked onto the edge of a desk behind the monitor. This allows increased control over the webcam orientation and circumvents the typical limitation on downward tilting observed when the webcam is mounted directly onto the monitor.

The reason for this operation was to allow the webcam hinges to extend and lower the webcam over the monitor frame, thereby reducing the distance between the lens and the gaze target and providing better control over camera orientation. The upside-down view was then corrected using the Zoom software settings. Second, the height of the desk chair was adjusted in order to elevate the individuals' eyes to at least the level of the webcam and closer to the top of the video feed. According to our testing, if individuals sit a little higher, their eye level will be slightly over the webcam, which can further reduce the gaze angle. Finally, individuals moved 30 cm farther from the monitor and webcams were oriented slightly downwards, cropping the view of their heads at the hairline. This final setup featured a gaze angle of approximatively 2.3° (measurement error notwithstanding; see Figure 4). Experimenters who gazed back and forth between the webcam and the other individual's eyes did not observe a change in eye contact perception. The setup was thus considered to preserve eye contact in VC calls.

This final setup can accommodate two variations of camera framing obtained by using the zoom feature accessible on most webcams without interfering with eye contact. By zooming out, the framing encompasses a large portion of the individuals' body (a "head-to-waist" framing), allowing body posture and gestures to be transmitted in VC. By zooming in, a "head-to-chest" framing can be obtained, which increases the saliency of facial expressions and gaze orientation while hindering the perception of body posture and gestures. To explore how each type of camera framing is experienced by clients and therapists, a pilot study was conducted using four therapist-client dyads.

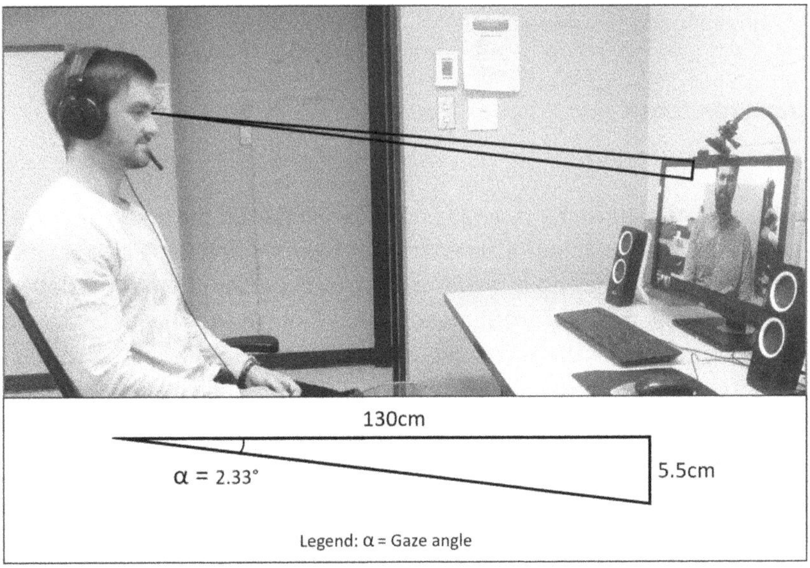

Figure 4. Final setup enabling eye contact and its measurements. Individuals are farther from the screen, sit higher in their chair, and a gooseneck webcam mount offers more flexibility in the positioning of the webcam. As shown in the figure, the individual's eyes can be positioned slightly higher than the webcam to further reduce the gaze angle. Alternatively, the individual's eyes can be lowered to the level of the webcam if the webcam is oriented slightly downwards.

Procedure

Upon their enrollment in the study, therapists and clients were paired in dyads with gender-matched therapists. Therapists and clients were greeted in separate rooms and filled their version of the consent form and the sociodemographic questionnaire. Clients were asked to choose a theme of discussion that they wanted to explore with the therapists for 20 min. Therapists and clients were informed that the session would be briefly interrupted at the 10-min mark to introduce a change in the VC session but were not informed that this change consisted of a variation in the camera framing and zoom. The order of the 10-min camera framing conditions (a head-to-waist vs a head-to-chest framing) was counterbalanced between the four dyads. In each room, experimenters logged the participants into the Zoom session and adjusted the desk chairs and the webcam orientation to enable eye contact. They also adjusted the camera zoom on each side so that participants experienced the same condition of framing at the same time. The Picture-in-Picture screen, or the miniature screen by which individuals can see themselves, was closed to avoid distracting the participants. Upon completion of the two 10-min camera framing conditions, participants (both therapists and clients) briefly met with the experimenter to discuss their experience of each camera framing condition. Specifically, the experimenter asked the following questions: "How did the session go?", "How did the session compare to usual, in-person sessions?", "What did you prefer between the 'zoomed-in' and the 'zoomed-out' condition?", and "Knowing how both conditions feel to you, would you want to make the switch from the less preferred framing to your preferred framing setting if you had the chance?". After this brief interview, participants completed other questionnaires as part of the larger research project. A debriefing concluded the experiment.

Participant feedback

Therapists

All therapists indicated having an overall positive feeling from the session and mentioned that this was their first meaningful experience of telepsychotherapy by VC. Opinions on the session ranged from having a similar feeling to in-person therapy sessions to being particularly aware that they did not share the same room as the clients. On the subject of the preferred condition, all therapists described that it impacted the perceived psychological distance with the clients, with half the therapist preferring a zoomed-in view because they felt closer to the clients. The other half indicated that they would choose the zoomed-out view because it was more reminiscent of an in-person session.

Clients

All clients mentioned that they quickly forgot about the use of the technology once engaged in the VC interaction, but reported different perceptions regarding their experience of the change of zoom in the session. The two clients who began with the zoomed-in framing reported that seeing the enlarged view of themselves on the monitor while the experimenters adjusted the desk chair and the webcam increased their level of self-consciousness, making them initially uncomfortable. These clients noted that this feeling diminished when the experimenters zoomed-out the cameras in the second half of the session. Like the therapists, they also noted that gestures and body posture were easier to see when the camera was zoomed-out, making the latter framing condition their preferred one. The two clients who began with the zoomed-out framing, on the contrary, preferred when the view was zoomed-in because they felt closer to the therapist, as if they were in the same room. They also mentioned feeling less distracted by the background in the zoomed-in condition.

Discussion

This article describes a simple procedure to enable eye contact in VC by decreasing the gaze angle down to approximatively 2.5°. This was done by asking participants to sit at 1.30 m from the computer monitor, by having the webcam positioned at eye level by adjusting the height of the desk chairs, and by angling the webcam slightly downwards, cropping the view of the participants' heads at the hairline. Although these parameters contrast somewhat with the typical VC setup, these adjustments allow users to make eye contact in VC sessions without needing expensive and complex technological systems. The described setup can be easily reproduced in telepsychotherapy sessions by therapists and clients, although it requires therapists to pre-emptively test their setup at least once before its use in actual sessions. Clients who attend to telepsychotherapy sessions in their home will also need to be guided through the steps to recreate this setup. For therapists and clients who plan on meeting multiple times over VC, setting up the equipment to enable eye contact is worth the effort since it would alleviate concerns regarding the perception of nonverbal behaviors (Connolly et al., 2020).

This article contributes directly to clinical practice by bridging the gap between experimental research surrounding eye contact in VC and clinical needs. However, the contribution of eye contact in telepsychotherapy sessions needs to be investigated further before recommending this setup for all clients in all situations. For example, eye contact can influence emotion attribution and perception of approachability, dominance, and pleasantness depending on cultural norms (Akechi et al., 2013). In comparison, VC systems which do not enable eye contact could allow users to look at the face on the monitor for a prolonged period of time without contravening social norms. Therapists are therefore encouraged to take these aspects into account when considering the possibility of enabling eye contact in VC sessions.

The procedure described in this study assumes therapists and clients have access to a desktop computer, a webcam, and a large enough monitor (22″ or more) to be able to stand farther from the screen and still easily see the other person's face and body on the monitor. Laptop users are likely to face some challenges when attempting to enable eye contact since their monitor is smaller but also because the webcam is merged into the laptop screen. This characteristic of laptops makes it awkward to elevate and then crop the video feed by tilting the screen since the laptop keyboard partly obstructs the view of the screen. Ideally, laptop computers should be placed on an inclined plane such as a cooler stand or a binder (Figure 5). The laptop screen could then be tilted to crop the view of the head above the hairline, therefor emulating the procedure for desktop computers. However, this setup has yet to be thoroughly tested across laptop dimensions and types of inclined planes to properly ascertain the desired configuration.

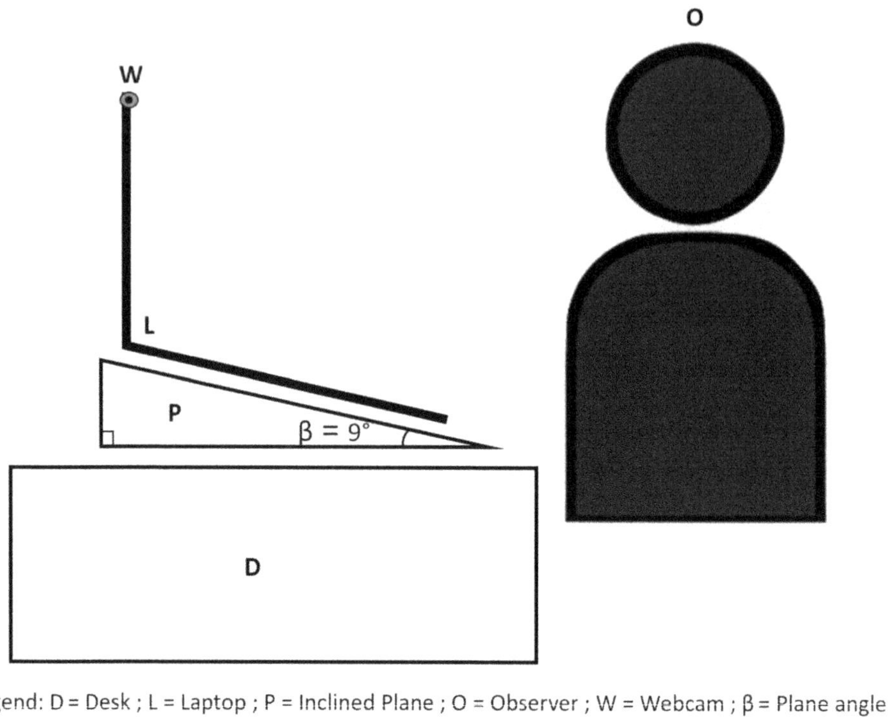

Figure 5. Schematic representation of the setup enabling eye contact when a laptop computer is used. An inclined plane of approximatively 9° is employed to bring the laptop camera closer to eye level. The screen is tilted back slightly until the head of the observer is seen on the screen. This adjustment results in the laptop being close to 90° in relation to the desk surface.

Participant feedback

Participant feedback regarding their VC session experience demonstrates that the choice of a certain camera framing (and zoom) was related to the desired psychological distance for both clients and therapists, with some therapists and clients feeling uncomfortable when the view was zoomed-in. Zooming-in when also enabling eye contact could have induced an uncomfortable level of self-awareness in therapists and clients (Baltazar et al., 2014), highlighting the importance of inquiring about a client's preference regarding zoom and framing in order to reach a satisfying setup for both parties.

When asked about their perception of the session, all therapists and clients indicated having a positive feeling of the session. While these results provide encouraging indications that VC sessions are overall appreciated by therapists and clients, there exists the possibility that participants, and more specifically therapists, could have answered more positively due to a social desirability bias. Such a bias could have arisen from the context of the interview, where therapists could have refrained from offering negative feedback during the piloting phase knowing that they are expected to conduct more sessions once the research project enters the actual recruitment phase. In addition, therapists shared the same graduate program as the first author (i.e., a doctoral degree in clinical psychology), which could have elicited a positivity bias in the responses to the interview.

Table 1. List of recommendations on materials, VC setup, and preparation for both therapists and clients to optimize telepsychotherapy sessions.

Materials (for each individual):

- A desktop computer able to easily run VC calls
- A large, high definition computer monitor (22" and more)
- A high definition webcam with good zooming capabilities
- An adjustable webcam mount
- An adjustable desk chair
- A noise-cancelling headset with microphone, with at least 6 foot of wire
- A desktop lamp to adjust lighting, if desired
- A stable high-speed Internet connexion
- Access to a free or paid secured subscription to a videoconferencing software for confidentiality and data security purposes
- An up-to-date antivirus software

VC Setup

Instructions to initially configure the setup:

(1) Affix the webcam to the adjustable mount and ensure the webcam can be lowered over the edge of the computer monitor. In some cases, this can require buying a gooseneck webcam mount and reversing the webcam as pictured in Figures 3 and 4. Use the VC software settings to reverse the image back to the appropriate orientation.
(2) Place yourself at approximatively 130 cm away from the computer monitor. You can draw marks on the floor using tape to easily realign yourself in-session.
(3) Adjust the height of your desk chair until your eyes are level with the webcam.
(4) By going into the VC software, enable self-view and expand the picture to easily see yourself when you're sitting away from the monitor.
(5) Adjust the orientation of the webcam in order to crop out the view at your hairline.
(6) When zooming in and out in the VC software, you should be able to produce any camera framing from a zoomed-out, head-to-waist framing when sitting away from the monitor to a zoomed-in, head-to-chest framing.
(7) The Picture-in-Picture screen can be turned off to avoid being distracted during the session.
(8) Maximize the viewing window so it fills the entire monitor.

Preparations going into a VC session:

- Make sure the room is well lit. However, avoid overexposing the webcam by sitting in front of a window during the day.
- Physical environments on both sides of the VC call should be secluded and devoid of noise. Likewise, precautions should be taken to avoid other individuals coming into the room during the session.
- Sources of off-screen distractions (such as cellphones) should be limited as would be expected in an in-person therapy setting.
- Sources of on-screen distractions should also be limited (e.g., auto notifications shut off, browser tabs closed, etc.)

Another interesting observation derived from the interviews was that every therapist and client preferred the second framing condition (used in the second 10-min segment of the 20-min session), regardless of the actual framing condition. Although these findings could be due to chance or to the progress of the conversation bringing participants closer in the second 10-min segment, these results could also derive from the fact that each framing condition facilitates the perception of some nonverbal cues at the expense of others: a zoomed-in view of the face increases the saliency of facial expressions and eye gaze but limits the perception of gestures and posture, and vice-versa. From the perspective of therapists and clients, changing the framing mid-session would provide the "missing" piece to the interaction and would therefore be perceived as preferable over the first framing condition.

Future studies should build upon the methodology described here to test the effect of eye contact on the perception of clinically relevant factors such as empathy and alliance. Eye contact has been associated with higher perceptions of empathy (Deladisma et al., 2007; Dowell & Berman, 2013) and thus enabling eye contact in VC sessions could contribute to optimizing the experience of empathy in teletreatments (Grondin et al., 2019). A replication of this study in actual telepsychotherapy sessions instead of simulations would enhance the generalization of the present results to broad clinical practice.

As an ending note, we present a set of recommendations on materials, VC setup, and room preparation that can benefit any teletreament conducted via VC (Table 1). These recommendations should be heeded by both therapists and clients for optimal efficacy.

Acknowledgments

This project was funded by a research grant from Natural Sciences and Engineering Research Council of Canada (Award number: RGPIN 341631-2013).

F.G. is the recipient of a graduate scholarship from the Social Sciences and Humanities Research Council (SSHRC) of Canada and from the Fonds de recherche du Québec – Nature et technologies (FRQNT). The authors would also like to thank Geneviève Belleville, Stéphane Bouchard, Marc-Antoine Linteau, Laetitia Reduron, and Vincent Poiré for their help and their comments on the project.

Disclosure statement

No potential conflict of interest was reported by the authors.

Funding

This work was supported by the Natural Sciences and Engineering Research Council of Canada [RGPIN 341631-2013].

ORCID

F. Grondin http://orcid.org/0000-0002-1290-9102
A. M. Lomanowska http://orcid.org/0000-0003-0847-6153
V. Békés http://orcid.org/0000-0003-3043-5155
P. L. Jackson http://orcid.org/0000-0001-8991-3217

Prior dissemination

These results were not presented elsewhere prior to the submission.

References

Akechi, H., Senju, A., Uibo, H., Kikuchi, Y., Hasegawa, T., & Hietanen, J. K. (2013). Attention to eye contact in the West and East: Autonomic responses and evaluative ratings. *PLoS One*, *8*, 3.

American Psychological Association. (2013). Guidelines for the practice of telepsychology. *The American Psychologist*, *68*(9), 791–800.

Backhaus, A., Agha, Z., Maglione, M. L., Repp, A., Ross, B., Zuest, D., & Rice-Thorp, N. M. (2012). Videoconferencing psychotherapy: A systematic review. *Psychological Services*, *9*(2), 111–131.

Baltazar, M., Hazem, N., Vilarem, E., Beaucousin, V., Picq, J. L., & Conty, L. (2014). Eye contact elicits bodily self-awareness in human adults. *Cognition*, *133*(1), 120–127.

Chen, M. (2002). Leveraging the asymmetric sensitivity of eye contact for videoconferencing. *SIGCHI Conference on Human Factors in Computing Systems*, Minneapolis, MN. doi:10.1145/503376.503386

Connolly, S. L., Miller, C. J., Lindsay, J. A., & Bauer, M. S. (2020). A systematic review of providers' attitudes toward telemental health via videoconferencing. *Clinical Psychology: Science and Practice*, e12311. doi:10.1111/cpsp.12311

Deladisma, A. M., Cohen, M., Stevens, A., Wagner, P., Lok, B., Bernard, T., . . . Lind, S. (2007). Do medical students respond empathetically to a virtual patient? *The American Journal of Surgery*, *193*(6), 756–760.

Dowell, N. M., & Berman, J. S. (2013). Therapist nonverbal behavior and perceptions of empathy, alliance, and treatment credibility. *Journal of Psychotherapy Integration*, *23*(2), 158.

Duff, C. T., & Bedi, R. P. (2010). Counsellor behaviours that predict therapeutic alliance: From the client's perspective. *Counselling Psychology Quarterly*, *23*(1), 91–110.

Elliott, R., Bohart, A. C., Watson, J. C., & Murphy, D. (2018). Therapist empathy and client outcome: An updated meta-analysis. *Psychotherapy*, *55*(4), 399–410.

Foley, G. N., & Gentile, J. P. (2010). Nonverbal communication in psychotherapy. *Psychiatry (Edgemont)*, *7*(6), 38–44.

Grayson, D. M., & Monk, A. F. (2003). Are you looking at me? Eye contact and desktop video conferencing. *ACM Transactions on Computer-Human Interaction (TOCHI)*, *10*(3), 221–243.

Grondin, F., Lomanowska, A. M., & Jackson, P. L. (2019). Empathy in computer-mediated interactions: A conceptual framework for research and clinical practice. *Clinical Psychology: Science and Practice*, *26*(4), e12298.

Hall, J. A., Harrigan, J. A., & Rosenthal, R. (1995). Nonverbal behavior in clinician-patient interaction. *Applied & Preventive Psychology*, *4*, 21–37.

Hill, C. E. (2014). *Helping skills: Facilitating exploration, insight, and action* (Fourth Ed.). Washington, DC: American Psychological Association.

Hilty, D. M., Ferrer, D. C., Parish, M. B., Johnston, B., Callahan, E. J., & Yellowlees, P. M. (2013). The effectiveness of telemental health: A 2013 review. *Telemedecine and e-Health,16*(6), 444–454. doi:10.1089/tmj.2013.0075

Leach, M. J. (2005). Rapport: A key to treatment success. *Complementary Therapies in Clinical Practice, 11*(4), 262–265.

Regenbrecht, H., & Langlotz, T. (2015). Mutual gaze support in videoconferencing reviewed. *Communications of the Association for Information Systems, 37*(1), 965–989.

Simpson, S. G., & Reid, C. L. (2014). Therapeutic alliance in videoconferencing psychotherapy: A review. *Australian Journal of Rural Health, 22*(6), 280–299.

Tam, T., Cafazzo, J. A., Seto, E., Salenieks, M. E., & Rossos, P. G. (2007). Perception of eye contact in video teleconsultation. *Journal of Telemedicine and Telecare, 13*(1), 35–39.

Topooco, N., Riper, H., Araya, R., Berking, M., Brunn, M., Chevreul, K., … Andersson, G. (2017). Attitudes towards digital treatment for depression : A European stakeholder survey. *Internet Interventions, 8*, 1–9.

Let's face it: video conferencing psychotherapy requires the extensive use of ostensive cues

Shimrit Fisher, Timur Guralnik, Peter Fonagy and Sigal Zilcha-Mano

ABSTRACT
The COVID-19 crisis has required many therapists to switch to video conferencing psychotherapy (VCP). Knowledge about the importance of epistemic trust and its determinants has been accumulating over the last few years, with important implications for psychotherapy and specific significance for the transition to VCP. The present paper provides a brief background on the concept of epistemic trust, research on the determinants of its development and the integrative framework it provides for some traditional concepts in psychotherapy, such as the therapeutic alliance. In particular, research on ostensive cuing, which requires significant modification in a remote delivery context, has important implications in the transition to VCP. We will advance some suggestions while illustrating the ideas with clinical case studies. This knowledge may be of value to psychotherapists, who are required to make substantial changes in the nature of the encounter with their patients, and may help them identify benefits and hindrances that might arise from this transition, as well as pointing out techniques that may encourage effective adaptation to the change.

The present paper was written as the COVID-19 outbreak raged worldwide, forcing many healthcare professionals and their patients to shift to remote therapeutic encounters. This paper proposes guidelines for making the transition from face-to-face therapeutic sessions to videoconferencing psychotherapy (VCP). The proposed guidelines are based on the theoretical framework of epistemic trust (ET), which has important implications for the aims and conduct of psychotherapy (Fonagy, Luyten, Allison, & Campbell, 2019). We argue that ET can be instrumental in facilitating the transition to VCP. Although many remote therapy platforms can be used, including emails, phone calls, on-line self-help modules, etc., (cf. Andersson et al., 2012; Johansson et al., 2012; King, Brooner, Peirce, Kolodner, & Kidorf, 2014; Kingsley & Henning, 2015), the present paper focuses on VCP, a live synchronized conversation in which two parties can hear and see each other (Backhaus et al., 2012). The guidelines proposed in this paper for making the transition to VCP can be applied to any situation in which therapists and their patients are required to switch to remote sessions, as may be the case following relocation of one of the parties, injury that restricts movement or requires confinement in the home, meetings during long vacations, and more.

The establishment of epistemic trust

Epistemic trust (ET) is defined as openness to acquiring social knowledge that is regarded as personally relevant and of generalizable significance (Bo, Sharp, Fonagy, & Kongerslev, 2017; Fonagy & Allison, 2014; Luyten, Campbell, & Fonagy, 2019). When new (social) information is regarded as personally relevant, one might consider permanently accommodating it, thus changing or elaborating some information already stored. A general predisposition to ET is developed throughout social interactions, beginning early in life, including the infant's experiences with their primary caregivers. Infants are generally open to receiving social communications, especially from their primary caregivers, but are also biologically predisposed to be epistemically vigilant (Fonagy & Allison, 2014; Fonagy, Campbell, & Bateman, 2017). Epistemic vigilance refers to the ability to be justifiably suspicious about socially transmitted information, in a manner that helps protect one against potentially deceitful or erroneous information (Fonagy & Allison, 2014; Sperber et al., 2010). The ability to selectively prioritize vigilance or trust, depending on the circumstances, will allow individuals to flexibly adapt to the social environment in which they live (Fonagy et al., 2019). When faced with an ambiguous situation, infants appropriately seek an available adult. Depending on the adult's signals, the infant judges whether to approach the situation or to avoid it (Campos & Stenberg, 1981; Camras & Sachs, 1991). More recently, developmentalists identified signals such as eye contact, baby talk, turn-taking contingent discourse, calling an infant by name, and marked mirroring of the infant as cues often used by the adult to indicate that new, specific, and relevant information is being conveyed (Egyed, Király, & Gergely, 2013; Gergely, 2013; Gergely & Csibra, 2005; Gergely, Egyed, & Kiraly, 2007). It has been suggested that these signals, referred to as *ostensive cues*, play a key role in triggering a pedagogic (learning) stance in the infant (Gergely, 2013). Ostensive cues typically lead the recipient to feel recognized as a subject (Fonagy & Allison, 2014); therefore, they reinforce the recipients' capacity to benefit from positive influences in their environment and encourage faster knowledge acquisition (Luyten, Campbell, Allison, & Fonagy, 2020). Such positive signals increase the likelihood that the information delivered is accepted and generalized to other circumstances or interactions (Schröder-Pfeifer, Talia, Volkert, & Taubner, 2018).

By contrast, when the infant's early environment is characterized by unreliable communications, the establishment of ET can become compromised. The individual's capacity to move flexibly between a stance of epistemic vigilance and ET is weakened. The consequences may be both an absence of appropriate openness to social learning or excessive credulity and inappropriate trust in unreliable informants. The compromised capacity to know when to trust and whom to trust might significantly distort interpersonal functioning. For example, children with histories of adversity may become limited in their ability to update their knowledge and understanding of social situations, and appear inflexible or even rigid in the face of rapid social change (Fonagy et al., 2019).

ET determinants in development throughout life

Children who have established a predisposition to ET, as opposed to those who have not, may demonstrate distinct developmental trajectories that may result in differing capacities to function in social and interpersonal contexts as adults. Those who successfully established ET as children are likely to be able to modify their inner position safely in the

Table 1. Examples of the ET markers sorted by the two categories of state-like vs trait-like.

State		Trait	
High	Low	High	Low
"I gradually shared more, and I said to myself – well this is a really good opportunity to stop pretending and start telling and sharing.";	"I tried to talk with my husband, but I could tell right away that he is not interested in listening to me.";	"I felt that sharing was inevitable in some way, because that's how I grew up and that's how I got used to it.";	"I don't think I have anyone in my life that I feel comfortable enough to really share openly with.";
"At the beginning I thought it's all fine. But after talking to the other student I felt a little uncertain. I started to think that maybe it's not all fine, maybe there is a bigger problem that I miss out here."	"I talked to him about that and he immediately made all kind of suggestions. But it was all rubbish! All those solutions didn't help, it only made things worse."	"I am trying to think about it . . . after talking to my wife I always ask myself if there is anything new that I didn't think of before."	"This is wrong. I can't relate to anything that you are saying, and I will not consider it. This thing is of great importance to my family, it has always been. I won't change the way I see it."

light of new information or experiences as adults (Fonagy, Luyten, Allison, & Campbell, 2018). As adults, they tend to be curious about outside information and have a tendency to use interpersonal interactions as an opportunity for learning. Because they are open to learning about themselves and others, they can make sure that communication remains advantageous for them by maintaining appropriate degrees of vigilance (Sperber et al., 2010). In contrast, in the absence of ET, the capacity to change diminishes or becomes excessive (Fonagy et al., 2018); hence, individuals may find it difficult to downregulate their natural vigilance, meaning that they cannot accept valuable new information, or, at the opposite extreme, respond with epistemic credulity and believe and accommodate information from untrustworthy informants (Luyten et al., 2019).

In either case, the strategy is fixed and not malleable to the current context. Thus, new information is not retained in the person's knowledge structure; it is not generalized to other settings, even if it is temporarily accepted as true. This rigidity dictates that individuals rely on the same models of relating to the self and others, even in an environment that may be rapidly changing (Luyten et al., 2019). This perspective on the development of ET over the course of life eventually creates a relatively stable behavioral pattern, which can be viewed as a trait-like characteristic of the individual. We have started to develop a framework for identifying high and low ET individuals, based on close textual study of their narratives in therapy. Table 1 (appendix) includes statements taken from actual therapies that may serve to illustrate all four categories of utterances.

Applications in psychotherapy

Although the process of establishing ET originates in early social relationships, it is subjected to other influences throughout life (Luyten et al., 2020), including those of teachers, peers, and even social media. Psychotherapists may also nurture (or hinder) the further development of ET. According to this theoretical conceptualization, a meaningful outcome or therapeutic change is possible only if the patient can use the therapy in a positive way (Fonagy & Allison, 2014). To allow this to happen, the therapy must be sufficiently supportive and facilitate state-like improvements in ET over the course of treatment. Even more importantly in this context, ET is seen as a valid goal of therapy that may enable an individual to change their long-term attitudes towards others in their social network, and move their approach to relationships from one of epistemic mistrust and an incapacity to adapt, to one of trust, flexibility and an extended capacity to be influenced by a social network.

Given their distinct developmental trajectories, different patients may enter treatment with a distinct trait-like tendency to consider the information offered by the therapist as relevant to them, and to remember, retain and readily generalize it to other social contexts. Patients who demonstrate high trait-like ET are skilled in learning new and useful information about themselves. These individuals are willing to openly share their feelings, thoughts, and experiences with the therapist. They are curious and inclined to learn from therapy, assuming that the therapist's intentions are beneficent, or at least benign. The willingness to share and learn enables both the therapist and the patient to seek, to understand, and to elaborate on one another's perspective, resulting in a strong alliance. Since implicit personal narratives may be more accessible for these individuals, therapeutic change becomes possible when the therapist recognizes and articulates their more nuanced self-experience, which emerges out of the primary content they share (Fonagy et al., 2019).

Some patients, however, begin therapy with low trait-like ET and may find it challenging to experience ET even when their personal narrative is appreciated (Fonagy et al., 2019). Their difficulty in reaching an agreement with their therapist stems from the fact that they distort the way others represent them, causing them to feel perpetually misunderstood and resulting in a poor alliance with the therapist. Interventions with epistemically mistrusting patients are, therefore, likely to be ineffective, unless the task of recognizing and jointly considering the subjective experience of the patient is achieved. Such recognition enables a shift in the direction of the general restoration of epistemic trust, which opens up the mind of the individual to benefitting from the routine sharing of social information within their social network; it encourages the patient to learn about themselves and others and update and adjust their knowledge structures, enabling improved functioning in the social world (Fonagy et al., 2019).

The transition to VCP

Experienced therapists are somewhat undecided about the efficacy of videoconferencing psychotherapy (VCP) compared to face-to-face psychotherapy (Simpson & Reid, 2014; Vincent, Barnett, Killpack, Sehgal, & Swinden, 2017), but psychotherapy trials seem to show similar efficacy for both intervention modes (Backhaus et al., 2012; Norwood, Moghaddam, Malins, & Sabin-Farrell, 2018). Randomized control trials (RCTs) show that VCP is equally effective as face-to-face psychotherapy in terms of patient satisfaction (Backhaus et al., 2012; King et al., 2014; Kingsley & Henning, 2015; Simpson & Reid, 2014), therapeutic alliance (Backhaus et al., 2012; Simpson & Reid, 2014), overall treatment outcome (Kingsley & Henning, 2015; Sucala et al., 2012), and improvement judged in terms of target symptoms (Backhaus et al., 2012). These promising effects of VCP have been found in the treatment of a variety of mental health disorders, such as depression (Backhaus et al., 2012; Berryhill et al., 2019; Chavooshi, Mohammadkhani, & Dolatshahi, 2016), anxiety and stress-related disorders (Backhaus et al., 2012; Chavooshi et al., 2016), pain and physical problems (Backhaus et al., 2012; Chavooshi et al., 2016), and addictions

(Backhaus et al., 2012; King et al., 2014). It has been suggested that, with appropriate training and knowledge, practitioners with little experience in VCP can adapt their communication style and adjust to the technology (Simpson & Reid, 2014). The literature suggests guidelines for instructing practitioners through the transition to VCP, including ethical considerations and concrete issues related to the treatment settings and boundaries, for both traditional dynamic psychotherapy (Scharff, 2018), and protocol-based interventions (Backhaus et al., 2012; Chavooshi et al., 2016).

Distinguishing reaction to the transition to VCP by ET trait-like characteristics

The literature on epistemic trust provides therapists with a theoretical framework to identify the patient's needs and to tailor the therapeutic techniques used in the treatment of such needs. Consistent with recent developments in psychotherapy research (Zilcha-Mano, 2018), a distinction between trait-like characteristics (individual differences between patients) and state-like changes (improvements occurring within the patient over the course of treatment) seems to be an important key in understanding how psychotherapy works, and how changes might occur in the wake of intervention (Zilcha-Mano, 2020). Drawing on our clinical experience and based on our work in the psychotherapy lab, we propose that the construct of ET can be considered as comprising these two distinct components. We have started to develop a framework for identifying high- and low-ET individuals, based on close textual study of their narratives in therapy. We found this process surprisingly easy and are in the process of formalizing this distinction into a coding system which can be reliably used with therapeutic texts from a range of therapeutic modalities.

Transition to VCP requires a stance of willingness to change flexibly to adapt to a changed external reality, and a sense that such a transition is, or will be, of personal benefit, even if this is not entirely clear at first. Patients whose life trajectories brought them to mistrust social information conveyed by others are likely to mistrust the therapist as well. Bringing such a tendency to the transition from face-to-face therapy to VCP, these patients may question the true intentions of the therapist in inviting them to make such a transition together, and there is a risk that they may attribute malicious intentions to the therapist's invitation. For example, a patient might say: "You know it doesn't suit me, you know I can't meet in video and if that's the only choice, it means we can't meet at all. You don't want to meet me, do you? This is simply your way to bring this treatment to an end." Although these patients may agree to give it a try, they are likely to expect disappointment, much like their original feeling concerning face-to-face therapy. This may result in severe ruptures in the alliance (Safran & Muran, 1996, 2000; Safran, Muran, & Eubanks-Carter, 2011), which may place the therapeutic relationship at risk and jeopardize the patient's ability to benefit from treatment, or even to remain in treatment. These patients may dismiss the therapist's efforts at reaching out, drop out of therapy, and question the future feasibility of therapy.

In contrast to patients with low trait-like ET, patients who show high trait-like ET find it is easier to make the transition to VCP. Over their life trajectory, these individuals have come to learn how to feel safe in the presence of a trustworthy person and may perceive the transition to VCP as an opportunity to learn about themselves and the way they function in a different social context. Transitioning from face-to-face therapy to VCP with openness to learn, they may find additional motivation to explore the medium, to find new methods that make it easier to share their feelings, thoughts, and experiences with the therapist, and connect with the therapist so they are able to feel mirrored and understood, even if the two are divided by a screen. This may result in a renewed and strengthened alliance that reflects the shared journey of transition as a collaborative process that may enhance the patient's potential to make beneficial use of the therapy.

Guideline for an effective intervention

Based on the ET literature and the various manifestations of high vs. low trait-like levels of ET, it is possible to derive a few tentative guidelines for making the transition to VCP. It has been suggested that ostensive cues are key indicators used in the context of a therapeutic process to revive or preserve ET (Fonagy et al., 2019). Ostensive cues signal to the patients that personally relevant information is being conveyed by the therapist. These may help them in the current context to adjust to the change to VCP. Below, we detail several suggestions of techniques for guiding therapists in the use of ostensive cues during transition to VCP.

(1) Ostensive cues as physical signals. As the transition to VCP can be challenging for both therapist and patient, physical signals must be emphasized to support its effectiveness. Therapists can use physical ostensive cues in a variety of ways, based on different modalities: facial expressions like raising eyebrows or showing marked surprise; body gestures and mannerisms, like sitting straight and leaning forward; maintaining eye contact continuously; exaggerating voice intonation or making marked changes in tone; and being meticulous in turn-taking by waiting for the patient to finish speaking and pause before beginning to speak. An example from a therapy session demonstrates how such ostensive cues can be used. The patient and therapist had to transition to VCP because of the COVID-19 epidemic, after having worked face to face for several months. At the first VCP session, the patient was talking about a fight she had with her coworker, which was very frustrating for her. When she described how "annoying" and inconsiderate her colleague was towards her, the therapist contracted his eyebrows (reflecting the patient's possible anger or frustration), rolled his eyes, and groaned out loud (expressing the patients' possible dissatisfaction). The patient then said: "Oh, I knew you would understand me! Isn't it nerve-racking?". Successfully projecting the feeling of being accurately mirrored and understood potentially sets the stage and prepares patients for learning new and useful information about themselves.

(2) Ostensive cues as identifying the patients' personal narrative. The patient's personal narrative is part of the construct of identity and is operationalized as a way of understanding oneself and others at a specific moment in time in relation to the world, in the past and the present (Fonagy et al., 2019). When the therapist recognizes and articulates the patients' more nuanced self-experience, which emerges from the primary content, shared intentionality is achieved. Maintaining continuity in the patients' personal narrative, bridging to

something that was identified before the transition and articulated during the VCP session serves as an ostensive cue. Its articulation during a VCP session in the same way as it was articulated in face-to-face sessions emphasizes its personal relevance. Thus, the therapist may use bridging statements that deliberately make the connection between themes that were processed previously in the face-to-face encounter. For example, the therapist may use phrases like "It's like we talked about a few weeks ago" or "This sounds to me quite similar to that incident you told me about when we met face-to-face." This modality of ostensive cueing helps patients experience themselves as being understood contiguously across settings, making them inclined to learn from the therapist.

(3) Ostensive cues as a direct reference to the change in setting. A variety of responses can be anticipated in the transition to VCP of patients with high vs. low trait-like ET, from an inquisitive stance to a vigilant and more skeptical one. The therapists should be sensitive to the individual response of the patient and refer directly to the change in setting in a way that is tailored for the specific patient. The therapist may invite the patient to explore feelings, thoughts and perceptions that arise from the transition to VCP, and work through them in a way that fits the needs and characteristics of the given patient. Given that the transition is a dyadic change, rather than an individual process, exploring its meaning for oneself together with the therapist can help the patient feel protected by the shared reality, and the therapy can again be a safe and low-arousal environment (Fonagy et al., 2019). The therapist should use plural pronouns when articulating the shared experience, like "This is all very new for us" or "I was wondering how it would be for us to meet this way." This technique may enhance the capacity of patients to regulate their affect through someone else, which is one of the building blocks of human self-organization (Fonagy & Target, 1997) and signals a restoration of ET. The objective is for the patient to apply the new regulation skills to other contexts.

Tailoring the intervention

The techniques described above are important for patients with either high or low trait-like ET. Nevertheless, they should be prioritized somewhat differently according to the patient's ET trait-like characteristics to achieve state-like changes. For patients with high trait-like ET, who tend to be easy to reach, the preferred ostensive cue is identifying their personal narrative. Their curiosity about the social environment and willingness to see the transition to VCP as an opportunity to elaborate their internal working model enables learning. One patient with high trait-like ET said at the beginning of the first VCP session, somewhat jokingly, "I guess this is a whole new way to see myself! And you know what? I look different than I expected. I kind of like this new perspective." Ostensive cues directly referencing the change in the setting work efficiently for such patients. They enjoy moments of mutuality with the therapist, feeling that they are safe together. Although physical ostensive cues are important in any human interaction, with patients with high trait-like ET, these are assumed to be less required.

Work with patients with high ET is demonstrated below, using a case study from an ongoing psychotherapy trial, in which patients diagnosed with Major Depressive Disorder receive 16 sessions of short-term psychodynamic treatment with either a supportive or an expressive focus. A detailed protocol of the trial appears elsewhere (Zilcha-Mano, Dolev, Leibovich, & Barber, 2018). The study was approved by the institutional ethics committee. The patients and therapists signed informed consent forms and agreed to be videotaped during the treatment. All background details are disguised to ensure the anonymity of the patients and therapists.

High ET case study

Jordan is a 32-year-old undergraduate student. He sought therapy shortly after being expelled for failing to meet academic requirements. Three years earlier, the long-standing but conflictual romantic relationship he was in, had come to an end. Although a few years had passed since then, he found it difficult to get his life back on track and kept grieving over the loss of this relationship. Jordan blamed himself for mistreating his girlfriend, causing himself significant distress that resulted in depression and anxiety.

Jordan was able to rapidly form a strong therapeutic alliance with his therapist. He shared his thoughts and feelings openly with the therapist, reflected inquisitively about himself and gained new insights. He tended to respond excitedly to statements from the therapist, when the latter articulated his latent narrative. Demonstrating openness to learning new information, that is, to reviving ET early in therapy, indicated Jordan's high trait-like characteristic. Jordan wanted to feel loved and desired, but most of the time he felt unworthy. Because of a sense of being undeserving and fear of being abandoned or left alone, he had several superficial relationships with women, making sure that he was not alone at any given time. But he still felt lonely, alienated, and rejected. Four weeks into the therapy, the therapist recognized and articulated Jordan's central personal narrative: "It seems to me that it's so important for you to feel secure in a relationship, that you sometimes take all kinds of measures that are aimed at giving you some confidence, but don't allow the relationship to be deep or long-lasting. Eventually, you end up feeling the way you had tried to avoid: lonely and alienated". Jordan was wondering out loud: "I've never thought about it this way before (pauses). You know, when I think of it, I can see how this might explain many things in my life, especially in recent years."

After nine weeks in therapy, the COVID-19 outbreak and the ensuing curfews ruled out face-to-face meetings. The therapist offered to change over to VCP meetings. Jordan accepted without hesitation because he was keen on attending the therapy sessions. Given his high trait-like ET, the therapist prioritized the use of ostensive cues for identification of Jordan's personal narrative, as this was articulated before the transition to VCP, in addition to explicitly referring to the change in setting:

T: "Jordan, how are you, given all the restrictions?"

J: "Well ... you know ... I've had better times. I'm sitting here in my pajamas."

T: "Right, this is quite different from what we are used to." [Regarding the dyadic need to adjust together].

J: "Yeah, I guess. But it's not bad, it has its advantages. After all, I can't complain, sitting here in the comfort of my home."

T: "There is no place like home, is there?"

J: "Absolutely, you got that right."

T: "Well, I'm very happy we can still meet despite these challenging times for us." [the therapist provides an ostensive cue regarding the dyadic need to adjust together].

J: "So do I. Yeah (sigh). I'm a bit confused ... I'm not sure what to talk about."

T: "Last week you told me about that new girl you met." [therapist helps with continuity].

J: "Right! So, I met this girl, and I felt it's going to be different this time. Now ... I'm not sure it's going to last. Anyway, it's probably dead. So maybe I'll call that girl from the bar, do you remember her?" [personal narrative emerges from the main content].

T: "Certainly."

J: "Say, do you think we can keep having our regular meetings even though we can't meet in person?" [manifestation of a state-like ET change, as the possible application of his somewhat renewed internal working model against feeling lonely].

T: "This is of great importance for you, isn't it?"

J: "Yeah ... It's like we are always saying – staying alone doesn't bring me closer to what I wish for [ability to refer to the therapeutic continuity and its collaborative aspects, and to retain themes that were previously processed].

T: "Right, Jordan. You're able to identify it while it's happening to you in real time!" [reinforcing the application of relevant information]. "I see what you're saying. Is it similar to what happened with your ex-girlfriend? Maybe fear is taking over again?"

J: "Oh, let's see. It might be (sighs). But what else can I do? How can I protect myself?"

This short vignette illustrates how Jordan's high trait-like ET influences the therapist's decisions about the techniques to be used during the transition to VCP, and how to choose the ostensive cues that are needed to reinforce state-like ET changes. His current crisis makes Jordan feel that he should be somewhat vigilant about others' intentions toward him, and he believes his new romantic relationship is going to end before it has properly begun. When he was working through the underlying narrative in face-to-face mode, Jordan appeared fearful about the possibility of being abandoned, and he took some steps to make sure this would not happen to him. Signaling to Jordan that his subjective experience has been recognized, encourages him to reply with further elaboration. Jordan shows interest in what the therapist has to say because he can recognize it as personally relevant to him. This promotes better understanding about the best way to navigate the social environment in the face of upcoming challenges (expecting the therapist to keep seeing him). This tendency reflects the restoration of ET in a challenging context: Jordan is willing to see the therapist as trustworthy and willing to try out different kinds of behaviors outside the therapy room. This means that state-like ET changes in the course of therapy revive trait-like ability to learn and adapt to our ever-changing environment.

Low ET case study

In contrast to patients with high trait-like ET, patients with low trait-like ET may be highly alert to small nuances in the therapist's reactions in the transition to VCP because of the past difficulties of these patients in trusting socially transmitted information. All too readily, hypervigilance may be activated, and the therapy is liable to deteriorate. To handle this situation effectively, therapists should convey to their patients that they understand their current narrative and validate their present subjective experience, even if this is divergent from that of the therapist and arguably "false" in relation to "objective" reality. Recognizing the patient as an agent, even with expectations and constructions wildly different from the therapist's own, has the potential to revive ET and make it more likely that learning from the therapist will be ultimately possible.

With these patients, the technique that prioritizes physical signaling and the simplest ostensive cues is most likely to be helpful. Therapists may consciously and deliberately make extended use of marked facial expressions, contingent turn-taking reactivity, marked mirroring, and continuous eye contact. This physical emphasis can help, to some degree, to allay the patient's vigilant stance. Validation of the patient's experience, paraphrasing to indicate understanding and only gently going on to ask for elaboration and expansion of statements made by the patient is necessary to (re-)establish trust after a shift to VCP.

Therapists should use physical ostensive cues to help their patients feel they are not alone, and, despite their natural hypervigilance, to be able to benefit from the possibility of a collaborative relationship with the therapist to make a successful transition to VCP.

Ostensive cues directly referencing the change in physical setting might be effective, as it is the physical aspect of the therapeutic environment that is most likely to be felt as shared by the patient. It is essential to empathically validate their declared experience, whether their feelings are positive or negative in nature. Considering the transition to VCP uniquely from the patient's point of view can eventually help revive ET to move beyond the change in physical environment and make learning from therapy once again possible. Attempts on the part of the therapist at re-presenting to the patient an overly detailed version of their personal narrative are unlikely to be helpful, as the patient (a) will likely fail to identify clearly the therapist's representation of their personal narrative and (b) even if they do, the distortions in both their representation of what they believe the therapist sees, and in their own self-image are likely to be so great that an epistemic match is not possible to achieve. Thus, elaborating the patient's personal narrative may be less effective in helping these patients adjust to the transition to VCP. Because the transition has the potential to trigger enhanced vigilance, even an accurate articulation of one's personal narrative might be experienced as inaccurate by the patient, causing a painful experience of interpersonal alienation to persist. A case study from the ongoing psychotherapy trial mentioned earlier (Zilcha-Mano et al., 2018) is used below to demonstrate work with patients with low ET.

Nicole, a 19-year-old student, sought therapy after several months of experiencing mild depressive symptoms. When she was 12, her father died of a sudden cardiac arrest, and she had to take care of her younger sister and her mother, who suffered from recurrent and persistent depressive episodes after losing her husband. After graduating from high school with honors, she enrolled in an academic excellence program for young engineers, and trained to integrate into the high-tech industry. Her choice was motivated by the desire for a good professional future and a steady income at an early age. Nicole began her studies with enthusiasm, but quickly became discouraged. She struggled with the highly intense curriculum, and tuition fees imposed a great financial burden. Moreover, because of her relatively young age, she had difficulty socializing with other students. At the first therapy session, she described harsh feelings of anger toward her high school teachers, who had recommended that course of study. She was also jealous of her friends, who enjoyed the support of their parents and were free to enjoy leisure activities.

Altogether, she had recently become impatient with people around her, and tended to erupt whenever she felt injustice being done. Nicole had never been in therapy before, and at the first session, she stated: "I highly doubt you can help me. This is the reality; you can't change it. Will you make my studies easier? Will I have more money in the bank? Will my father come back into my life? No. So maybe it's a waste of time. Any way, you can't understand." After several meetings, her internal narrative became clear. Nicole wanted others to validate the injustice done to her in life and become witnesses to it. She wanted them to be able to see and understand what makes her so angry and to justify her. Although she wanted them to understand, this wish conflicted with her difficulty in honestly sharing her feelings and thoughts with them. She seemed to fear that, if she shared her feelings, she would be criticized and judged, and as a result, she avoided it. When sensing injustice, she became angry and flew into a rage. After each outburst, however, she felt guilty and self-critical, and regretted her rude behavior. As the weeks passed, Nicole attended the sessions but showed resistance to change. Although she had occasionally been able to feel understood and began to contemplate the possibility of restructuring her life story in response to other perspectives, she was not able to apply new insights outside the therapy room. It was clear, however, that the social reality was changing and that the COVID-19 outbreak required transitioning to the VCP. Therefore, an opportunity was created within the protected framework of therapy to experience the significance of learning new information from the therapist. After coordinating the change in the therapeutic setting, from session 8 onward, therapy carried on through the VCP mode. Given Nicole's low trait-like ET, the therapist prioritized the use of physical ostensive cues, in addition to explicitly referring to the change of setting.

N: "Well, well. How did you manage to coax me into such a session? It's unbelievable! Do you really think it's worth something?" [Nicole exhibits low trait-like ET, as manifested in her doubtful attitude toward VCP].

T: [Smiling and moving closer to the camera to send a physical ostensive cue]. "Yes, this change is really tough!" [Validating]. "I'm very impressed, you know. Even though you said video conversation is not your cup of tea, you agreed to give it a try." [Reinforces the potential of a learning experience]. "How are you doing, Nicole?" [Addressing by name].

N: "I'm fine. Now that everyone around me is anxious and depressed about the situation, I'm no longer exceptional. Say, what are you doing there?" [Refers to the therapist moving her gaze downward].

T: [Opens eyes wide, raises eyebrows in wonder] "You're sharp! you don't miss a thing! Well, I looked down to move my mic closer. I wasn't sure it was placed correctly. What did you think I was doing?" [First validating her reality testing, then indirectly inviting a joint investigation of the vigilance around the nature of the meeting].

N: "To tell you the truth, I thought you could now do a million other things and pretend to be listening to me, and I'd never know. I'll be talking like an idiot, and you'll nod while answering your emails."

T: "I see. You're absolutely right; you can't be sure what I'm doing behind the screen. That probably feels awful!" [Empathic validation with contingent facial expression and a bit exaggerated intonation, keeping constant eye contact].

N: "It's awful indeed."

T: "It's really important for you to feel that I'm 100% with you. When we met at the clinic last week, you told me video calls were not your cup of tea". [Maintaining continuity between face-to-face and VCP contexts and use of the patient's language as ostensive cues]. "But Nicole, maybe now that we're here, you can share with me a little bit how it is for you?" [Inviting a joint exploration of feeling, and making the connection to the pre-transition sequence].

N: "It makes me feel you're not bearing with me here, and it makes me a bit angry."

T: "Angry? I'm curious." [Contracting eyebrows, slightly nodding to communicate interest in her subjective feeling].

N: Look, all this Corona Virus thing is weighing down on me. I can't learn, can't work, can't work out. It's not fair. It's a lot to take. This session is another challenge I must face now, you know, it's not that easy to find a quiet place in my house [A possible narrative emerges, but the therapist must be careful not to relate to it at this point].

T: "All these changes demand a great deal from you. It doesn't sound simple at all. There are always tasks you are required to do, and a video call with me is one of them, right? [The therapist is being supportive, and shares her best understanding to make Nicole feel she is with her].

N: "True, another task to manage, and I'm not even sure it's worthwhile. I'm so overloaded that every little thing burdens me. At least you can understand it, it's more than my mom and sister are able to do." [Conveying the feeling of being understood can be achieved because of prior extensive use of ostensive ques].

T: "It's very impressive that you have not given up trying. And here we are, together. For a moment it may also feel that it's not so bad." [Reinforcing parts of effective coping].

N: "I admit it's a little encouraging to see you smile at me like that. And it does feel good to share my feeling without being judged."

T: "Recently, you've been trying all kinds of new things." [Reinforcing the learning process].

N: "Totally. At least I try. Maybe seeing you every week will be worth something, in the end."

T: "that's a different way of seeing things compared to the way you started therapy."

Nicole's case illustrates how patients with low trait-like ET enter the transition to VCP in a state of hypervigilance, conducting themselves in similar ways to other situations in their lives. For Nicole, and other patients like her, with low trait-like ET, to be able to successfully make this transition and continue the therapeutic work, the therapist is required to use more distinct and clear ostensive cues.

Although the covert narrative may emerge from the main content, any reference to it during the transition phase might cause patients to feel that their subjective experience is being dismissed. Rather, extensive ostensive physical cues, such as marked facial expressions, contingent reactivity, maintaining constant eye contact, etc., can help patients with low trait-like ET recognize the therapist as trustworthy. This, in turn, enables the revival of ET and makes it possible for state-like changes to occur. Trusting what the therapist has to offer in the course of psychotherapy stimulates curiosity and enables the patient to continue acquiring social information that is personally relevant for coping. After Nicole's internal working model has been elaborated within the therapeutic context, there is a good chance that she might try to further apply it outside the therapy room.

Discussion and conclusions

The present paper was written while the COVID-19 pandemic imposed a substantial change in the way psychotherapy was delivered. The proposed suggestions, however, are most likely applicable to any situation in which it is necessary to switch to a remote mode of therapy. The guidelines suggested here may contribute to steps therapists follow to tailor the transition to VCP to their patients' trait-like ET characteristics, which can help therapists navigate the transition and choose the techniques that are expected to be most effective.

The techniques are based on a set of guidelines for the use of ostensive cues (a) as physical signals, (b) for identifying the patients' personal narrative, and (c) as a direct reference to the change in setting. These techniques may enable therapists and patients to achieve the desired state-like ET improvements. However, the State-like vs Trait-like distinction and its adaptation to the context of epistemic trust is very preliminary. Further in-depth research needs to be carried out to validate this distinction and to strengthen its application in the therapeutic context.

The primary focus of the present paper was the transition to VCP for an ongoing course of treatment. There are cases, however, in which psychotherapy is initially conducted through VCP, prior to establishing the therapeutic alliance and without the opportunity to assess a patient's ET in advance. Nevertheless, similar considerations should be taken into account in commencing therapy. In such cases, the therapist should prefer to use physical ostensive cues, such as eye contact, marked facial expressions, etc. These cues are a basic point of reference that can be effective for any patient and has no harmful potential for the therapeutic relationship.

The present paper focuses on adult therapy, but can also be adapted to guide therapists in the transition to VCP with children. Because children rely heavily on physical ostensive cues from the adults around them, it is important to consider using such cues first and foremost. In psychotherapy with children, these cues can be used playfully and in an exaggerated manner to signal to children that their subjective experience has been identified by the therapist. For example, children are sometimes expected to relate to the change in setting through a hide-and-seek game, to help them process the breakup and reconnection experience. Although they are in different rooms, wondering aloud about the child's whereabouts when hiding, searching for the child in the room, and showing excitement when the child is discovered are important signals that may support a sense of agency.

The present paper focuses on psychodynamic therapy, but the proposed suggestions can also be relevant to making the transition to VCP in other therapeutic orientations. Because they contribute to the therapeutic alliance, these guidelines are not unique to a given therapeutic approach. It has been suggested that the therapeutic alliance is not merely a product of successful treatment or the context in which successful treatment is provided, but rather it can serve as an active ingredient in itself, relevant to all types of therapies (Zilcha-Mano, 2017). Cognitive behavioral therapy, for example, can use homework given before switching to VCP as a way of maintaining continuity in the patient's narrative. In other protocol-based therapeutic approaches, continuity is maintained by being more meticulous about treatment goals at each meeting.

As the guidelines suggested here are being applied to the COVID-19 situation, as with any other global or local disaster, it is important to take into account the mental health effects of the situation on both the patient and the therapist. Under a shared traumatic reality (Boulanger, 2013), both therapist and patient are exposed to the same public risk factor. When both sides are at similar risk, a strong symmetry may be created between their experiences in adversity. To continue to support patients in a positive way and to contain feelings of anger, rejection, need, or anxiety, therapists must find sources of support and resilience for themselves, otherwise they may overidentify with their patient and possibly fail to recognize the patient's distress signals.

In the ever-changing reality of our lives, as the world is increasingly moving online, it seems important to preserve the characteristics of human communication as we know them from face-to-face encounters, and embrace them as we are going online. Under such circumstances, ET can provide healthcare professionals a tentative framework to meet this challenge. Being able to address the dialectic of remote care that meets human proximity needs is an important challenge, and how therapists meet it, may determine the continued relevance of the field in the face of global change.

Disclosure statement

No potential conflict of interest was reported by the authors.

Funding

This work was supported by the Israeli Science Foundation [186/15].

ORCID

Peter Fonagy http://orcid.org/0000-0003-0229-0091

References

Andersson, G., Paxling, B., Roch-Norlund, P., Östman, G., Norgren, A., Almlöv, J., … Silverberg, F. (2012). Internet-based psychodynamic versus cognitive behavioral guided self-help for generalized anxiety disorder: A randomized controlled trial. *Psychotherapy and Psychosomatics*, *81*(6), 344–355.

Backhaus, A., Agha, Z., Maglione, M. L., Repp, A., Ross, B., Zuest, D., … Thorp, S. R. (2012). Videoconferencing psychotherapy: A systematic review. *Psychological Services*, *9*(2), 111–131.

Berryhill, M. B., Culmer, N., Williams, N., Halli-Tierney, A., Betancourt, A., Roberts, H., & King, M. (2019). Videoconferencing psychotherapy and depression: A systematic review. *Telemedicine and e-Health*, *25*(6), 435–446.

Bo, S., Sharp, C., Fonagy, P., & Kongerslev, M. (2017). Hypermentalizing, attachment, and epistemic trust in adolescent BPD: Clinical illustrations. *Personality Disorders: Theory, Research, and Treatment*, *8*(2), 172.

Boulanger, G. (2013). Fearful symmetry: Shared trauma in New Orleans after Hurricane Katrina. *Psychoanalytic dialogues*, *23*(1), 31–44.

Campos, J., & Stenberg, C. R. (1981). Perception, appraisal and emotion: The onset of social referencing. In M. E. Lamb & L. R. Sherrod (Eds.), *Infant social cognition: Empirical and theoretical considerations* (pp. 273–314). New Jersey, USA: Lawrence Erlbaum Associates.

Camras, L. A., & Sachs, V. B. (1991). Social referencing and caretaker expressive behavior in a day care setting. *Infant Behavior & Development*, *14*(1), 27–36.

Chavooshi, B., Mohammadkhani, P., & Dolatshahi, B. (2016). A randomized double-blind controlled trial comparing Davanloo intensive short-term dynamic psychotherapy as internet-delivered vs treatment as usual for medically unexplained pain: A 6-month pilot study. *Psychosomatics*, *57*(3), 292–300.

Egyed, K., Király, I., & Gergely, G. (2013). Communicating shared knowledge in infancy. *Psychological Science*, *24*(7), 1348–1353.

Fonagy, P., & Allison, E. (2014). The role of mentalizing and epistemic trust in the therapeutic relationship. *Psychotherapy*, *51*(3), 372.

Fonagy, P., Campbell, C., & Bateman, A. (2017). Mentalizing, attachment, and epistemic trust in group therapy. *International Journal of Group Psychotherapy*, *67*(2), 176–201.

Fonagy, P., Luyten, P., Allison, E., & Campbell, C. (2018). Reconciling psychoanalytic ideas with attachment theory. In P. Shaver & J. Cassidy (Eds.), *Handbook of attachment* (3rd ed., pp. 780–804). New York: Guilford Press.

Fonagy, P., Luyten, P., Allison, E., & Campbell, C. (2019). Mentalizing, epistemic trust and the phenomenology of psychotherapy. *Psychopathology*, *52*(2), 94–103.

Fonagy, P., & Target, M. (1997). Attachment and reflective function: Their role in self-organization. *Development and Psychopathology*, *9*(4), 679–700.

Gergely, G. (2013). Ostensive communication and cultural learning: The natural pedagogy hypothesis. In H. S. Terrace & J. Metcalfe (Eds.), *Agency and joint attention* (pp. 139–151). England: Oxford University Press.

Gergely, G., & Csibra, G. (2005). The social construction of the cultural mind: Imitative learning as a mechanism of human pedagogy. *Interaction Studies*, *6*, 463–481. https://doi-org.ezproxy.haifa.ac.il/10.1075/is.6.3.10ger

Gergely, G., Egyed, K., & Kiraly, I. (2007). On pedagogy. *Developmental Science*, *10*(1), 139–146.

Johansson, R., Ekbladh, S., Hebert, A., Lindström, M., Möller, S., Petitt, E., … Andersson, G. (2012). Psychodynamic guided self-help for adult depression through the internet: A randomised controlled trial. *PloS One*, *7*(5). doi:10.1371/journal.pone.0038021

King, V. L., Brooner, R. K., Peirce, J. M., Kolodner, K., & Kidorf, M. S. (2014). A randomized trial of web-based videoconferencing for substance abuse counseling. *Journal of Substance Abuse Treatment*, *46*(1), 36–42.

Kingsley, A., & Henning, J. A. (2015). Online and phone therapy: Challenges and opportunities. *The Journal of Individual Psychology*, *71*(2), 185–194.

Luyten, P., Campbell, C., Allison, E., & Fonagy, P. (2020). The mentalizing approach to psychopathology: State of the art and future directions. *Annual Review of Clinical Psychology*, *16*, 9.1–9.29.

Luyten, P., Campbell, C., & Fonagy, P. (2019). Reflections on the contributions of Sidney J. Blatt: The dialectical needs for autonomy, relatedness, and the emergence of epistemic trust. *Psychoanalytic Psychology*, *36*(4), 328.

Norwood, C., Moghaddam, N. G., Malins, S., & Sabin-Farrell, R. (2018). Working alliance and outcome effectiveness in videoconferencing psychotherapy: A systematic review and noninferiority meta-analysis. *Clinical Psychology & Psychotherapy*, *25*(6), 797–808.

Safran, J. D., & Muran, J. C. (1996). The resolution of ruptures in the therapeutic alliance. *Journal of Consulting and Clinical Psychology*, *64*(3), 447–458.

Safran, J. D., & Muran, J. C. (2000). The therapeutic alliance. Introduction. *Journal of Clinical Psychology*, *56*(2), 159–161. http://dx.doi.org/10.1002/(SICI)1097-4679(200002)56:2%3C159::AID-JCLP2%3E3.0.CO;2-D

Safran, J. D., Muran, J. C., & Eubanks-Carter, C. (2011). Repairing alliance ruptures. *Psychotherapy*, *48* (1), 80–87.

Scharff, J. S., (Ed.). (2018). *Psychoanalysis online: Mental health, teletherapy, and training.* England: Abingdon. doi:10.4324/9780429478833

Schröder-Pfeifer, P., Talia, A., Volkert, J., & Taubner, S. (2018). Developing an assessment of epistemic trust: A research protocol. *Research in Psychotherapy: Psychopathology, Process and Outcome*, *21* (3), 123–131.

Simpson, S. G., & Reid, C. L. (2014). Therapeutic alliance in videoconferencing psychotherapy: A review. *Australian Journal of Rural Health*, *22*(6), 280–299.

Sperber, D., Clement, F., Heintz, C., Mascaro, O., Mercier, H., Origgi, G., & Wilson, D. (2010). Epistemic vigilance. *Mind & Language*, *25*(4), 359–393.

Sucala, M., Schnur, J. B., Constantino, M. J., Miller, S. J., Brackman, E. H., & Montgomery, G. H. (2012). The therapeutic relationship in e-therapy for mental health: A systematic review. *Journal of Medical Internet Research*, *14*(4), 175–187.

Vincent, C., Barnett, M., Killpack, L., Sehgal, A., & Swinden, P. (2017). Advancing telecommunication technology and its impact on psychotherapy in private practice. *British Journal of Psychotherapy*, *33*(1), 63–76.

Zilcha-Mano, S. (2017). Is alliance really therapeutic? Revisiting this question in light of recent methodological advances. *American Psychologist*, *72*(4), 311–325.

Zilcha-Mano, S. (2018). Major developments in methods addressing for whom psychotherapy may work and why. *Psychotherapy Research*, *29*(6), 693–708.

Zilcha-Mano, S. (2020). Toward personalized psychotherapy: The state-like/trait-like model of therapeutic change. *American Psychologist*, in press. doi:10.1037/amp0000629.

Zilcha-Mano, S., Dolev, T., Leibovich, L., & Barber, J. P. (2018). Identifying the most suitable treatment for depression based on patients' attachment: Study protocol for a randomized controlled trial of supportive-expressive vs. supportive treatments. *BMC Psychiatry*, *18*(1), 362.

Appendix

We have started to develop a framework for identifying high- and low-ET individuals. We start by distinguishing momentary experiences of epistemic vigilance, which we consider normative low state-like ET. Other individuals make statements that imply longstanding mistrust and hypervigilance, which we would regard as indicators of having low trait-like ET. Both low and high trait-like ET individuals will manifest instances of low state-like ET, as evidenced by statements that apply to specific situations within delimited settings. It is our expectation that low trait-like ET individuals will evidence a greater number of low state-like ET statements and fewer high state-like ET statements than high trait-like ET individuals. As an illustration, Table 1 includes statements taken from actual therapies that may serve to illustrate all four categories of utterances.

Part III

Working with Emotions

Clinical recommendations for psychotherapists working during the coronavirus (COVID-19) pandemic through the lens of AEDP (Accelerated Experiential Dynamic Psychotherapy)

Hillary L. McBride, Andrew J. Joseph, Peter G. Schmitt and Brett M. Holtz

ABSTRACT

The coronavirus (COVID-19) pandemic created an unprecedented physical and mental health crisis on an international scale. Clients and therapists alike navigated the fears and uncertainty surrounding the virus, often in an environment of social isolation. The following paper presents a brief overview of the unique stressors and psychosocial factors impacting therapeutic work in the time of the coronavirus pandemic, including fears of the virus and social transmission, relational stressors due to isolation, grieving in isolation, fear of death, financial challenges, and the transition to telehealth. In addition, this paper aims to provide specific interventions and helpful approaches for psychotherapists navigating the novel challenges and demands to their clinical work through an AEDP (Accelerated Experiential Dynamic Psychotherapy) perceptive. This includes finding an entry point for accessing the pain: undoing aloneness; moving through the pain: dyadic affect regulation; and paying close attention to vitality within suffering: searching for transformance. Recommendations for the health and care of the clinician are also discussed, such as attuning to self-needs, anticipating and detecting dysregulation, staying with the good, meaning-making, identifying and responding to burnout, and the importance of receiving personal therapy and clinical supervision.

Due to the rapid spread across several countries and high rate of infection, the coronavirus (COVID-19) was declared a global pandemic by the World Health Organization (WHO) on 11 March 2020 (WHO, 2020). Communities around the globe have isolated and social-distanced in ways never before seen in order to slow down the infection rate. To promote the utilization of telehealth so that those in need are supported, on 30 March 2020 the U.S. Department of Health and Human Services published a statement empowering medical advisors to serve patients wherever they are during this public health emergency.

The drastic lifestyle changes required to protect public health have touched each ecological system level impacting human experience (Bronfenbrenner, 1979). This includes changes at a macrosystem level, such as social and cultural attitudinal changes towards illness, public spaces, the limitations and necessity of household resources, media use, and collective distress. At an exosystem level, there have been changes to economic stability, changes in access to education and school closures, and closure of non-essential businesses. At a mesosystem level, there are new dangers in the workplace or the inability to go to work, changes in access to parahealth professionals, closures of places of worship, and limited access to extended family members and social supports. At a microsystem level, parents have faced the burdens of working from home while trying to educate their children, families have experienced grief over ill or deceased members, and many have dealt with loss of income and increased financial stress, the need to protect vulnerable family members, and the existential threat of illness or death.

Communities have responded in coordinated behavioral efforts to minimize the spread of the virus, with a focus on protecting the most vulnerable populations, the health care providers treating them, and the medical material resources needed to do so (Collins, 2008). Social changes have been occurring rapidly across the globe, and individuals and those supporting them therapeutically have felt the psychosocial consequences. Psychotherapists providing clinical support to their existing patient population may find themselves suddenly facing the emergence of unique stressors within their patient population, needing to adapt their clinical approaches overnight to fit their patients' changing presenting concerns, and anticipating or noticing their own biopsychosocial indicators of burnout, vicarious trauma, or caregiver fatigue (Cook, Schwartz, & Kaslow, 2017; Pulido, 2012). Research conducted during the SARS (severe acute respiratory syndrome) outbreak identified that the psychosocial and physical impact on those providing care to others during an infectious disease outbreak must be considered (Brooks, Dunn, Amlot, Rubin, & Greenberg, 2018). Given the significance of the coronavirus outbreak, the impact on individuals and their psychological supports will also be significant (Brooks et al., 2018, 2020). Psychotherapists must be prepared for how their clinical work will continue to change, and how that will impact them personally.

This paper presents a brief overview of the unique stressors and psychosocial factors which may impact therapeutic work or patients' presenting concerns, offers specific AEDP clinical interventions and approaches which psychotherapists may find helpful in their changing clinical work, and discusses recommendations for the health and self-care of the psychotherapist.

"clinical recommendations" and "self-resourcing, and care for the person of the therapist" and "conclusion"

Whether working with new or existing patients, the concerns felt by individuals impacted by the coronavirus are likely new, unfamiliar, and thus require adaptation and experiential learning on the part of the therapist. As is the case when experiencing something new and unfamiliar, feeling accompanied by a skilled other may reduce the sense of aloneness or fear about traversing the unknown (Fosha, 2006; Wallin, 2007). It may be helpful for some therapists to anticipate concerns represented in their patient population, while having the stressors in their clinical work normalized. The following ideas are presented to support other clinicians to feel seen, equipped, and supported to accompany their patients through whatever they might be experiencing.

The Realness of Threat and Fears

Due to the coronavirus, there is a wide-scale threat of illness and death resulting in understandable and neurobiologically appropriate fear responses (Shultz et al., 2016). The extent of the devastation of the virus, how long it will take for things to regain a semblance of normalcy, and what will be lost are unknown and unpredictable. Patients who are unable to regulate their fear, are unfamiliar with processing emotion, or do not have the social resources to be attuned to and accompanied through their emotions, are at risk for the development of anxiety, depression, or maladaptive defensive behaviors and strategies (Fosha, 2009).

The Shared Experience

It is not unusual for therapists to work with a presenting concern or population with which they identify or have received support for in the past. However, it is less likely for a therapist to be facing a concern at the same time as those with whom they are working. Although cities are being hit with varying degrees of severity, therapists and patients alike are currently experiencing the effects of COVID-19. A therapist might have an elderly relative intubated in hospital, when the patient discloses that they are afraid for an elderly relative intubated in hospital, or a patient might disclose fear of financial loss, while the therapist is also struggling with patient retention. They may share similar emotional experiences, as both therapist and patient may be experiencing anxiety, fear, and growing uncertainty.

Often, the recommendation for therapists experiencing the same concern as their patients is to seek additional consultation, supervision or personal therapy (Macran & Shapiro, 1998; Redinger & Gibb, 2020). In addition to the challenge of experiencing a parallel concern, there also lies the opportunity for therapists to better understand their patient's experience and potentially build stronger rapport or intimacy through sharing in the experience together (see clinical recommendations below) (Boulanger, 2013; Boulanger, Floyd, Nathan, Poitevant, & Pool, 2013).

Therapy Through a Screen

To adhere to recommendations of physical distancing, and to continue a therapeutic relationship where one person may need to be in quarantine, therapists have been recommended to shift from traditional in-person clinical work to telehealth (HHS Office of the Secretary, Office for Civil Rights, & OCR, 2020). This is a necessity both for creating continuity of care and for engaging in societal efforts to minimize the spread of the virus. However, it presents additional challenges: insecure network connections, inaccessibility for individuals who do not have access to appropriate technology or are unfamiliar with how to work the necessary software, distractions in the home environment of the patient or therapist, and securing platforms which do not present any additional security or confidentiality measures. This may also result in limitations in which kinds of clinical interventions are used, such as those requiring more somatic or touch-based processes. These challenges may get in the way of establishing therapeutic flow, or noticing what is happening in the body – a tapping foot or fidgeting fingers may not be visible. Even with modern technology, much of the sensory experience is lost.

Pivoting to Crisis Work

While existing clients may go through crisis from time to time, crisis work requires a different skill set and approach to treatment than ongoing therapeutic work (Hoff, Hallisey, & Hoff, 2009). Instead of working on a patient's initial goals for treatment, the therapist may need to adapt their work to support a patient through a new crisis related to job loss, a death of a loved one, new intimate partner violence, illness, or financial hardship. This will require clinicians to suspend existing treatment goals, adjust to meet the present needs of the patient, and familiarize themselves with evidence-based approaches to crisis intervention.

Population Concerns Based on Occupation or Socioeconomic Status

Individuals may present with population-specific concerns based on their socioeconomic status, race, or occupation. The Navajo Nation, the largest land area retained by an indigenous tribe, is being ravaged by COVID-19 (Romero, 2020). Blacks and Hispanics are also hit harder by COVID-19, and experts say that social factors are to blame (Nania, 2020). Health care workers may be more likely to be contemplating and preparing for their own death, present with symptoms of post traumatic stress disorder (PTSD) or acute stress disorder, or feel inner conflict between their sense of duty to protect and support their families and their responsibilities to coworkers and patients. Individuals who work in the service industry or in the arts may feel devastated due to loss of income, but be better able to stay at home, practice social distancing, and protect themselves and their families physically. Religious leaders may feel overwhelmed with their congregations' need for support, and consequently neglect their own self-care, or experience compassion fatigue and burnout (Flannely, Roberts, & Weaver, 2005). Ceasing to meet in person may be experienced as a lack of faith or religious disobedience, while others might find meaning in staying home, seeing it as a way to express faith and care for the vulnerable in the community.

Exasperation of Existing Relational Stressors

The effort to engage in isolation and physical distancing presents an increased psychosocial challenge for individuals who have been experiencing ongoing intimate partner violence (Dubus, 2020), struggle with parenting, have children with high needs for educational or psychosocial support, or are negotiating relationship issues. Existing communication challenges may feel intensified, as individuals within the same household do not have the same autonomy or space with which to regulate themselves or engage in self-care. Although there is the opportunity that couples or families may experience the time as an invitation to attachment and increased intimacy, it is possible that being in the same household will result in more conflict, challenging interpersonal behavior, and the possibility of abuse and violence in the home.

Payment for Sessions

Patients who previously were able to pay for therapy, either out-of-pocket or through employment-provided extended health insurance, may not be able to pay for therapy at the time when they are experiencing new stressors, such as unemployment. Patients may request treatment on a sliding scale, delayed payment, or may need to forgo treatment altogether, rendering them with less social support through the connection and secure attachment with a therapist at a time when their symptoms or degree of suffering are increasing.

Isolation and Terror around Being Outside of their Home

Individuals who have been in quarantine or self-isolation for an extended period of time may experience increased fear and anxiety when leaving their home, even when taking reasonable precautions (Brooks et al., 2020). This may be more acute for people who live in highly populated spaces, and/or those with a severe outbreak, such as Wuhan Province, New York City, London, or Milan.

Grief and the Inability to Grieve with Ritual or in Community

Grieving with loved ones, grief rituals, and communal faith practices are important avenues to support the processing of grieving, which in many cases have not been available at a time when death counts are rising. Patients, mourning the loss of someone they love, are unable to hold memorials, and may struggle to navigate a way forward not having the opportunity to say a final goodbye. Additionally, patients may experience distress knowing a loved one is in critical condition, and may soon die, but be unable to be near them as they take their final breaths. The rituals associated with death are an important part of someone processing the loss, and with this taken away, it is an opportunity for therapists to create a space wherein patients can process and grieve the loss of their loved one (Rycroft & Perlesz, 2001).

Clinical recommendations

Just as we normalize the patient's feelings around the world's uncertain state, this paper aims to normalize the challenges and feelings associated with practicing psychotherapy through a pandemic. Common presenting concerns during this pandemic, unsurprisingly, are feelings that result due to isolation. Additionally, presenting concerns that patients were originally bringing to treatment are now exacerbated as patients are removed from the social support which may have previously kept them stable. Accelerated Experiential Dynamic Psychotherapy (AEDP) is presented in this paper for three main reasons: (1) its fundamental aim is to undo aloneness, (2) it provides a thorough framework which works actively with both positive and negative emotions (Fosha, Thoma, & Yeung, 2019) with systemic interventions that upregulate the positive affect systems to bring about positive neuroplasticity and flourishing session by session (Fosha & Thoma, 2020), and (3) its clinical outcomes appear promising in alleviating a range of symptoms including depression and maladaptive cognitions in 16 or fewer sessions (Iwakabe et al., 2020, submitted for publication).

AEDP is a psychotherapeutic model of treatment developed by Diana Fosha and colleagues (Fosha, 2000, 2004, 2005; Fosha, Gleiser, & Ford, 2009; Fosha et al., 2019; Russell, 2015), which describes psychopathology and suffering as the patient's best attempts to cope with "unwilled and unwanted aloneness in the presence of overwhelming emotion[al experience]" (Fosha et al., p. 182). Due to the theory's emphasis on explicit and authentic interpersonal connection, the attention to processing and savouring enjoyable emotion (e.g., excitement and joy) as in-depth as painful emotion (e.g., sadness and anger), and the orientation towards strength and thriving, this treatment model is apt for treating the unique issues facing patients during the pandemic. Below is a description of several AEDP skills and interventions useful for therapists. The interventions outlined below can be used in conjunction with any theoretical framework to deepen the attachment between patient and therapist, and support the flourishing of patients, while navigating the coronavirus pandemic (Fosha, 2009, 2017a, 2017b).

Entry Point for Accessing the Pain: Undoing Aloneness

To support patients moving in the experience of difficult emotions, they need to know they are accompanied – in other words, their aloneness must be undone (Fosha, 2017). In the current context of the coronavirus pandemic, we provide a brief introduction to the relational stance of the therapist within AEDP, as well as the following interventions and approaches: paying attention to and exploring the changes in the relational dynamic as therapy moves online or onto the phone, metatherapeutic processing of the continuity of relationship amidst change, making the implicit explicit, self-disclosure of shared experience, and attention to processing and repairing therapeutic ruptures.

AEDP theory and the relational therapist

A central tenet of AEDP is the focus on relational accompaniment to undo aloneness. Instead of the prototypical position of the therapist at a distance, or as a blank slate, in AEDP the therapist is a non-neutral other and endeavours to draw emotionally close to the patient. Closeness between the patient and the therapist is not assumed, inferred, nor is it thought to be a by-product of the therapy process. Rather, closeness is constantly made explicit through authentic relating and the therapist's checking in with the patient to process what is transpiring in the relational matrix. The therapist might say, "you know, when you just expressed your anger toward me for being late, I actually felt more connected to you."

At the heart of transformational therapy is a patient who feels safe and a therapist who is brave (Fosha, 2000). The avenue through which transformation takes place is the relationship. The depth of that relationship is initiated by a brave therapist who, through attunement and care, takes mindful relational risks with the intention of secure attachment. With warmth and acceptance, the therapist helps the patient access and move through their difficult emotions. The therapist aims to creates a corrective relational experience by using moment to moment tracking to notice the patient's emotional expression and withdrawal ("I noticed you light up when you mentioned that," or "I felt like there was sadness in what you just expressed, could we stay with that for a moment?"), and using verbal and non-verbal expressions of compassion and warmth to communicate to the patient that they are with them in each moment, and have not abandoned them, and always checking with the patient to explore how the therapist's expressions are being received.

Relational risk-taking on the part of the therapist is an invitation for growth within the therapeutic dyad, and a model for the patient's own risk-taking in their relationships. The therapist can exercise bravery through their own "judicious self-disclosure" (Prenn, 2009), and in doing so, model vulnerability which can be a powerful tool to support the patient in accessing their own deeply-held emotions.

During a recent session, one of the authors of this paper (Andrew Joseph) virtually met with his patient. As they began, his patient noticed a grin on the therapist's face, and asked, "Do you have something to tell me?" The therapist, surprised, responded, "No, what do you mean?" The patient reiterated – "It looks like you have something to tell me. I see you smiling over there." The therapist took a moment to reflect on his affect that the patient was observing, recognized within himself a feeling of excitement that the patient was drawing attention to. This opened the door for a vulnerable self-disclosure, as the therapist stated honestly, "I don't see you every week, and when I saw that we had an appointment today in my calendar, I felt excited. That's what you're seeing on my face." There was a brief pause in the conversation before the therapist asked, "What is it like for you to know that I'm excited to see you?" This self-disclosure allowed the patient to move into a state of emotional processing. The patient's face flushed and he burst into tears. The patient recognized a feeling and shared, "I had no idea that what I have been missing over the last eight weeks while I have been isolated, was somebody being excited to see me." The patient, due to their self-isolation in their NYC apartment, had found himself in a painful state of aloneness. In disclosing their own feelings of excitement, the therapist was able to create a tangible sense of connection that surfaced a deeply human need within the patient – the need to feel like others are excited to see them. The patient looked up at the screen, after his wave of emotion, and said, "It feels good to hear you say that, and I feel relieved."

Noticing and exploring relational changes as therapy moves online or onto the phone

The switch to online or phone sessions may present challenges for patients to feel the therapist with them and to experience the therapist's care and attunement in the same way. Patients may want reassurance that their therapist is not only present with them on the other side of the phone-line or screen, but will stay with them through the continued changes and uncertainty about what will happen in the future (Prenn & Halliday, 2020a). Therapists can provide space to address these challenges by beginning sessions with the question, "What is it like for us to meet together in this new way?" For patients who found comfort in the ritual of leaving their daily routine to enter a space for the sole purpose of being seen and accompanied, there may be a sense of loss as they do therapy at home with children, a partner, or the associations of home-life demands lingering in the background. Instead of dismissing these concerns as peripheral, therapists are encouraged to make space within sessions to grieve the changes with patients, and to make self-disclosures about how they experience the change in format. For example, the therapist might say, "I feel the loss too. I enjoy the experience of sitting together in the same room. I always like noticing what shoes you are wearing, or seeing how you relax when you come in and sink down onto the couch. What is it like for you to know that I miss being in person together too?"

Metatherapeutic processing of the continuity of relationship amidst change

For therapists seeing new patients online, it is still important to explore the experience of doing online or phone therapy. This might include asking, "What is it like to do therapy while in your home," or even "What is it like to have me with you while at home?" Some patients, new or continuing, may experience comfort with being home. If previously driving or taking the subway, or entering a new space provoked fear or anxiety, they may now experience comfort in conducting therapy within their familiar environment. If this occurs, therapists are encouraged to stay with this positive affect, a step explored in more detail in the section below titled *Deepening and Magnifying the Good: Metatherapeutic Processing to Upregulate Positive Affect Systems.*

While the changes and losses need to be named and explored, it is important for the therapist to emphasise the continuity of the relationship even though the dyad now takes place over the phone or computer screen. Many of the comforting accoutrements of therapy may be gone – the waiting room, the check-in process, tasteful and soothing office decor, or comfortable furniture. Yet the core aspect of therapy, the therapist/patient dyad, remains. Drawing attention to the ability of the dyadic connection to persist in spite of change is important for supporting the patient to experience the strength of the connection built through previous work. This might include asking patients the question, "What is it like for you to know that even in the midst of change, we are still connecting?"

Making the implicit explicit

The technology that allows therapists to meet with their patients also limits what the therapist is able to see and attend to, such as some somatic markers. Video calls allow the therapist to see the patient's face, but not somatic markers occurring off-screen. Phone calls can bring more awareness to changes in vocal tone, but have no visual information about facial affect. To demonstrate moment-to-moment tracking of affect in their patient, the therapist can further prioritize the importance of making the implicit explicit when it comes to present moment awareness about the patient's affect. Therapists can first verbally state their queries and noticings about their patients' facial expression (e.g., "I think I'm seeing some sadness on your face," or "It looks like you are having some tears," or "Wow, a big deep breath"). Therapists can then get consent to be more explicit about monitoring affect ("Is it ok if we notice together how emotions are emerging in us"), followed by metatherapeutic processing the continuity in tracking through a different format ("What is it like for you that even though I can't see your face, I can still feel, hear, and notice your sadness about this?").

Self-disclosure of shared experience

With awareness of their shared experience, some patients may be more curious about how their therapist experiences and navigates the changing world. Some therapists may notice that, unlike in the past, they are sharing and living through the same experience as their patients. As therapists may have already experienced, some patients are more curious than usual about the wellbeing of their therapist, beginning sessions by prioritizing asking, "how are *you* doing?" Dismissing the patient's question, or responding with another question ("What about that is important for you to know?") may have the effect of thwarting the patient's attempt to (re-)establish connection, or locate the humanness of the therapist in a way that offers themselves the permission to be human (Prenn, 2009).

Instead, therapists are encouraged to answer concisely and honestly, followed by metatherapeutic processing of the self-disclosure. They might say, "I have noticed feeling more tired than usual," or "I'm feeling afraid for some of my family members, and grieving the losses of others close to me." This is to be followed by exploring how the self-disclosure is experienced by the patient. A therapist might ask, "What is it like for you to know that, like you, I am also feeling fear?"

Attention to processing and repairing therapeutic ruptures

Attention to therapeutic ruptures and their repair is essential for helping the patient experience being seen, cared for, and attended to, and for strengthening the therapeutic attachment bond (Lipton & Fosha, 2011; Prenn, 2011). Ruptures can be experienced as a break in attunement or connection. When processed and repaired, ruptures can lead to a deepening of the attachment experience between therapist and patient, helping the patient feel even more seen and cared about, and creating a corrective experience of when ruptures in attachment relationships occurred in the past but were not repaired. Some examples of rupture can include misreading or missing the patient's affect altogether, rushing through or trying to fix a situation, and technological glitches where calls drop or video is delayed when the patient is sharing about an experience of isolation, disconnection, or other painful emotions. Due to patients' perceptions of changes in connection (through moving sessions online or to the phone) working with ruptures may be even more rewarding and therapeutic than usual. Repairing a rupture includes the therapist noticing that it occurred, the therapist taking an appropriate level of responsibility for their part in the rupture, exploring what it was like for the patient to experience that break in attunement, and staying with the affect that emerges in the patient because of the rupture. Therapists can ask their patients questions such as, "What is it like that I misunderstood," and "What does it feel like for you when I get it wrong?" Once both the therapist and patient feel a reestablishment of the sense of connection between them, AEDP emphasizes the importance of the therapist asking, "What is it like that we can find our way back to connection?" Naming and processing the repair and resulting reconnection is as important in AEDP as naming and exploring the rupture of the connection (Fosha, 2017b). Asking this question can help the patient remember the strength and continuity of the connection which persists through changes and challenges, stay with and better understand the experience of re-connection, and know implicitly and explicitly that they are not alone.

Moving Through the Pain: Attention to Affect and Dyadic Regulation

To support patients moving through pain, we provide a brief presentation of the theoretical approach within AEDP when working with emotional pain, followed by a description of specific approaches and interventions. These include bringing attention to defensive coping, slowing down to experience emotion in the body, dyadically regulating and effectively accompanying their patients, and noticing and supporting the repair of historical wounds. This process may serve a particularly important function for patients currently experiencing loss, grief, fear, anxiety, or other painful emotions due to the COVID-19 outbreak.

AEDP theory and working with emotional pain

The relational interventions outlined in the previous section create the pathway to access deep emotion. When the patient feels securely attached and explicitly accompanied, emotion which was previously unbearable becomes bearable, and the processing of it becomes the natural pathway towards healing (Rubinstein, 2015). Unlike cognitive-focused approaches, the focus of AEDP is supporting the patient to experience emotion, accompanied moment to moment through the somatic experience of affect, pulling them towards the sensing and feeling dimensions of emotion and away from the thinking about the emotion (Russell, 2015). Doing this releases the body's natural ability to self-right, prevents the thwarting of the adaptive action tendencies, and allows the person to experience psychobiological release, decreasing allostatic load and increasing the experience of present-moment wellbeing (Fosha, 2009).

Once the patient begins to experience emotion, not only simply talking about it, the therapist's role is to support them to stay with the wave of emotion until completion. A slow pace is important while moving through the emotion so that the patient and the therapist can assiduously notice what is happening for the patient and process it accordingly ("I'm noticing anger in your voice and body as you talk about losing your job due to the pandemic, can we stay with that feeling for a moment?"). Explicitly letting the patient know that the therapist sees and is tracking their experience cues the patient that it is safe to move deeper into the painful elements of their experience. An emotion processed to completion is often signaled by the patient looking up at the therapist, smiling, exhaling, or blowing their nose (Prenn & Halliday, 2020b). This becomes the invitation to process what has just taken place, which becomes therapeutic in and of itself (Fosha, 2013, 2017b).

Bringing attention to defensive coping

Due to the immediacy and magnitude of the individual and societal changes experienced by patients during the current pandemic, the intensity of the stress and emerging emotions may feel unfamiliar or overwhelming, resulting in the emergence of new or historical defensive coping strategies. Patients may reflect that they are drinking more, eating more, engaging in more restrictive or controlled eating behaviors, spending hours combing media for new information about the virus, or trying to stay busy to stop themselves from experiencing the fear, sadness, or anger in response to what is happening. Individuals may find themselves minimizing their distress, sense of loss, or fears, because they perceive others to have it worse. They may find themselves minimizing their experiences of gratitude, connection, and vitality, because of their awareness of the magnitude of others' suffering. Feelings of isolation or hopelessness due to COVID-19 may trigger memories or flashbacks to past trauma and associated defenses. Patients who are developing new defences against emotion will need to be guided to identify them, and empathically invited to learn to experience and regulate their emotions. Therapists are encouraged to normalize and communicate the limited helpfulness of defensive coping to patients, reminding them that this part of them has emerged to protect them from the pain of feeling, but that in the safety of the therapeutic relationship they could experience the emotion in such a way that was not overwhelming (Prenn & Halliday, 2020a, 2020b). The therapist might say, "I heard you say that being aware of other's suffering makes you feel guilty for being sad that your graduation ceremony was cancelled. But I'm wondering if that is also a way to get away from the significance of the loss for you. What would it be like for us to stay with some of your sadness together?" Alternately, "I hear that you are worried I will think you are selfish for feeling so connected to your partner while other people are hurting. I know how much you are treasuring that connectedness. Would it be alright with you if we stayed with that experience of connectedness, together?" They may encourage patients to experience the sadness that comes with their losses, moving into the emotion underneath the minimization defense, or invite patients to stay with and savor their experiences of joy and delight (Fosha & Thoma, 2020).

Slowing down to experience emotion in the body

While some patients may need more psychoeducation about their defenses (for example, an introduction to the change triangle), some patients will be able to circumnavigate the defense when invited by the therapist, to drop into the somatic experience of the emotion (Hendel, 2018). Reassured that they will not be judged, that they are safe, and that they will not be abandoned, patients may begin to experience the emotion which was previously too much to experience alone. This may include attending to patient's fears of death, sadness about the loss of meaningful opportunities or anticipated experiences, the profound loneliness that has come with social distancing, and grief about being unable to be near loved ones who are sick or have died. Therapists can encourage patients to begin to feel by inviting them to slow down (Fosha, 2013). When affect markers are noted in the voice, on the face, or through the body of the patient, signaling that emotion is present, therapists can begin to direct the patient using questions, tentative language, or polite commands, e.g., "Let's notice what is happening right now as you share that," or "Can we stay with what's coming up? It seems so important." When the patient struggles to experience the emotion, the therapist is encouraged to scaffold the patient by noting affect markers or querying about sensations. For example, "I saw something around your eyes that made me wonder if there was sadness there," or "You mentioned you felt angry. Whenever I feel angry I notice feeling heat coursing through my body; can you notice that?" or "Why don't we go really slow, and pay attention to any areas where you might sense energy moving in you". When a patient is sharing an emotionally charged account of what they have experienced or survived, yet is unable to be in touch with their emotion, the therapist may find himself solely holding the emotion in the dyad. When this takes place, the therapist could say, "When you shared this story with me, I felt so angry. How is it to know that you've had this impact on me?"

Dyadically regulating and effectively accompanying their patients

When the patient is able to notice and stay with the emotional experience, therapists can affirm and encourage the patient so they know they are not alone, and can continue to ride the experiential wave of emotion from beginning to end (Prenn & Halliday, 2020c). Therapists will need to be more explicit than usual to help the patient feel empathically accompanied through the intensity of emotion. Therapists might say, "I'm right here," or "You are doing so well, let's let it come," "I can hear there is more," "Stay with it and stay with me," or "Let's keep feeling this together" (Fosha, 2017b; Prenn, 2011). If patients become emotionally dysregulated, typically eye contact would be helpful for bringing them back into the window of tolerance (if using a video call, the therapist might need to look into the computer's camera to appear as if they are making eye contact on the patient's screen). To demonstrate their presence and attention to what is being processed, the therapist can also make explicit affective self-disclosures, such as, "I'm feeling sad with you. If we were in the room together you would see tears in my eyes as well." After the emotion has been processed to completion, there is often the emergence of a new emotion in which the patient experiences hope, relief, or the fatigue that comes with release. The new emotion can be accompanied by new information about themselves or the situation that they could not previously access. Therapists are encouraged to metatherapeutically process with the patient what it was like to experience the emotion, and what they are currently experiencing (Fosha, 2013). This could include making explicit relational statements about emotion processing, such as, "Wow, what is it like for us to be able to do such deep work together over the phone?" Therapists could also offer encouragement about the change process, in light of circumstances which feel unchanging: "You had mentioned before that you would only feel ok when things went back to normal, but here I can see how settled, present, and relieved you look. What is it like for you to know that the world doesn't have to change for you to feel at rest?"

Noticing and supporting the repair of historical wounds

Living through the global pandemic may reactivate historical trauma in some patients who have a history of neglect or social isolation, fear and uncertainty about circumstances or medical outcomes, or have been separated from loved ones because of political circumstances. Additionally, some patients might be surprised by their responses, unaware of implicit memory storage, or the impact of previously traumatic experiences which were minimized, dissociated, or pre-verbal. Some patients might benefit from having their therapist normalize their responses and provide psychoeducation about the implicit storage of traumatic memory. The current circumstances provide an opportunity for patients to reprocess and correct the experience of past trauma. Within AEDP this is referred to as a portrayal, similar to a retrieval used in other theoretical approaches. Using vivid imagery to return to a scene with emotional valence, and having the patient enter the scene as an agent to provide something corrective or assertive, the patient can experience a powerfully contrasting emotional experience which transforms the original traumatic memory (Ecker, 2015; Fosha, 2000; Fosha, Paivio, Gleiser, & Ford, 2009). Portrayals can be used to complete unprocessed emotion about a past experience, have a longed for experience that was interrupted or blocked, or to facilitate a reunion and relationship of care and attunement between the patient's adult self and their imagined younger self (Fosha, 2000; Fosha et al., 2009). In this case, the therapist might support the patient to return in their mind to the scene in the past that they are being reminded of due to the pandemic. The therapist might say, "This feels so much like when you were left alone as a kid all on your own for days. I'm wondering if you can imagine little you all alone. What is that like? What do you feel for that kid? What would you like to say or do that was needed but was never done then?" As always, once the portrayal has been completed, metatherapeutic processing about the experience can occur.

Detecting and Magnifying The Good: Searching for Transformance and Metatherapeutic Processing to Upregulate Positive Affect Systems

To support patients beyond distress into wellbeing and thriving, the following is a brief presentation of the theoretical approach within AEDP to supporting patient flourishing, followed by a description of specific approaches and interventions such as noticing and then metaprocessing evidence of transformational experience.

AEDP theory and supporting patient flourishing

Within the AEDP frame, a goal for a patient is not just symptom reduction, but magnifying positive affect through the metatherapeutic processing of the experience of successful and growth oriented change within therapy. Fosha (2008) has defined transformance as the motivational drive to heal, self-right, and flourish, manifested for example as moments of vitality in the midst of defensiveness or demoralization, it's manifestation, big or small, invariably marked by positive somatic/affective markers, such as a brightening of the eyes, or a relaxation of tension. The role of the therapist is to detect evidence of this drive and bring it from the background to the foreground, helping the patient see what the therapist sees. Markers of transformance may be visible as actions, thoughts, or emotions, characterized by hope, openness, curiosity, or the courage to risk or micro-expressions of positive affect.

The metatherapeutic process helps the patient access positive emotion, as well as positive energy that had previously been latent within them (Fosha, 2009, 2017a). A moment of transformation or change becomes an opportunity to create an upward spiral within the patient (Fosha & Thoma, 2020), and challenges them to construct and express new imagery around their transformation that reframes their positive change in a way they can see and feel. Through rounds of inquiry (e.g., "And what's that like?"), layers of new imagery around the positive transformation are formed, and the narrative becomes richer and brighter. New colors and textures are formed around the experience, like adding music to an image, and then introducing smell and taste to that image. A positive transformation begins as a single new note that feels on point, and through further processing of that note, develops into a symphony that feels congruent, consistent and yet somehow new.

Noticing transformation

Within the experience of the coronavirus pandemic, patients and therapists alike may find particular challenges in continuing to experience (or feeling permission to experience) positive affect. Patients may block off their experience of growth or change because of guilt, perhaps sensing that it is inappropriate or selfish to find moments of goodness within a time where there is so much suffering in the world. The patient may experience ambivalence or confusion towards positive affect ("I wake up to the sound of birds outside my window") that is intertwined with a painful reality ("due to the lack of cars on the road"). Moments of peaceful reflection are colored by the experience of loneliness, and feelings of communal resilience and pride are inextricably linked to deep feelings of sorrow and grief.

The first task of the therapist is to notice the evidence of transformance manifested in the positive affect. The patient is invited to direct their attention to the moment, and the feelings, thoughts, and emotions present. The therapist might ask the patient to slow down and be present with what is occurring. The patient is encouraged to stay with this feeling of change, and the sensations of pleasure, delight, or pride that may accompany it. This staying with the feeling provides the opportunity for the patient to reflect on the change, its impact on the self, and the emotions emerging through the process. The therapist may then reflect on and disclose their own experience (a shared joy, pride, or experience of being moved), and explore the impact of their self-disclosure on the patient.

Examples of transformance in action that therapists may notice include a patient who found it scary to cook but since being in isolation has found a way to try new recipes and experienced mastery in the process; a patient whose need for self-care enabled boundary settings with anxious family members; a patient who has rediscovered an old hobby and noticed a resurgence of creativity. Therapists can be looking for evidence of transformance, and when they see it bring it to the patient's attention:"I heard you talk about how afraid you are, and how you describe these moments of bliss in your day when you are cooking for yourself. Can you tell me more about the part of you that comes alive when you're cooking?"

Metaprocessing transformational experience

If the patient also recognizes the experience of change, and change for the better at that, the next step is to explore how that change is experienced, perhaps through a simple, "And what is that like for you?" The exploration may be expanded to somatic feelings and sensations within the patient's body. The therapist, attuned to the patient's experience, will direct their own energy towards a joining with the patient, allowing them to share in the patient's affective experience, while outwardly matching the patient with their non-verbal expressions. At this point, the role of the relationship is brought to the surface – what is it like for a patient to feel joined, witnessed, or moved with their therapist? If the therapist has an emotional reaction, what is it like for the patient to notice their impact within the relationship?

The therapist supports the patient in fully experiencing their positive and negative emotions, allowing space for both the entirety of their grief and the entirety of their joy. The complexity of patients' emotional experiences during a moment of crisis such as COVID-19 serves to heighten the importance of the therapist creating space for moments of transformance, and transformational experiences, and creating an atmosphere of safety in which a patient can fully allow themselves to connect with their experience of positivity or growth. Transformational experience of transformance can be deepened and expanded when the patient and therapist experience it together: "What is it like for me to notice that?" or "What is it like to stay with that experience of aliveness right now?"

A recent example of transformance detection and processing of the resulting positive change (transformational change) during the coronavirus pandemic occurred with one of the authors of this paper (Hillary McBride). The patient is a physician working in the Intensive Care Unit (ICU) at the hospital designated for treating COVID patients in her city. She had previously successfully received treatment for an eating disorder, but described herself as still struggling with body-hatred, and the inability to care for her body or notice interoceptive cues. Within the session, she expressed her anger in a recent meeting at the hospital when the status of personal protective equipment was discussed. She told her therapist that for the first time since she started in her position, she spoke up in a meeting to state authoritatively that her body, and her colleagues bodies, were valuable, and worth protecting. After the patient said this somewhat matter-of-factly in the session, she was ready to move on. Instead, the therapist invited her to pause, and slow down, and notice what she was experiencing in the moment. The patient paused, and with a confused expression she said "Maybe for the first time, well the first time that I can remember as an adult, I can feel my worth. It's confusing, it feels new, but I feel like I know, deep in my bones, that my voice matters, and I have to use it". Knowing that within AEDP phenomenology, feeling confused in response to new experiences is a marker of the tremulous affects associated with positive and novel experiences that are at the edge of the patient's previous capacity (Fosha, 2006, 2013), the therapist with excitement asked: "And what is *that* like?" The patient, this time without hesitation, answered that she felt powerful and steady.

After two more rounds of metatherapeutic processing, and staying with this powerful and important new set of experiences, the therapist returned to a statement the patient had previously made when telling the story about being in the meeting and asserting that her body was valuable and worth protecting. The therapist said, "it really struck me when you used the word valuable to talk about your body. When we started working together you told me that your body seemed like such a burden to you. It seems that working in the ICU during the pandemic has really helped you know in a new way that your body is worth protecting". As the therapist shared her noticing of the patient's emerging transformation, the patient began to cry and said, smiling to the therapist, "you are so right, I didn't see that till you pointed it out. Something about being in this crisis has made me feel so connected to protecting myself, my actual physical body, in a way that I never have before". After pausing to metatherapeutically process this experience, the patient said with brightness in her eye, "I knew the pandemic would change me, but I didn't realize it would help me heal this thing I thought I'd carry around forever." She laughed and then said "if I think about it that way, I don't feel so scared to go to work anymore, I actually feel like it is part of how I can heal myself." This moment is reflective of the broaden-and-build theory of positive emotion, which identifies positive emotion as a tool to build upon our innate capacities to grow and flourish (Fredrickson, 2001). AEDP's methodology provides the how-to for bringing about these innate capacities (Fosha & Thoma, 2020).

Self-resourcing, and Care for Person of the Therapist

Demarcating personal and work life

With their clinical practice moving onto screens and into their homes, therapists who typically see patients at an office may sense the loss of a commute, or a separate space, and how those spatial distinctions offer them a boundary to further separate work life and personal life. Therapists working from the home office are encouraged to find other ways to demarcate their work, and what they energetically carry from sessions, into their home life. This may include a change of clothing following the work day to signify that work is finished, and now it's time to rest, beginning and ending the day with a mindfulness practice, visualization to signify the end of the work day (imagining closing files and placing them in a cabinet), washing hands or taking a shower, or going for a walk to then have the experience of "coming home" after the day of work.

Noticing and staying with the good

In the same way that therapists notice and encourage positive affect, moments of connection, and moments of vitality in their patients, therapists are encouraged to pay attention to these experiences within their personal life to put positive neuroplasticity into action (Hanson, 2018). As identified above, therapists may also notice that patients are more curious and attuned to their therapist's wellbeing than usual. While it can be habitual to deflect the patient's inquiry as irrelevant or a distraction, therapists too need to connect and know they are held in the heart and mind of their patients (Fosha, 2000). This is the ideal opportunity to model receptive affect, demonstrating to the patient how to take in concern and affection, while also feeling the closeness to their patients. Individuals can take time throughout the day, between sessions, and at the end of the day, to reflect on moments they feel proud of, or where they felt connected and seen by others. As recommended by Hanson (2013), to activate positive neuroplasticity, when something positive or meaningful occurs, individuals can allow themselves to drop into the sensory elements of the experience and expand it, stay with and sink into the experience, and link the positive content with something painful from the past. Hanson summarized his approach using the acronym HEAL (Have the experience, Enrich it, Absorb it, and Link it).

Experiencing dysregulation

Therapists will also likely be experiencing similar fear, sadness, grief, and anger that their patients are experiencing. While this is to be expected outside of session, as therapists encounter changes and losses in their every-day lives, therapists may be surprised to experience such dysregulation in session. When this happens during a session, therapists are encouraged to notice their emerging emotions, pause to ground themselves (perhaps using breathing or other somatic anchors), and use immediacy and modelling with their patients when appropriate. For example, the therapist may state, "I am noticing my own fear as you share about your own; this is impacting all of us. I am going to take a moment here to support myself so that I can be here in this moment with you; we can do that together if you like." After taking a moment to self-regulate, the therapist could make this experience more therapeutic by metatherapeutic processing the expression of their own fear (Fosha, 2017b), by asking the patient to notice what it was like for them to witness the therapist's experience of and attention to their own emotion. For therapists familiar with "parts" work from the Internal Family Systems school of practice, they may identify these as the emergence of a protective part, or younger child part, and thank those parts for emerging in the moment but ask to step aside to allow the therapist to continue to access their core self while attending to the patient (IFS; Schwartz, 1995; Schwartz & Sweezy, 2019). Taking note of which emotions, defenses, or parts, make themselves known in session can help the therapist identify the concerns to bring to their own therapist or supervisor.

Attuning to the self

The demands of caring for others in the pandemic, while also living through it themselves, cannot be understated. As therapists often suggest to their patients, when distress, pain, or suffering increase, there is an equal need for increased time to process, space for caring for the self, boundaries to be set, receiving care from others. Therapists are encouraged to note their level of fatigue, the quality of their inner dialogue, their sense of obligation to care for others, and the tasks and activities which were previously quotidien but now seem burdensome. What may have been an average day of seeing clients, may now seem too demanding. Adapting to new ways of living and conducting clinical work may require more opportunities to pause, check in, and mindfully observe one's inner experience. As therapists are skilled at supporting others in doing, the invitation is to notice the inner experience with curiosity, kindness, and compassion.

Making meaning through social engagement

Viktor Frankl's words and life experience remind us that we always have a choice about how to respond to situations, and have a choice about finding or making meaning out of situations that otherwise seem absurd and chaotic. Therapists are uniquely positioned to skillfully support people through a time of uncertainty, and may find meaning in their ability to help others, perceiving themselves and their training as useful to individuals and the broader community. For some, managing the daily duties may seem ample and even overwhelming. But for those who are energized through community involvement, and engagement in social discourse, there may be an opportunity for meaning making in speaking more publicly about mental health, and navigating the stressors and uncertainty of what lies ahead. Although not as clearly outlined in the APA code of ethics, the CPA code of ethics identifies that principle 4 is a responsibility to society – where psychologists are encouraged to participate in shaping the social construction of mental health, and decrease the barriers to access to therapy for those who are excluded from traditional forms of support because of socioeconomic, racial, or accessibility issues. Some therapists may consider this change in the social landscape as the right time to begin speaking more publicly about mental health, offering psychological resources and practices to their community as a way to find or make meaning.

Noticing and anticipating burnout

Maslach and Leiter (2016) identified the three key dimensions of job burnout as *exhaustion*, where workers feel overextended and depleted, *cynicism*, where workers experience negative, callous, or excessively detached relationship to work, and *inefficiency*, where workers self-identify as incompetent and lacking achievement. They also identified that lack of control, work overload, insufficient rewards, breakdown of community, inequity and lack of fairness, and value conflicts (such as conflict between personal goals and job demands) are conditions which create burnout, all variables which may impact therapists due to the changes in work because of the global pandemic. Leiter and Maslach (2014) identified that evidence based strategies for preventing and treating burnout across helping professions with high rates of burnout include mindfulness skills training, group and individual psychotherapy, expressive and dynamic approaches to psychotherapeutic interventions, increased peer support, and organization-wide changes. Their review of the literature has also suggested that intervention is immediate, specifically targeted for the person or organization, collaborative, and ongoing. Because of the isolating nature of providing psychotherapy from one's home office, therapists are encouraged to be in peer supervision groups, where they are noting signs of exhaustion, cynicism, and the sense of inefficiency.

Therapy and supervision

As client's presenting concerns change, as therapists themselves struggle with new concerns in their personal lives, or experience the isolation of working from home offices, therapists may also need to adapt the ways that they get support, including the frequency with which they receive supervision or their own therapy. Those experiencing the isolation of working from home may choose to coordinate online peer supervision to share resources and decrease the sense of carrying a clinical load alone. Therapists who are used to orienting their lives around the experiences of others might notice their own emotions and inner experiences impossible to ignore, are in need of more attention, or emerging indirectly through defensive coping behavior or thinking. Peer consultation, individual supervision, or therapy can be a place for therapists to discuss how they are faring personally, where others may be able to identify signs of burnout, compassion fatigue, or vicarious trauma invisible to themselves.

Conclusion

The rapid global changes occurring because of COVID-19 have dramatically impacted each level of the ecological system (Bronfenbrenner, 1979). It is anticipated that the impact on individuals and the therapists who support them will be profound. Through identifying the emerging concerns experienced by patients through this pandemic, therapists can be better prepared to offer support. These concerns centre around emotions such as fear, grief, and sadness, and a sense of isolation and disconnection unique to the current global events. The experience of social isolation and acute emotional experiences uniquely positions AEDP as an appropriate approach for working with clients at this time, by paying attention to emotional pain and undoing aloneness, moving through pain with dyadic affect regulation, and deepening and magnifying the good. However, for effective and meaningful clinical work to occur, self-care of the therapist must also be considered.

For individuals and communities to navigate through this unprecedented time, with the ability to experience goodness and connection intact, it will be important for deep relational therapeutic work to continue. As we physically distance, and move through the uncertainty of the future, we can be certain that we do not have to truly be or feel alone.

Disclosure statement

No potential conflict of interest was reported by the authors.

References

Boulanger, G. (2013). Fearful symmetry: Shared trauma in New Orleans after Hurricane Katrina. *Psychoanalytic Dialogues, 23*(1), 31–44.

Boulanger, G., Floyd, L. M., Nathan, K. L., Poitevant, D. R., & Pool, E. (2013). Reports from the front: The effects of Hurricane Katrina on mental health professionals in New Orleans. *Psychoanalytic Dialogues, 23*(1), 15–30.

Bronfenbrenner, U. (1979). *The ecology of human development*. Cambridge, MA: Harvard University Press.

Brooks, S. K., Dunn, R., Amlot, R., Rubin, G. J., & Greenberg, N. (2018). A systematic, thematic review of social and occupational factors associated with psychological outcomes in healthcare employees during an infectious disease outbreak. *Journal of Occupational and Environmental Medicine, 60*(3), 248–257.

Brooks, S. K., Webster, R. K., Smith, L. E., Woodland, L., Wessely, S., Greenberg, N., & Rubin, G. J. (2020). The psychological impact of quarantine and how to reduce it: Rapid review of the evidence. *Lancet, 395*(10227), 912–920.

Collins. (2008). Preventing health care–associated infections. Retrieved from https://www.ncbi.nlm.nih.gov/books/NBK2683/

Cook, S. C., Schwartz, A. C., & Kaslow, N. J. (2017). Evidence-based psychotherapy: Advantages and challenges. *Neurotherapeutics, 14*(3), 537–545.

Dubus, S. (2020, April 18). *Reports of domestic violence rise in recent weeks amid coronavirus outbreak* (S. Simon, Interviewer). National Public Radio.

Ecker, B. (2015). Understanding memory reconsolidation. *The Neuropsychotherapist* (10), 4–22. doi:10.12744/tnpt(10)004-022

Flannely, K. J., Roberts, S. B., & Weaver, A. J. (2005). Correlates of compassion fatigue and burnout in chaplains and other clergy who responded to the September 11th attacks in New York City. *The Journal of Pastoral Care & Counseling, 59*(3), 213–224.

Fosha, D. (2000). *The transforming power of affect: A model for accelerated change*. New York: Basic Books.

Fosha, D. (2004). "Nothing that feels bad is ever the last step:" The role of positive emotions in experiential work with difficult emotional experiences. *Clinical Psychology & Psychotherapy, 11*(1), 30–43.

Fosha, D. (2005). Emotion, true self, true other, core state: Toward a clinical theory of affective change process. *Psychoanalytic Review, 92*(4), 513–551.

Fosha, D. (2006). Quantum transformation in trauma and treatment: Traversing the crisis of healing change. *Journal of Clinical Psychology/In Session, 62*(5), 569–583.

Fosha, D. (2008). Transformance, recognition of self by self, and effective action. In K. J. Schneider (Ed.), *Existential-integrative psychotherapy: Guideposts to the core of practice* (pp. 290–320). New York, NY: Routledge.

Fosha, D. (2009). Emotion and recognition at work: Energy, vitality, pleasure, truth, desire & the emergent phenomenology of transformational experience. In D. Fosha, D. J. Siegel, & M. F. Solomon (Eds.), *The healing power of emotion: Affective neuroscience, development, clinical practice* (pp. 172–203). New York, NY: Norton.

Fosha, D., Paivio, S. C., Gleiser, K., & Ford, J. (2009). Experiential and emotion-focused therapy. In C. Courtois & J. D. Ford (Eds.), *Complex traumatic stress disorders: An evidence-based clinician's guide* (Chapter 14, pp. 286–311). New York: Guilford Press.

Fosha, D. (2013). Turbocharging the affects of healing and redressing the evolutionary tilt. In D. J. Siegel & M. F. Solomon (Eds.), *Healing moments in psychotherapy* (Chapter 8, pp. 129–168). New York: Norton.

Fosha, D. (2017). How to be a transformational therapist: AEDP harnesses innate healing affects to re-wire experience and accelerate transformation. In J. Loizzo, M. Neale, & E. J. Wolf (Eds.), Advances in contemplative psychotherapy: Accelerating healing and transformation (p. 204–219). Routledge/Taylor & Francis Group. https://doi.org/10.4324/9781315630045-18

Fosha, D. (2017a). How to be a transformational therapist: AEDP harnesses innate healing affects to re-wire experience and accelerate transformation. In J. Loizzo, M. Neale, & E. Wolf (Eds.), *Advances in contemplative psychotherapy: Accelerating transformation* (Chapter 14, pp. 204–219). New York, NY: Norton.

Fosha, D. (2017b). Something more than "something more than interpretation:" AEDP works the experiential edge of transformational experience to transform the internal working model. In S. Lord (Ed.), *Moments of meeting in psychoanalysis: Interaction and change in the therapeutic encounter* (Chapter 15, pp. 267–292). New York: Routledge.

Fosha, D., & Thoma, N. (2020). Metatherapeutic processing supports the emergence of flourishing in psychotherapy. *Psychotherapy*. doi:10.1037/pst0000289

Fosha, D., Thoma, N., & Yeung, D. (2019). Transforming emotional suffering into flourishing: Metatherapeutic processing of positive affect as a trans-theoretical vehicle for change. *Counselling Psychology Quarterly*, *32*(3–4), 563–593.

Fredrickson, B. L. (2001). The role of positive emotions in positive psychology. The broaden-and-build theory of positive emotions. *The American Psychologist*, *56*(3), 218–226.

Hanson, R. (2013). *Hardwiring happiness: The new brain science of contentment, calm, and confidence*. New York, NY: Harmony.

Hanson, R. (2018). *Resilient: How to grow an unshakable core of calm, strength, and happiness*. New York, NY: Harmony.

Hendel, H. J. (2018). *It's not always depression: A new theory of listening to your body, discovering core emotions and reconnecting with your authentic self*. New York, NY: Spiegel and Grau.

HHS Office of the Secretary, Office for Civil Rights, & OCR. (2020, March 30). Notification of enforcement discretion for telehealth. Retrieved from https://www.hhs.gov/hipaa/for-professionals/special-topics/emergency-preparedness/notification-enforcement-discretion-telehealth/index.html

Hoff, L. A., Hallisey, B. J., & Hoff, M. (2009). *People in crisis: Clinical and diversity perspectives*. New York, NY: Routledge.

Iwakabe, S., Edlin, J., Fosha, D., Gretton, H., Nakamura, K., Joseph, A. J., … Thoma, N. (2020). The transdiagnostic effectiveness of Accelerated Experiential Dynamic Psychotherapy (AEDP) in private practice settings: A practice-research network study. Submitted for publication.

Leiter, M. P., & Maslach, C. (2014). Interventions to prevent and alleviate burnout. In M. Leiter, A. Bakker, & C. Maslach (Eds.), *Burnout at work: A psychological perspective* (pp. 145–183). New York, NY: Psychology Press.

Lipton, B., & Fosha, D. (2011). Attachment as a transformative process in AEDP: Operationalizing the intersection of attachment theory and affective neuroscience. *Journal of Psychotherapy Integration*, *21*(3), 253–279.

Macran, S., & Shapiro, D. A. (1998). The role of personal therapy for therapists: A review. *British Journal of Medical Psychology*, *71*(1), 13–25.

Maslach, C., & Leiter, M. P. (2016). Understanding the burnout experience: Recent research and its implications for psychiatry. *World Psychiatry: Official Journal of the World Psychiatric Association (WPA)*, *15*(2), 103–111.

Nania, R. (2020, April 9). Higher covid-19 incidence in minority communities. Retrieved from https://www.aarp.org/health/conditions-treatments/info-2020/minority-communities-covid-19.html

Prenn, N. (2009). I second that emotion! On self-disclosure and its metaprocessing. In A. Bloomgarden & R. B. Mennuti (Eds.), *Psychotherapist revealed: Therapists speak about self-disclosure in psychotherapy* (pp. 85–99). New York, NY: Routledge.

Prenn, N. (2011). Mind the gap: AEDP interventions translating attachment theory into clinical practice. *Journal of Psychotherapy Integration*, *21*(3), 308.

Prenn, N., & Halliday, K. (Directors). (2020a). Kate & Natasha: AEDP therapy in the age of corona episode 2 [Video file]. https://www.youtube.com/watch?v=U8goSFvTTN8

Prenn, N., & Halliday, K. (Directors). (2020b). Kate & Natasha: How to do AEDP therapy online episode 3 [Video file]. https://www.youtube.com/watch?v=7ZVTxLnDRbo

Prenn, N., & Halliday, K. (Directors). (2020c). Kate & Natasha: How to do AEDP therapy online episode 7 [Video file] https://www.youtube.com/watch?v=0aYW2MPbZdg

Pulido, M. L. (2012). The ripple effect: Lessons learned about secondary traumatic stress among clinicians responding to the September 11th terrorist attacks. *Journal of Clinical Social Work*, *40*(3), 307–315.

Redinger, M., & Gibb, T. (2020). Counter-transference and the clinical ethics encounter: What, why, and how we feel during consultations. *Cambridge Quarterly of Healthcare Ethics*, *29*(2), 317–326.

Romero. (2020, April 9). Checkpoints, curfews, airlifts: Virus rips through Navajo nation. Retrieved from https://www.nytimes.com/2020/04/09/us/coronavirus-navajo-nation.html

Rubinstein, T. (2015). Relational theory: A refuge and compass. *Clinical Social Work Journal*, *43*(4), 398–406.

Russell, E. M. (2015). *Restoring resilience: Discovering your clients' capacity for healing*. New York, NY: Norton.

Rycroft, F., & Perlesz, A. (2001). Speaking the unspeakable: Reclaiming grief and loss in family life. *Australian and New Zealand Journal of Family Therapy*, *22*(2), 57–65.

Schwartz, R. (1995). *Internal family systems therapy*. New York: The Guilford Press.

Schwartz, R. C., & Sweezy, M. (2019). *Internal family systems therapy* (2nd ed.). New York, NY: Guilford.

Shultz, J., Cooper, J., Baingana, F., Oquendo, M., Espinel, Z., Althouse, B., ... Rechkemmer, A. (2016, November). The role of fear-related behaviors in the 2013–2016 West Africa Ebola virus disease outbreak. Retrieved from https://www.ncbi.nlm.nih.gov/pmc/articles/PMC5241909/

Wallin, D. (2007). *Attachment in psychotherapy*. New York, NY: Guilford Press.

World HWorld Health Organization. 2020. WHO director-general's opening remarks at media briefing on covid-19 March 11. https://www.who.int/dg/speeches/detail/who-director-general-s-opening-remarks-at-the-media-briefing-on-covid-19-11-march-2020

Work with emotions in remote psychotherapy in the time of Covid-19: a clinical experience

Alexine Thompson-de Benoit and Ueli Kramer

ABSTRACT

Objective: Face-to-face experiential work with emotions is effective, but it remains unclear what the feasibility of teletherapeutic work with emotions is. The current Covid-19 worldwide situation represents an opportunity for psychotherapists to test new ways of working with clients, including from an emotion-focused and emotionally focused perspective.

Methods: The present brief report describes a clinical experience based on 6 weeks, so far, of telepsychotherapeutic work focused on emotions via online tools, during the Covid-19 partial confinement in Switzerland.

Results: We found a certain feasibility of remote work with emotions in psychotherapy, for individual clients, and for couples. Specific challenges represent relationship and contextual factors (clear communication, using tone of voice, regular check ins, setting up a clear frame, technical aspects of communication, the Self of the therapist), accessing and deepening emotions and managing dysregulated experience and interpersonal escalation.

Discussion: Based on this initial clinical experience, we propose that Integrative experiential practice partially delivered via a computer screen be studied in controlled settings by psychotherapy research in the future.

Introduction

Accessing, expressing, describing, regulating, accepting and transforming emotion are described as central processes for outcome in psychotherapy (Peluso & Freund, 2018). Beyond the general consensus that emotion is important in psychotherapy, there is a growing acceptance that the in-session *experience*, within a warm and prizing therapeutic relationship, is key for successful processes and outcome (Auszra, Greenberg, & Herrmann, 2013; Fosha, 2000; Greenberg, 2019). Experiential-humanistic therapy approaches have revised and refined their tasks and techniques over the past five decades, moving towards specific, and more and more differentiated, steps of productively working with emotions from an integrative perspective (Elliott, Watson, Greenberg, Timulak, & Freire, 2013; Greenberg, 2019; Johnson et al., 1988; Pascual-Leone, 2018). The current Covid-19 situation challenges experiential practice in psychotherapy to some extent, and poses the challenge of transiently working remotely, via teletherapy, in effective ways with emotions in psychotherapy, assuming that there will be a time of face-to-face meetings again in the future. However, in light of the fact that it is not clear how long the pandemic will be around for, but also of the large percentage of clients who do not have access to experiential therapists, this situation also provides an opportunity to ask ourselves whether one can do experiential therapy remotely, for the entirety of the treatment. Our experience so far is conclusive.

Since the 1980s, experiential couple's therapies, developed initially by Greenberg and Johnson (1988) as an integration of experiential, Person-Centered and Gestalt therapy, have differentiated today into several models of psychotherapy, including emotion-focused therapy for couples (Greenberg & Goldman, 2008; Greenberg & Woldarsky Meneses, 2020) and emotionally focused couple therapy (Johnson, 2019a/b). Emotionally focused couple therapy (EFCT; Johnson, 2019a) focuses on attachment-related emotions triggered in partner interactions and understands their dysfunctional dynamic in terms of a fundamental separation distress. The emotions that ensue – fear, panic, sadness, anger – are understood as secondary defensive or protective reactions, rather than a primary emotion that aims to reach out to each other from a vulnerable place and asking for needs to be met in a clear, non-threatening manner. EFCT helps partners access their more vulnerable emotions and attachment-related needs, and fosters, through enactments, the creation of a new dynamic in which vulnerability is possible, safety is restored, and needs are clearly expressed and responded to within the couple's relationship.

Emotion-focused approaches differentiate in their assessment between primary adaptive, maladaptive and secondary emotional experiences (Greenberg, 2019). In the current context of Covid-19, primary adaptive fear is core to many clients' experience ("I am afraid of being infected/unwillingly infect others, and death may ensue") which orients the person's decisions, actions and cognitions. While fear has been discussed as a cognitive coping strategy with the current crisis (Schimmenti, Billieux, & Starcevic, 2020), from a differentiated perspective focused on emotion, primary adaptive fear is a freshly experienced core emotion that has a high adaptive value (i.e., the social distancing serves survival), thus needs to be differentiated from singular experiences of primary maladaptive fear (i.e., "I am afraid of remaining lonely and disconnected amid the pandemic") and from secondary fear (i.e., "I am afraid of being overwhelmed by too much information related with the pandemic"). From an emotion-focused viewpoint, while the primary adaptive experiences need to be acknowledged, deepened and completed, primary maladaptive and secondary fear experiences call for specific experiential interventions (Greenberg, 2019) requiring in addition emotion transformation. Similar elaborations may be proposed for helplessness, loneliness, anger and shame, all possible human emotional responses to a pandemic.

In the context of work with couples, EFCT is an evidence-based approach, supported by a number of outcome and process studies (e.g., Bradley & Furrow, 2004; Cloutier, Manion, Gordon Walker, & Johnson, 2002; Couture-Lalande, Greenman, Naaman, & Johnson, 2007; Halchuk, Makinen, & Johnson, 2010; Johnson & Greenberg, 1988), and providing a clear map of the therapeutic processes of change.

At the time of writing this paper (May, 14th, 2020; source: corona-data.ch), Switzerland presents with one of the highest formally reported numbers of infections per capita, with 30 364 nominally reported infected cases and 1870 fatalities in a small country of approximately 8.57 millions inhabitants (as of 2019). Yet, emotion-focused work is intensively practiced in Switzerland, mostly by psychotherapists in private practice, in particular in the context of a currently ongoing national practitioners-researchers network study (PRN; Castonguay, Barkham, Lutz, & McAleavey, 2013; Kramer & Woldarsky Meneses, 2019). The question whether working remotely with emotions is feasible, and effective, given the current Covid-19 situation, has arisen among this network of clinicians. Similarly, the current situation also raises the question whether there is a "good-enough" level of depth of emotional processing which can be achieved via teletherapy. While from a larger perspective we can conclude that teletherapy was demonstrated to be effective according to a recent meta-analysis (Varker, Brand, Ward, Terhaag, & Phelps, 2019), the more differentiated work with emotions remains a clinical challenge in the current context.

There has been conversations in the past among practicing clinicians whether experiential approaches are compatible with teletherapeutic work, whether it is possible to access emotions in a good-enough manner, or as deeply as in the face-to-face interactions one has in their private practice office, whether enactments are as powerful when done through a computer screen, and whether couple interactions are manageable when the therapist is not in the same room. The current brief paper offers a subjective experience of work with emotions, from an emotionally focused work with couple's perspective, and suggests that, under certain circumstances, such work is feasible.

From our experience across the past weeks of therapeutic work in the context of Covid-19 situation, we offer here principles of an effective and safe teletherapeutic process focused on emotion. While these principles stem from EFCT, we think that they may hold true for many integrative therapists interested to evoke, describe and deepen, support and foster adaptive emotional experiences when working with clients via teletherapy in the context of Covid-19. We need to note that all experiences crystallized in the present paper are transient and based on real clinical material with clients that had consulted in face-to-face meetings before, as well as during the current situation. We do not know if these experiences hold true in therapies conducted exclusively via teletherapy, or in other contexts of confinement, but we may speculate that they may be relevant in the broader context of experiential therapy delivered remotely.

The main challenges, from our perspective, are bundled into three categories: (a) relationship and contextual factors, (b) accessing and deepening emotions, and (c) managing dysregulated experience and interpersonal escalation. We will speak to these one by one in the present account.

Relationship and contextual factors

A core task of emotion focused work in psychotherapy concerns the building of a therapeutic alliance, using empathic stance and techniques, and creating an in-session safety space by a therapist's presence in the here and now (Elliott, Bohart, Watson, & Murphy, 2019; Geller et al., 2012). Face-to-face sessions allow therapists to communicate warmth and safety through many different sensory channels: direct eye contact, tone of voice, open posture, body movements, synchrony and attunement, all of which are much harder to coordinate via a screen, but not impossible.

Clear communication

Informed consent about the risks, benefits and differences of teletherapy is important. Clients need to be informed about how therapists maintain safety and confidentiality, which encrypted platform we use online (different options like zoom business account, doxy.me, doctolib and such seem to offer secure options). We think therapists may communicate with clients about what they cannot see during the session, such as the fact that when the therapist looks down to his/her right, it may be that he/she is taking notes. It may also be important to render explicit that the therapist is in a closed room, all alone, so that privacy is maintained. Addressing what to do if the internet connection fails is also essential.

Using tone of voice

Direct eye contact is slightly compromised, because looking at the person on the screen will make the therapist look slightly down from the camera. Hence, the client does not necessarily know the therapist is looking at him/her. When working with couples, it is important to say the first name of each partner when addressing them and to let them know that we are looking at them. Tone of voice, as the polyvagal theory suggested (Porges, 2011), may be an unequivocal signal of safety communicated to the brain. This channel becomes a potential asset during online sessions and is part of the process of emotional attunement.

Regular check ins

Making process inquiries may be familiar to many process-oriented psychotherapists. With teletherapy work, these inquiries are emphasized through making sure the client is comfortable, asking him/her how this experience is going and checking in at the end of the session to see how the session felt.

Setting up a clear frame

Transparency about the therapist's work, how difficult moments, crisis, or interpersonal escalation will be handled, why therapist may use enactments, why the therapist may interrupt the process at specific moments, will ensure not only a safer process, but also a smoother one.

> For example, a couple's therapist may say: "I am not interrupting you to be rude, I am interrupting you because I can see you are starting to spin into your typical interpersonal cycle right now, and since I am not in the room with you, I have no other way than to stop you from getting taken into this destructive pattern. So when I see this is starting to happen, I will stop you, we will slow down the process, and we will zoom in on what is happening in the moment so we can gain understanding and control over this pattern. Does that make sense?".

In particular in emotion-focused work, the therapist takes a humble position, adopts and models an authentic curiosity for the other's experience and suffering (Buber, 1958), and in couple's therapy, shows interest in understanding the inner world of *both* partners. Transparency is an important part of that humble stance in particular when working remotely.

Technical aspects of communication

Having a good online connection and a good microphone, proper lighting, setting up the camera at eye level to maximize the precision of eye contact, logging out of other programs on the computer, turning off all notifications so as to avoid distractions, having everything the therapist needs during the session only a few inches away and dressing up professionally are key in conducting a successful teletherapy session.

The self of the therapist

Relationship and affective attunement in session is central for working with emotions. It was suggested that self-awareness, in the sense of therapist presence, is important in order to do good-quality work and remain truly open-minded and welcoming to the ongoing process (Geller & Greenberg, 2012; Zeytinoglu-Saydam & Nino, 2018). Doing remote work may require even more than usual self-awareness on part of the therapist. Staying attuned to one's energy level, need for breaks and time between sessions, as well as time before sessions to ground oneself in the moment and review progress notes from previous sessions will help therapists be ready to use all their senses and skills to connect to their clients. Remote sessions seem to require more focus for many therapists and having to rely more heavily on the use of one's voice, as mentioned above, can be tiring. However, it can also be extremely rewarding when the use of interventions such as leaning in, mirroring, validating, empathic-evocative responding and enactments create comparable processes than can be observed face-to-face.

Accessing and deepening emotions

Experiencing emotion is key to productive work in psychotherapy (Johnson & Greenberg, 1988; Pascual-Leone & Yeryomenko, 2016): it does go further than just "talking about the emotion", but it involves a bodily felt sense that informs the person about what he/she needs and what their innermost goals are. Change in therapy was linked with the depth of experiencing of emotions in session (Johnson & Greenberg, 1988), therefore, it makes sense that therapists may be reluctant to use online tools when working with emotion, based on a fear that emotions cannot be accessed at a deep enough level. In the context of EFT for couples, reflecting the moment-by-moment process, along with the secondary reactive emotions expressed in the interpersonal dynamics, and slowing down and zooming in on each partner's experience of the dynamic, in order to access more vulnerable attachment-related emotions underlying the defensive posture each one takes in the cycle may be indicated. From our experience, this requires a good reading of non-verbal cues so they can be noted and explored, and a sharp attunement to the inner world of each partner.

One could argue that a lot of information is lost when trying to do that via a screen. Our experience is that emotions can still be accessed at a deep level, even through a screen, at least to a certain extent. It can even, at times, be more powerful. Part of the powerfulness might come from the fact that a large part of the world population currently lives in a climate of fear and uncertainty, locked into their homes and doing their best to cope with these exceptional circumstances. This can definitely bring to a boil, not only secondary reactive emotions of irritation, frustration and impatience, but also more vulnerable emotions such as fear, sadness, loneliness, and isolation. Therefore, the current Covid-19 situation may be an opportunity to sharpen the therapist competencies in deepening and transforming emotions in therapy, in order to be able to help clients access, process and interpersonally disclose these emotions with their loved ones with whom they currently share a limited space.

We observe that it is important, more than ever, to slow down the process, and create a space where we can stop and feel. The therapist may have to choreograph that moment with precise directives.

> He/she may say: "Can we slow down here? You just talked about your sadness and the loneliness you feel when she doesn't hear you and seems stuck on her tracks, moving on without you. And yet as you talk about this sadness, you are still pretty energetic in your voice and the pace of your words. Can we slow down here and just see if you can feel the sadness? In your body, right now, if we stop here, how does the sadness feel? (silence, give time to answer). What would the sadness say, if it could talk?".

One could use the image of stopping the car one is currently driving, getting off the car, and choosing a spot to observe it, take in the view, breathe in the air, seeing how it feels to be stopped here, outside of the car, to have turned the engine off and just take it all in. From our experience, it might happen a bit less organically than in a face-to-face session, but with the therapist gentle direction, repetition, use of images, soft voice, slow pace, and using the clients' words, clients will follow into that space and allow themselves to access what is bubbling under the surface. Surprisingly, we find that being "forced" to be more directive via teletherapy may contribute to potentially positive results. The remote therapist will need to be more determined to stay away from content, because specific content may contribute to unmanageable experience and interpersonal escalation. More frequent interruptions seem to be necessary while making the implicit explicit to the clients and letting them know why we are stopping them.

> The therapist may say: "I'm sorry, I need to stop you because I see you going back into your head right now, and we are getting lost in examples, and that is exactly what happens, isn't it? When you get into your typical interpersonal cycle, it becomes about who's right and who's wrong, and you guys start spinning in circles, so I am going to stop you right here. I would like to go back to what you said a moment ago, because it was really important. You said ... ".

As therapists, we take here an assertive position of leading the session and interrupting clients. When such interruptions are done from a stance of emotional attunement unconditional positive regard and responsiveness (Bozarth, 2013), clients tend to be grateful and the process may become smooth.

Managing dysregulated experience and interpersonal escalation

Momentary dysregulated experience may be specifically related with finding oneself in quarantine, or semi-quarantine, as it is the case in the current Covid-19 situation in many places in the world. Clients may present with heightened levels of expressed emotions in the sessions and may feel the need to have a downregulating experience while talking to a therapist. While in certain cases, it may be advised to activate resourceful coping strategies to downregulate emotion in the telehealth session – because the therapist has less control of the session and is not physically present to provide support and help regulate the client – we point out to the underlying ethical dilemma when working with emotion: by proposing coping strategies in the face of apparent momentary dysregulated experience, the therapist may fail to acknowledge the underlying pain and deeper emotional vulnerability present in the moment (Kramer & Elliott, 2019). Such focus on coping may therefore contribute to the invalidating experience many clients have had in their personal history with regard to primary adaptive experiences. By focusing on down-regulating, the therapist may potentially undermine a productive therapeutic process. During teletherapy, the therapist may consider reflecting on this process, but also he/she may aim at "meeting" the client on an interpersonally deeper level, by offering empathic reflections and prizing, thus opening a space of shared experience via the screen. From our experience, this may also be feasible in the context of teletherapy.

In couple's therapy, it may be the case that partners engage in unproductive cycles in front of the camera. By interrupting such interpersonal cycles, the therapist maintains safety in the session. This is particularly important for teletherapy, given that the therapist cannot use the body to interrupt the couple's cycle, such as by getting up, moving closer or sitting between them. For example, therapists can prepare their couples at the beginning of the session, by setting some ground rules and explaining how such instances will be managed.

The therapist may say:

- "We all need to make an effort to listen to each other. Since I am not in the same room, if you start talking over each other, I cannot hear anything and will quickly get lost. Therefore, I will have to interrupt you right away if you start doing that."
- "If one of you starts feeling triggered, please let me know. If one of you leaves the room, we will interrupt the session until that person comes back."
- "We will end all sessions together, no matter what happens during the session. Your commitment to letting me bring closure to the session in a peaceful manner is extremely important."

If despite these instructions, couples still escalate, the therapist can use his or her voice to help regulate them, calling them by their first name, asking them to redirect their attention onto the therapist, and validating their reactive emotions so as to make them feel heard and seen, which may contribute to calming their nervous system. Later, the therapist can reframe what happened in terms of attachment and separation distress, highlighting the cycle they just got into, and normalizing how hard it is not to get into it, given how much is at stakes, how important this relationship is, and how much additional stress it is under, in this season of confinement.

Conclusions

Though doing experiential work remotely as psychotherapists may not have been what brought us into this profession in the first place, we can cautiously encourage mental health professionals to make their services available via an online platform, and try it out, and learn from the process. Health care needs for effective remote therapeutic work focused on emotion will most likely increase, and we believe that though some information is lost via an interposed screen, there are possibly ways of working around it, that still allow for emotions to be accessed, processed and transformed in powerful ways. The future will tell what psychotherapists may learn from this experience of confined work context, as well as their clients, that could be formulated in more precise recommendations on how to work with emotions in teletherapy. In the future, it may be useful to formulate specific research questions that can solidify our knowledge on the effectiveness, the relevance, and the specific conditions for therapeutic success in emotion and emotionally focused work partly delivered via teletherapy. Both couple's teletherapy and individual teletherapy should be studied, helping to enlarge the evidence base of experiential work in a great variety of human interactions.

Disclosure statement

No potential conflict of interest was reported by the authors.

References

Auszra, L., Greenberg, L. S., & Herrmann, I. (2013). Client emotional productivity – Optimal client in-session emotional processing in experiential therapy. *Psychotherapy Research*, *23*(6), 732–746.

Bozarth, J. (2013). Unconditional positive regard. *The handbook of person-centred psychotherapy & counselling* (pp. 180–192). doi:10.1007/978-1-137-32900-4_12

Bradley, B., & Furrow, J. L. (2004). Toward a mini-theory of the blamer softening event: Tracking the moment-by-moment process. *Journal of Marital and Family Therapy*, *30*(2), 233–246.

Buber, M. (1958). *I and thou* (2nd ed.). New York: Charles Scribner's Sons.

Castonguay, L., Barkham, M., Lutz, W., & McAleavey. (2013). Practice-oriented research. Approaches and applications. In M. J. Lambert (Ed.), *Handbook of psychotherapy and behavior change* (6th ed., pp. 85–133). Hoboken, NJ: John Wiley.

Cloutier, P., Manion, F., Gordon Walker, I. G., & Johnson, S. M. (2002). Emotionally focused interventions for couples with chronically ill children: A 2-year follow-up. *Journal of Marital and Family Therapy*, *28*(4), 391–398.

Couture-Lalande, M.-E., Greenman, P. S., Naaman, S., & Johnson, S. M. (2007). La thérapie de couple axée sur l'Émotion (EFT) pour traiter les couples dont la femme a le cancer du sein: Une étude exploratoire. *Psycho-Oncologie, 1*(4), 257–264.

Elliott, R., Bohart, A. C., Watson, J. C., & Murphy, D. (2019). Empathy. In J. C. Norcross & M. J. Lambert (Eds.), *Psychotherapy relationship that work*. (pp. 245-664), New York: Oxford University Press.

Elliott, R., Watson, J. C., Greenberg, L. S., Timulak, L., & Freire, E. (2013). Research on humanistic-experiential psychotherapies. In M. J. Lambert (Ed.), *Bergin and Garfield's handbook of psychotherapy and behavior change* (pp. 495–538). New York: Wiley.

Fosha, D. (2000). *The transforming power of affect: A model of accelerated change*. New York: Basic Books.

Geller, S. M., & Greenberg, L. S. (2012). *Therapeutic presence. A mindful approach to effective therapy*. Washington, D. C.: American Psychological Association.

Greenberg, L. S. (2019). Theory of functioning in emotion-focused therapy. In L. S. Greenberg & R. N. Goldman (Eds.), *Clinical handbook of emotion-focused therapy* (pp. 37–59). Washington, D. C.: American Psychological Association.

Greenberg, L. S., & Goldman, R. (2008). *Emotion-focused couples therapy: The dynamics of emotion, love and power*. Washington, DC: American Psychological Association.

Greenberg, L. S., & Johnson, S. M. (1988). *Emotionally focused therapy for couples*. New York: Guilford Press.

Greenberg, L. S., & Woldarsky Meneses, C. (2020). *Forgiveness and letting go in emotion-focused therapy*. Washington, D. C.: American Psychological Association.

Halchuk, R. E., Makinen, J., & Johnson, S. M. (2010). Resolving attachment injuries in couples using emotionally focused therapy: A three-year follow-up. *Journal of Couple & Relationship Therapy, 9*, 31–47.

Johnson, S. M. (2019a). *Attachment Theory in Practice: Emotionally Focused Therapy (EFT) with Individuals, Couples and Families*. New York: Guilford Press.

Johnson, S. M., & Greenberg, L. S. (1988). Relating process to outcome in marital therapy. *Journal of Marital and Family Therapy, 14*(2), 175–183.

Kramer, U., & Elliott, R. (2019). Ethical considerations in emotion-focused therapy. In M. Trachsel, S. Tekin, N. Biller-Andorno, J. Gaab, & J. Z. Sadler (Eds.), *The Oxford handbook of psychotherapy ethics* Oxford: Oxford University Press. doi:10.1093/oxfordhb/9780198817338.013.47.

Kramer, U., & Woldarsky Meneses, C. (2019). *Practitioner-researcher network on emotion-focused therapies: An example from Switzerland*. Discussion at the Biannual Meeting of the international society for emotion-focused therapy (isEFT). Glasgow.

Pascual-Leone, A. (2018). How clients change emotion with emotion: A programme of research on emotional processing. *Psychotherapy Research, 28*(2), 252–262.

Pascual-Leone, A., & Yeryomenko, N. (2016). The client's experiencing scale as a predictor of treatment outcomes: A meta-analysis on psychotherapy process. *Psychotherapy Research, 27*(6), 653–665.

Peluso, P. R., & Freund, R. R. (2018). Therapist and client emotional expression and psychotherapy outcomes. A meta-analysis. *Psychotherapy, 44*(4), 461–472.

Porges, S. W. (2011). *The polyvagal theory: Neurophysiological foundations of emotion, attachment, communication and self-regulation*. New York: W.W. Norton.

Schimmenti, A., Billieux, J., & Starcevic, V. (2020). The four horsemen of fear: An integrated model of understanding fear experiences during the COVID-19 pandemic. *Clinical Neuropsychiatry, 17*(2), 41–45.

Varker, T., Brand, R. M., Ward, J., Terhaag, S., & Phelps, A. (2019). Efficacy of synchronous telepsychology interventions for people with anxiety, depression, posttraumatic stress disorder, and adjustment disorder: A rapid evidence assessment. *Psychological Services, 16*(4), 621–635.

Zeytinoglu-Saydam, S., & Nino, A. (2018). A tool for connection: Using the person-of-the-therapist training (POTT) model in emotionally focused therapy supervision. *Journal of Marital and Family Therapy*. doi:10.1111/jmft.12349

Emotion-focused and video-technology considerations in the COVID-19 crisis

Allan Abbass and Jasen Elliott

ABSTRACT
The coronavirus or COVID-19 crisis has forced counsellors and therapists around the globe to use online videoconference programs to provide psychotherapy treatment, teaching, and supervision. Some varieties of psychotherapy have historically used video technology for these purposes. Intensive short-term dynamic psychotherapy (ISTDP), one such method, is built on activating intrapsychic crises that lead to emotional experiencing and change. In the current context, external or extrapsychic crises can also be a launchpad for personal growth. The treatment method relies on detailed examination of verbal and nonverbal cues as markers of unconscious avoidance processes and unconscious emotional experiences. Adopting video technology and online treatment presents some unique challenges and benefits. At the same time, the current COVID-19 crisis results in common treatment themes that therapists will encounter. In this review, we will examine common crisis response patterns, some client characteristics based on attachment trauma, and common themes emerging due to this crisis and the related social changes it brings. We will also review some technical issues and tips for those now pressed into using video technology, often for the first time.

Introduction

Videoconference technology is crucial to maintain counselling and psychotherapy services amid the isolating effects of the COVID-19 pandemic. Closed-circuit television and video link technologies for diagnostic and treatment efforts date as far as the 1960s, but, widespread clinical use of these has been ushered in by more recent technological, financial and other advances. (LeRouge & Garfield, 2013). The recent COVID-19 context is certainly pushing many clinicians out of their comfort zones to engage with clients online and incorporate this technology into routine clinical practice. Pros, cons, and other issues related to using this technology have been reviewed previously (e.g. Abbass, 2004; Elliott, Abbass, & Cooper, 2015; Elliott, Abbass, & Rousmaniere, 2018; Rousmaniere, 2014; Rousmaniere & Renfro-Michel, 2016). We provide a practical overview of videoconference technology and session recordings within the clinical context of a specific therapy approach – Intensive short-term dynamic psychotherapy (ISTDP; Abbass, 2015; Davanloo, 2001b).

ISTDP has a metapsychology that many common psychological problems are driven by unprocessed feelings from early attachment adversity that get reactivated in current relationships. The model incorporates video recording of sessions in training and routine practice for quality improvement and ongoing professional development. Given the limitations of memory and bias, a major advantage of using this technology is the opportunity for careful examination of verbal and nonverbal responses of both therapist and client through self-study, peer-consultation, and supervision.

When original reviews were written almost 20 years ago, videoconferencing and review of session recordings were not as common as they are today. Some initial challenges of using this technology include clinician and client discomfort with the technology. However, now, given the widespread use of social media and the fact that almost everyone has a camera in the form of a cell phone, people are generally more accustomed to being recorded. Thus, it is relatively easier to transition to recording and videoconferencing treatment sessions now than it was before the turn-of-the-century. Nonetheless, we recommend you take some extra time while orienting clients to the quality control rationale of using video recordings and the value of being able to see each other while connecting with videoconferencing technology.

If you have not been recording your counselling sessions or using videoconferencing, you may find this technology to be a challenge. Among other issues, you may for example, have discomfort or worry about how you will appear and perform on video or how others will perceive you while using recordings for peer review or supervision. These things may take some getting used to. However, once the initial discomfort passes, you will benefit from consultation and support from peers that this technology allows.

Videoconferencing issues

Secure videoconference applications are now more commonly used in clinical settings. However, there are certain issues that may arise while transitioning to this technology. Beyond ethical issues that we review in the above papers, some of the other emerging issues are as follows.

A change in the frame

Beginning to have online treatment sessions changes the treatment frame. First, you may be in your own home and you are seeing clients in their own homes while providing treatment. At the time of this writing, the vast majority of counselors in the Western world are housebound and not using their offices for clinical care because of the risk of spreading infection inside small offices. Now you are working from your house and your dog might be pawing at your door seeking food. You are only a few feet from post-work activity you will be doing later. You may be one room away from your children or partner. The context is a bit different and something to get used to. In the same way, your client maybe in a living room having shuffled both spouse and children out of the house for that hour. Otherwise, your client may be in a car, bedroom, or even a closet trying to find privacy. Another change in the context may include using a different administrative contact to arrange appointments and provide some orientation to the videoconference technology. We recommend being patient with yourself and clients while navigating this unusual situation. If there are feelings or other responses that come up about the change in frame or the technology; then, we recommend examining these feelings as a part of the therapeutic process so they do not become a treatment obstacle.

Comfort with technology

Although many videoconferencing applications are relatively simple to use, it is important for the therapist to be comfortable with the use of a computer and application while maintaining backup phone access to clients. It is not uncommon for therapists who finished their training in the 80s or 90s even to have some discomfort with these types of technologies. It is a good opportunity to speak to your younger relatives or friends who will be more than happy to give you an update on how current computers and these software programs work. It is also advisable to consult with your professional organization and current online application tutorials while conducting some trial runs.

Security and confidentiality

Both you and the client need to be comfortable with the security of the technology you use while negotiating the limits to confidentiality. For this reason, you require related professional procedures and secure videoconferencing applications that are encrypted and recommended by your professional licensing bodies for these purposes. It is important to recognize that sessions could be recorded by the client without your consent. While this is possible, it would be highly unlikely for this to happen inside of a trusting therapeutic relationship. It is important that there is an adequate level of trust both ways to have such an exposed process. Both of you need to be willing to work together to establish a reasonable level of comfort within this format in order to have a therapeutic impact rather than becoming distracted by related worries.

New client at a distance

Because you're not in the same location as your client, be prepared for unforeseen difficulties. If your client is new to you, then be sure to get personal phone numbers and a backup phone number (e.g. name and phone number of emergency contact, physician, or local urgent services). If you are seeing a new person, then you may not know what type of psychological or psychiatric difficulties are present in advance so these backups are important. Having the phone numbers is also important in case the technology breaks down and the session must be continued on the telephone.

Looking into a computer

With most videoconferencing applications you are typically looking at a computer screen at a person who is doing the same on the other end. Collaborate with your client to ensure adequate lighting and sound for a therapy session. Headphones are advisable along with adjusting your typical speech and turn-taking rates to the available Internet speed at the time of your videoconference. Even under the best conditions, the sound and appearance of the client will obviously differ from an in-person session. Getting used to these differences is important and it can help to imagine or think of the client in three dimensions while attempting to connect via a two-dimensional image. It can also be helpful to normalize the context and to begin referring to the videoconference space as "here with me" or "here together" while attempting to reach through any technological barriers to connect with your client.

Where is the eye contact?

If you're used to working in a therapy model where eye contact is encouraged and expected, such as ISTDP, it can be a challenge to maintain eye contact or even to know whether or not the client is looking at your eyes on their screen. Using a computer, it is useful to position the image of your client in the videoconference application just below your computer web camera so that you are looking in the general direction of the camera while viewing your client's image. Also, positioning your computer so that the web camera is at your eye level and sitting back from your computer slightly can enable good approximation of direct eye contact so you can detect breaks in eye contact and other nonverbal distancing maneuvers. We recommend coaching your client to set up a similar arrangement.

Seeing the upper body and gestures

Ideally, it is best to have your client sit far enough back from the computer web camera so that you can see them from the waist up or at least the gestures of their arms and upper body. This arrangement allows you to detect changes in muscle tension (e.g. hand clenching, sighing respirations) and other markers of emotional activation. Similarly, it is best for you to back up enough so that the client can see your emotional responses, arm gestures, and other nonverbal responses. Therapists also have a unique opportunity for increased self-reflection during sessions by periodically noticing their own emotional and nonverbal responses on the screen.

Recording sessions

After obtaining written consent to video record sessions, it will be a good opportunity to begin to record sessions if you have not been doing so before. This may be the first time that you record sessions and are able to review them for the benefit of yourself and your client. This may be one of the big advantages of this online treatment wave on future clinical practice. In order to get a more usable recording, it is best to set up a side-by-side image of you and your client for review purposes. Split screen is superior to having a smaller picture-in-picture configuration where the therapist is barely visible–making it difficult to examine your own responses to the therapy work under way. Some videoconferencing applications allow for secure and straightforward session recording whereas others require you to record from your computer screen, often with larger video file sizes.

Self review of video sessions

Different treatment methodologies emphasize different psychological processes. However, common themes across therapy models include the establishment of a conscious therapeutic alliance, emotional attunement, collaboration, shared goals and tasks, and an alive, engaged process bolstering various cognitive, interpersonal, and emotional capacities. While doing self-review from video recordings, you can self-reflect on areas of the interview that seemed challenging or where the process seemed to get stuck. You can then try to put yourself in the position of your client or see if you can detect any emotional or psychological responses in yourself that gives insight into what you may do differently the next time you meet together. You can also use the same technology for deliberate practice in targeted areas of your clinical work over time (Elliott et al., 2018). The advantages of this type of review are immense.

Peer review of video sessions

Peer review of video sessions offers an opportunity to have another pair of eyes and another person's emotional structure to provide an independent look at your treatment processes. This can be invaluable on so many different levels. First of all, it can assist you to feel more confident about what you are doing. It reduces the isolation that you may feel in private practice with often challenging clinical situations. It allows validation of various experiences that you may be having in your treatment sessions. Thus, in many ways, peer review contributes to your ongoing professional development. Beyond this, there are some client populations (e.g. severe personality disorder) and clinical situations (e.g. psychiatric inpatients) where none of us should be working entirely on our own without the support of a colleague.

Indeed, many peer review groups are already conducted online through videoconferencing applications and some include consultation and learning based on review of actual therapy session video recordings rather than discussion without any video. So, you will be sitting together, online, watching each other watch videos that were recorded online. All of these aspects are things to get used to compared to in-person meetings and case conferences. We have also used this technology to review the process of video-based supervision online, adding another layer to it all (Abbass et al., 2011; Elliott et al., 2018). A few advantages to think of include easier access to peers and supervisors from abroad as well as savings on parking costs, gas, and travel time.

Responses to the COVID-19 crisis

The responses that your client will have to a major crisis like the COVID-19 pandemic will depend on various factors such as the nature of her individual experience (e.g. duration, severity, and predictability of external stressor, degree of social isolation) combined with her psychological makeup, attachment history, early adversity, anxiety tolerance, and personality structure (e.g. Ford, Grasso, Elhai, & Courtois, 2015). Using an ISTDP framework (Abbass, 2015), we can categorize response patterns to external stressors such as COVID-19 in several ways: tense and busy, weak and depleted, and frightened and guarded response patterns (Table 1).

In the tense and busy response pattern, the person is fairly well adapted, keeping up on news, staying busy, mentally focused, and ready to respond to the environment. She may lose some sleep and complain about being tense. She is reaching out for information and supports. She aims to lend support to others and has energy to do so. She may tend to worry and obsess resulting in distraction.

In the weak and depleted response pattern, the person will be fatigued and note weak muscles. He may want to stay in bed. He may have stomach upset, headaches, and other somatic symptoms. He may be pessimistic and very depressed. He feels overwhelmed and defeated by the stressor, akin to a state of learned helplessness. In the extreme, he may have suicidal ideation. He is quite prone to substance use at this time.

In the frightened and guarded response pattern, the person is acutely preoccupied with the threat from the stressor. He may be obsessed with the risks of infection and be

Table 1. General stress response patterns.

	Tense–busy	Weak-depleted	Frightened-guarded
Cognitive	Realistic view on the crisis or obsessions about the crisis	Depressive view of the crisis, suicidal ideation	Paranoid ideas, preoccupied with threats, risks
Behavior	Staying educated, active, engaged, some compulsive behaviour	Low activity, avoidant due to low energy and drive	Hypervigilance, monitoring excessively
Interpersonal	Connect to others to help and get help, but tend to over-control	Avoiding support from others due to pessimism or become overly passive-dependant.	Avoiding others due to suspicion and mistrust
Emotional	Nervous, irritable, but able to grieve losses that arise	Weepiness, helplessness, hopelessness	Irritability, fearfulness
Physical	Tension in muscles. May have muscle aches. Some sleep loss	Stomach upset, migraines, fatigue, hypersomnia or insomnia	Tend toward mental clouding and confusion, insomnia

extremely vigilant to prevent it. He will have a lot of difficulty sleeping due to fear. He will have difficulty trusting others not to contaminate him so will likely avoid people and become more socially isolated. He may become overly irritable and hostile toward perceived threats. His senses are all on high alert, noting sounds smells and even tastes he would not otherwise detect. He may be too afraid to use a substance or medications to calm down.

Note that these response patterns can all be considered adaptations to external stressors and threats. All of these patterns have certain advantages and disadvantages. A person may move between these patterns as the nature or intensity of the threat changes. However, some of these patterns may reflect a serious mental illness reactivated by the stressors. For example, a person with schizophrenia may have a psychotic episode with delusions and other psychotic features. In this context, we should be monitoring and staying in supportive contact with more vulnerable individuals in such difficult times.

Intensive short-term dynamic psychotherapy

Intensive short-term dynamic psychotherapy (ISTDP) is a relatively brief treatment approach that was developed by Dr. Habib Davanloo at McGill University (Davanloo, 1990; 2001a; 2001b). He developed the approach and related metapsychology from detailed case studies of hundreds of recorded therapy sessions beginning in the 1970s and continuing into the 2000s. The method has been taught and researched using video technology for over 40 years. ISTDP and treatment methods derived from it called Experiential Dynamic Therapies (WWW.IEDTA.NET) have empirical support from 50 randomized controlled trials and a large number of case series for the full spectrum of common mental disorders, including personality disorders, anxiety, depression, and somatic symptom disorders. There is also evidence ISTDP can be helpful with clients with more severe mental disorders, including treatment-resistant depression, bipolar disorder, psychotic disorders and substance addiction (Abbass, 2016; Abbass, Bernier, Kisely, Town, & Johansson, 2015; Frederickson, DenDooven, Abbass, Solbakken, & Rousmaniere, 2018; Town, Abbass, Stride, & Bernier, 2017).

The ISTDP model has a dynamic, emotion-focused framework emphasizing the close study of nonverbal and verbal communication as well as unconscious anxiety and emotional pathways in the body. The ultimate objective of the treatment is handling unconscious defensive patterns or resistances that prevent emotional closeness with the therapist and the subsequent experience of unprocessed complex feelings related to the client's early attachment disruptions or adversities. In this framework, symptoms and behavior problems related to current and past attachments and attachment disruptions are the central focus (Malan, 1995; Figure 1).

Davanloo was influenced by the work of Lindemann (1944), an early grief researcher who worked with clients from the Cocoanut Grove fire tragedy in which almost 500 people perished. One of Lindemann's findings were that the psychological impact of the fire crisis appeared to create a window of opportunity in which some clients' past trauma-related feelings were activated and more accessible. It was partly from this work that Davanloo recognized a therapeutic opportunity could be achieved for clients who were not currently in a crisis by facilitating a type of internal or intrapsychic crisis. Specifically, this crisis involved more resistant clients being put face-to-face with the current destructiveness of their defensive response patterns that had been developed to cope with their attachment difficulties in childhood. Through developing treatment interventions specifically timed and geared to help the client recognize and rise above the defeating defensive patterns, Davanloo (1990) and his clients described a process of "unlocking the unconscious" wherein emotions, memories, and images related to previous attachment trauma were mobilized in the treatment relationship and then processed in a healing manner.

A major emphasis of the ISTDP model is on evaluating attachment patterns as identified by defensive response patterns to the clinical interview (Neborsky & Bundy, 2013). Clients are categorized along two major spectra in the ISTDP metapsychology (Figure 2). First, the psychoneurotic spectrum includes clients who have somatic anxiety mediated primarily through voluntary muscle tension along with the capacity to isolate affect and use formal defenses to distance and detach from the therapist. On one end of the psychoneurotic spectrum are low resistant clients who have had a loss with grief that is not resolved. They do not have any unprocessed rage or guilt about rage towards attachment figures and they have a secure attachment style. On the other end of the spectrum are highly resistant clients who have had major disruption of attachments inside the first 5 years of life (e.g. loss, parental divorce or depression). These clients have rigid defensive patterns that prevent closeness with the others, including the therapist, resulting in self-sabotaging behaviors and that prevent access to their own feelings. These

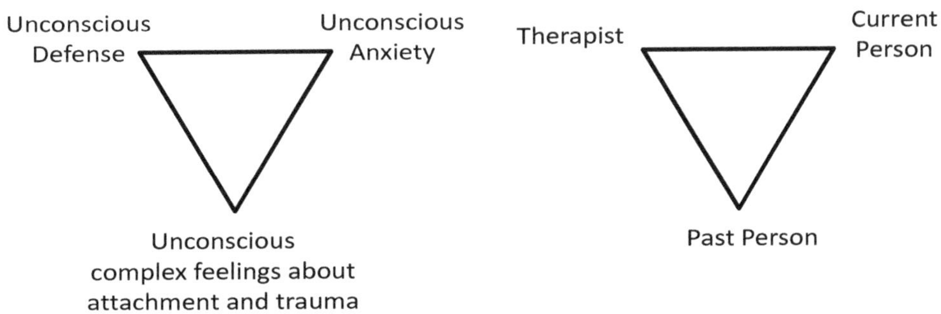

Figure 1. The two triangles.

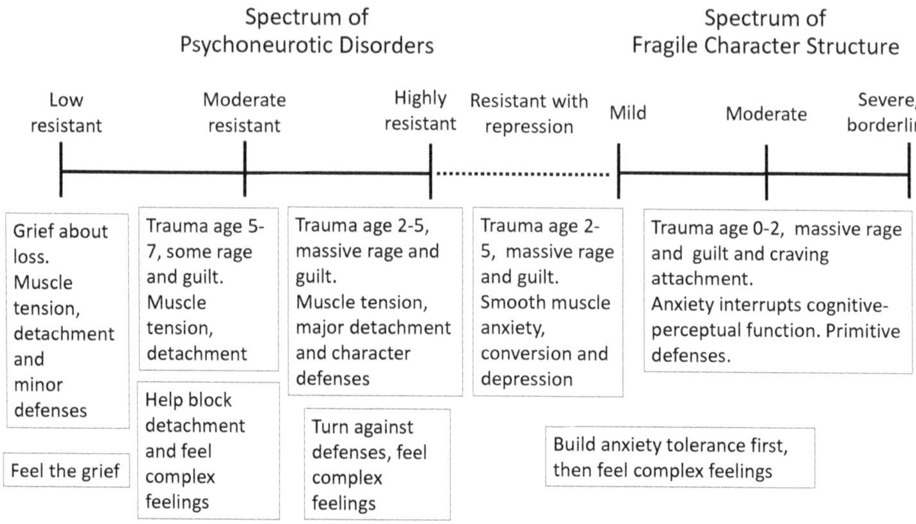

Figure 2. Spectra of clients suitable for ISTDP.

defenses are so fixed and automatic that the client himself cannot see them anymore. These clients have intense painful feelings, rage, and guilt about the rage toward attachment figures. In the middle of the spectrum are moderately resistant clients who have had later attachment trauma, typically from age 5 to 7. They have a moderate level of intensely held defenses to prevent the experience of mixed painful feelings, rage, and guilt about rage related to these attachment interruptions (Figure 2).

The second major spectrum, fragile character structure, includes clients with limitations in anxiety tolerance and reflective capacity, resulting in cognitive-perceptual disruption and primitive defenses at some level of rise in anxiety. Mildly fragile clients experience cognitive perceptual disruption and use primitive defenses at a high rise in anxiety while severely fragile clients have the same experiences at a low rise in anxiety. These clients have insecure attachment or disorganized attachment styles. The more severe fragile clients have dissociative disorders and borderline personality features (Figure 2).

In between these two spectra of clients are those who have resistance involving repression. These clients have also had major trauma in the first 4 years of life and the main manifestations of this are chronic repression of the emotions into the body. The result is fatigue, irritable bowel syndrome and migraine headaches, major depressive disorder, and motor conversion disorder with episodic weakness and paralysis (Figure 2).

Interventions to match response patterns

The treatment process for these different categories of clients varies according to client capacity to reflect and tolerate anxiety and related underlying attachment feelings. Low resistant clients and moderate resistant clients have good anxiety tolerance and reflective capacity, and generally only need encouragement to be emotionally present and to identify and feel their emerging complex feelings. The treatments with these clients are relatively short, ranging from one to 10 meetings. More highly resistant clients have robust defensive patterns that function as a barrier to emotional closeness with the therapist and their own underlying complex attachment feelings. These clients require considerable work to help them consciously recognize, evaluate and then turn against these defensive patterns in order to be emotionally present while identifying and experiencing their emerging attachment-related feelings. Treatment with these clients is longer, ranging from 20 to 40 meetings. Clients who have significant repression require a graded treatment process to build anxiety tolerance first before they are able to effectively tolerate their underlying mixed feelings. Treatment for clients with significant repression is typically longer, requiring 20 to 40 meetings. Fragile clients also require a gradual process of capacity building prior to being able to self-reflect, tolerate anxiety, and feel their underlying attachment-related feelings. Treatment with fragile clients can range from 20 sessions for symptom reduction to as much as 2 to 3 years in the case of severe fragility.

The Coronavirus crisis and the multiple resulting stressors involving quarantine, extended isolation, financial loss, inadequate communication, and stigma (Brooks et al., 2020) will interface and produce different responses with these different categories of clients. Some types of responses that an individual will have were described above. Your client's attachment history and his psychological makeup will have some impact on where he will land in terms of acute and longer-term response to a crisis. A person can fluctuate between these different response patterns as well. As a therapist, our first objective is to help stabilize the client, if needed, and hopefully help him make some gains or growth from the crisis so that he emerges stronger than he was before the crisis.

Common themes emerging around the Coronavirus crisis

The following are some common clinical themes seen with cases since the emergence of the COVID-19 crisis and the social, emotional, economic and behavioral impacts it has had on people (Brooks et al., 2020).

Loss

Ultimately, the most salient threat of the Coronavirus is illness and death of the self or others. Such a threat of loss will mobilize any unresolved grief about lost loved ones or lost relationships in the past. This may manifest as a preoccupation with death accounts, media of people who have died and the responses of their loved ones, or simply a preoccupation with one's own death. Depending on the characteristics of the client, a loss preoccupation may take the form of a high degree of somatic symptoms, exhaustion and depressive symptoms, tension and irritability, or emotional detachment (See Table 2).

Forced confinement

Quarantining and pressure from governments to stay at home is a type of externally imposed confinement. Clients report strong mixed feelings about the system trying to take care of people by confining them. In one recent case a person describing extreme irritability and rage coming up about government-imposed restrictions. When focusing on these feelings, the client was able to experience intense rage and also remorse for having such an intense rage towards the regional leadership. After experiencing these complex mixed feelings, the client was immediately reminded of times of control and physical brutality by a parent. The client was then able to experience intense rage in the body, sadness, and guilt about the rage related to this "confinement" by his parents. The

Table 2. Client categories using ISTDP meta-psychology.

Category	Treatment duration	Common symptoms	Common themes	Process
Low resistant	1–2	Worry and mild tension	Loss	Experience grief about recent and past losses
Moderate resistant	2–10	Tension and anxiety, sleep loss	Loss of control, fear of death of self or loved ones	Override detachment and feel underlying complex feelings
Highly resistant	20–40	Irritability and defensiveness, isolating self, sleep loss	Loss of control, control by others, fear of death of self or loved ones	Turn against firmly held defences then experience and process underlying feelings
Resistant with repression	20–40	Diarrhea, migraines, fatigue, muscle weakness and depression	Helplessness, hopelessness, resigned to death or welcome death	Build anxiety tolerance, then process underlying complex feelings
Fragile character structure	20–150	Confusion, fearfulness to paranoia, functional neurological symptoms or paradoxical calmness/ dissociation	Rage about abandonment, fear, preoccupation with conspiracies or calm resignation to possible death, Rotating themes	Build anxiety tolerance then process underlying complex feelings

end result of this session was a marked relief and reduction of defensive responses and symptoms. The client had moved from more "frightened and guarded" to more "tense and busy" as a result of this session.

Control by others

Similar to confinement, the experience of being controlled by others commonly mobilizes feelings about power use in previous relationships. One client described a great deal of rising tension and power struggle taking place in the home in relationship to being controlled by the spouse who was now at home full time. With the focus on these feelings, the client was able to experience strong complex feelings, including sadness, rage and guilt about the spouse. This immediately linked to memories of times of intense parental mental control and manipulation during the client's childhood. The client was then able to experience these strong complex feelings from the past and make a therapeutic gain out of it.

Stuck with the family

Another emerging theme is that of being "stuck" with family members in homes in a much more intense way than prior to the COVID-19 crisis and government restrictions. For all the upside of being present in the home with family members, clients describe the emergence of a lot of emotions tied to relentless interactions where they are forced to maintain their role in the family structure without any breaks. For example, a parent who was used to having days to herself while the children were in school is now confronted with constant parental duties, 24 hours a day, without any let up. This situation mobilized unprocessed complex feelings around having to assume a caretaking role for her parents when she was a child.

Economic losses

There is already a great deal of fear about what people are going to do financially as time goes on in this crisis. Will they lose their jobs, their house, their pension, their family savings? People are clambering to secure unemployment assistance or government assistance. Inevitably the loss of income and loss of role are major stressors for individuals and family members. Long-term economic downturn is linked to a range of adverse health effects and increased rates of suicide. The emotional impact of economic loss will inevitably become a focus for clients over 6 months to 2 years after a crisis.

Uncertain future

The unpredictability of the COVID-19 situation in terms of what is going to happen to society, jobs, roles, school, and other facets of life raises many elements of insecurity within the person. Any clients who have experienced nonsecure attachment will be reminded of childhood times when there has been chronic family instability. One client with severe fragile character structure described an increase in concentration difficulties and a sense of desperation. It was as if he was grasping for a piece of wood to hold onto while adrift in the ocean. A focused, reflective process aimed at reducing his anxiety and the security of the therapeutic relationship had a marked effect on him during these treatment sessions.

More closeness

The impact of social isolation and people having more time together in the home gives the opportunity for more emotional and physical closeness. This, on its own, is a positive thing so long as the person does not have a major history of trauma by close relationships in the past. If there is such a history and related attached feelings are stirred up, then there may be increased anxiety, somatic symptoms, depression or irritability, and defensiveness activated by this increased potential for closeness and intimacy. One client described with a great deal of muscle tension that she now has more time with her husband of 25 years. She described that she was tenser and was having sleep disruption even while in some ways she was enjoying having more time with her husband. When focusing on her responses there were a lot of underlying feelings related to accumulated emotions in that relationship and her childhood that had not yet been processed.

Less closeness

The impact of social isolation has meant disruption for some family members where they cannot even visit other family members. This is a painful process that can mobilize feelings about relational disruption in the past. The manifestation of this as with the other type of themes will depend on the characteristics of the individual client and the stress response they are having (Table 2).

Calm and indifferent

Some clients who have a tendency toward self-destructiveness may respond to these stressors with a paradoxical calmness, somewhat akin to "la belle indifference" seen with some conversion patients. They feel relaxed under what they see as "abusive" threats from the virus and controls by others. One patient, for example, noted that she no longer felt the urge to cut herself and felt oddly relaxed. In these cases, it is important to help the person turn against the pattern of passive submission and avoidance of emotions being mobilized in a difficult situation, in order to make further therapeutic gains.

Conclusion

There are a range of response patterns that all people can have under such a stressful period of time and with the unique features of this crisis. As we are also pressed into using videoconferencing to work with clients, it is best for us to be armed with information so that our efforts do not become an added stressor for our clients or ourselves. Certain themes related to attachments and risks of loss appear central in activating a range of somatic anxiety responses and defensive patterns to handle old feelings about attachment disruptions. There are notable advantages and disadvantages to transitioning to online treatment and we have described these above. Our experience is that most challenges of videoconferencing and video recording use diminish over time and you gradually feel as if you're sitting together in the same room with your clients once again. Until such time as we can meet back with our clients in person, we wish you the best in your clinical care and in your own adjustment to this crisis and any future crises that you may experience during your career.

Acknowledgments

This work was supported by the Dalhousie University Department of Psychiatry and the Department of Health and Wellness, Nova Scotia, Canada.

Disclosure statement

No conflicts of interest.

References

Abbass, A. (2004). Small-group video training for psychotherapy skills development. *Academic Psychiatry*, *28*, 151–155.

Abbass, A. (2015). *Reaching through resistance: Advanced psychotherapy techniques*. Kansas City, MO: Seven Leaves Press.

Abbass, A. (2016). The emergence of psychodynamic psychotherapy for treatment resistant clients: Intensive short-term dynamic psychotherapy. *Psychodynamic Psychiatry*, *44*(2), 245–280.

Abbass, A., Arthey, S., Elliott, J., Fedak, T., Nowoweski, D., Markovski, J., & Nowoweski, S. (2011). Web-conference supervision for advanced psychotherapy training: A practical guide. *Psychotherapy*, *48*, 109–118.

Abbass, A., Bernier, D., Kisely, S., Town, J., & Johansson, R. (2015). Sustained reduction in health care costs after adjunctive treatment of graded intensive short-term dynamic psychotherapy in clients with psychotic disorders. *Psychiatry Research*, *228*(3), 538–543.

Brooks, S. K., Webster, R. K., Smith, L. E., Woodland, L., Wessely, S., Greenberg, N., & Rubin, G. J. (2020). The psychological impact of quarantine and how to reduce it: Rapid review of the evidence. *Lancet*, *395*, 912–920.

Davanloo, H. (1990). *Unlocking the unconscious: Selected papers of Habib Davanloo, MD*. New York, NY: John Wiley and Sons.

Davanloo, H. (2001a). Intensive short-term dynamic psychotherapy: Extended major direct access to the unconscious. *European Psychotherapy*, *2*(1), 25–70.

Davanloo, H. (2001b). *Intensive short-term dynamic psychotherapy: Selected papers of Habib Davanloo MD*. Chichester, England: John Wiley & Sons.

Elliott, J., Abbass, A., & Cooper, J. (2015). International group supervision using videoconferencing technology. In T. Rousmaniere & E. Renfro-Michel (Eds.), *Using technology to enhance clinical supervision* (pp. 191–202). Alexandria, VA: American Counseling Association. doi:10.1002/9781119268499

Elliott, J., Abbass, A., & Rousmaniere, T. (2018). Technology-assisted deliberate practice for improving psychotherapy effectiveness. In J. J. Magnavita (Ed.), *Using technology in mental health practice* (pp. 163–180). American Psychological Association. doi:10.1037/0000085-010

Ford, J. D., Grasso, D. J., Elhai, J. D., & Courtois, C. A. (2015). *Posttraumatic stress disorder* (2nd ed.). San Diego, CA: Elsevier. doi:10.1016/C2013-0-19408-1

Frederickson, J., DenDooven, B., Abbass, A., Solbakken, O. A., & Rousmaniere, T. (2019). Pilot study: An inpatient drug rehabilitation program based on intensive short-term dynamic psychotherapy. *Journal of Addictive Diseases*, *37*(3–4), 195–201.

LeRouge, C., & Garfield, M. J. (2013). Crossing the telemedicine chasm: Have the U.S. barriers to widespread adoption of telemedicine been significantly reduced? *International Journal of Environmental Research and Public Health*, *10*(12), 6472–6484.

Lindemann, E. (1944). Symptomology and management of acute grief. *American Journal of Psychiatry*, *101*, 144–148.

Malan, D. H. (1995). *Individual psychotherapy and the science of psychodynamics* (2nd ed.). London: CRC Press.

Neborsky, R. J., & Bundy, C. (2013). Prediction of attachment status from observation of a clinical intensive psychotherapy interview. *American Journal of Psychotherapy*, *67*(1), 47–71.

Rousmaniere, T. (2014). Using technology to enhance clinical supervision and training. In C. E. Watkins & D. Milne (Eds.), *The Wiley international handbook of clinical supervision* (pp. 204–237). New York, NY: John Wiley & Sons.

Rousmaniere, T., & Renfro-Michel, E. (Eds.). (2016). *Using technology to enhance clinical supervision*. Alexandria, VA: American Counseling Association.

Town, J. M., Abbass, A., Stride, C., & Bernier, D. (2017). A randomised controlled trial of intensive short-term dynamic psychotherapy for treatment resistant depression: The Halifax depression study. *Journal of Affective Disorders*, *214*, 15–25.

Index

Note: Figures are indicated by *italics*. Tables are indicated by **bold**. Endnotes are indicated by the page number followed by 'n' and the endnote number e.g., 20n1 refers to endnote 1 on page 20.

For Product Safety Concerns and Information please contact our EU representative GPSR@taylorandfrancis.com
Taylor & Francis Verlag GmbH, Kaufingerstraße 24, 80331 München, Germany

www.ingramcontent.com/pod-product-compliance
Ingram Content Group UK Ltd.
Pitfield, Milton Keynes, MK11 3LW, UK
UKHW021507240926
475702UK00035B/542
* 9 7 8 1 0 3 2 3 9 9 6 3 8 *